AF597870

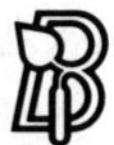

AAS
Agents and Actions Supplements
Vol. 36

Series Editors
K. Brune, Erlangen
M. J. Parnham, Bonn

Birkhäuser Verlag
Basel · Boston · Berlin

Contributions to Autacoid Pharmacology

A Festschrift in Honour of Maurício Rocha e Silva

Edited by

A. M. Rothschild

1992

Birkhäuser Verlag
Basel · Boston · Berlin

Volume Editor's Address:

Prof. Dr. A. M. Rothschild
Department of Pharmacology
School of Medicine
Ribeirão Preto, 14049 SP
Brazil

Deutsche Bibliothek Cataloging-in-Publication Data

Contributions to autacoid pharmacology: a Festschrift in honour of Maurício Rocha e Silva / ed. by A. M. Rothschild. –
Basel ; Boston ; Berlin : Birkhäuser, 1992
(Agents and actions : Supplements ; Vol. 36)
ISBN 3-7643-2617-4 (Basel ...)
ISBN 0-8176-2617-4 (Boston)
NE: Rothschild, Adolfo M. [Hrsg.]; Rocha e Silva, Maurício: Festschrift; Agents and actions / Supplements

Printed in Germany on acid-free paper, directly from the films provided by the Editor.

ISBN 3-7643-2617-4
ISBN 0-8176-2617-4

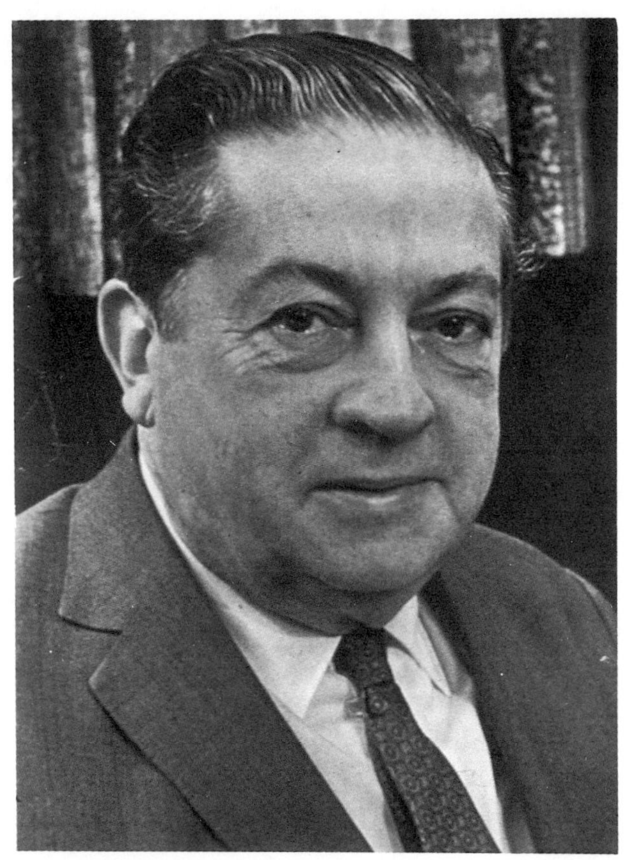

MAURICIO ROCHA E SILVA

CONTENTS

FOREWORD

In October 1990, a group of friends and former collaborators of the late Professor Maurício Rocha e Silva, met in São Paulo, Brazil, to honour his memory in the year of his 80th birthday. Scientific papers on Histamine and Bradykinin, his major fields of research, as well as biographical recollections were presented. They are reproduced in the present volume of Proceedings of the Academy of Sciences of the State of São Paulo, who sponsored the Symposium. Major Brazilian research-supporting agencies as well as several local branches of the international pharmaceutical industry were financially helpful. Their names are detailed elsewhere. The organizers were fortunate to be able to secure the collaboration of Birkhäuser Verlag Basel, to publish a special supplement of Agents and Actions, dedicated to this event. An invaluable source of inspiration to young scientists, the achievements of Professor Rocha e Silva in fostering the cause of science in general and pharmacology in particular will not soon be equalled in Brazil. His incessant toil, unshakeable belief in his country and brilliant victories in science and education must not be forgotten. History is not built but from its own records.

ADOLFO MAX ROTHSCHILD, Editor
Professor of Pharmacology
School of Medicine of Ribeirão Preto
University of São Paulo, Brazil

ACKNOWLEDGEMENTS

The organisation of the Symposium and the publication of its Proceedings would not have been possible without the financial support of the following: Financiadora de Estudos e Projetos (FINEP), Fundação de Amparo à Pesquisa do Estado de São Paulo (FAPESP), Secretaria de Ciência, Tecnologia e Desenvolvimento Econômico do Estado de São Paulo (SCTDE), University of São Paulo and, Ciba-Geigy, Hoechst, Pharmacia, Sandoz, Schering-Plough, Smith-Kline of Brazil.

Drs. Eleni L. Gomes, Eletra Greene, Elizabeth Farrelly Frota-Pessoa, Hanna A. Rothschild, Madhavarao N. Rao and Wayne A. Seale kindly helped with text proofreading. Mrs. Maria I. Rocha e Silva, Dr. and Mrs. Lewis J. Greene and Mrs. Solange Jorge provided valuable historical material.

Special motions of thanks are due to Professor Shigueo Watanabe, Executive-Director of the Academy of Sciences of the State of São Paulo (ACIESP) for his untiring interest and effort, to Miss Izabel T. Yokomizo for expert preparation of laser-printed manuscripts and to Dr. Cesar D. Nahoun for collaboration.

The Editor

AAS 36
Contributions to
Autacoid Pharmacology

OPENING LECTURE

MAURICIO ROCHA E SILVA: MAN AND WORK

A.M. Rothschild

Department of Pharmacology, School of Medicine of Ribeirão Preto, University of São Paulo, 14049 Ribeirão Preto, SP, Brazil

The brief visual and auditory contact we just had with Mauricio Rocha e Silva through this video-tape, brings back fond memories. Scientific, philosophical, political and humanistic discussions with him reappear; they enriched our lives when Rocha e Silva generously shared his intellectual creativity with those who looked for it. We are now repaying what he gave us during his life: are the records of this Symposium opening more doors of immortality to him? Or, rearranging a famous phrase: "We come, not to bury Cesar, but to praise him"?

Although I was a member of the Department of Pharmacology of the Medical School of Ribeirão Preto during 20 of Rocha e Silva's 26 years of activity there, it was during earlier years, at the Biological Institute of São Paulo that I, an emerging Master in Biochemistry, received, dazzled and incredulous, the impact of his rich, plethoric personality as a man and a scientist.

Although a witness to the enthusiastic work on bradykinin which pervaded his laboratory, it was in research on histamine, in particular anaphylatoxin, that I shared some of the victories and defeats of Rocha e Silva's work. Anaphylatoxin, described by Bordet in 1913, had emerged as an important factor in anaphylaxis by the demonstration of its capacity to release large amounts of histamine from the guinea-pig lung. The characterization of the process of activation of rat plasma anaphylatoxins paved the way for the subsequent demonstration by others, of anaphylatoxin's relationship to the C_3 and C_5 components of complement.

The many other contributions of Rocha e Silva to research on histamine can be well illustrated by his nomination as an honorary member of the American Academy of Allergy, in 1954 as well as by his books, "Histamina e Anafilaxia", published in Brazil in 1946, "Histamine, its Role in Anaphylaxis and Allergy" (1955), in the American Lecture Series of C.H. Thomas Ed. and, most significantly, by the two volumes on "Histamine and Anti-Histaminics" (1966 and 1978) of the Handbook of Experimental Pharmacology Series of Springer Ed.

It is a characteristic of good research to never exhaust a subject, but on the contrary, to sow the field for the emergence of new findings. Thus, a publication on "Histamine and Proteolytic Enzymes: Liberation of Histamine by Papain" by M. Rocha e Silva and S.O. Andrade, in 1943, may have led to the publication, 47 years later, of "Compound 48/80 – induced secretion of histamine depends on a tryptase controlled step also leading to chymase activity" by a Ph.D. candidate and myself; obviously, only one of the innumerable profits which research has gained from Rocha e Silva's pioneering work.

The theory of the residual occupancy (or interaction) of receptors with antagonists developed using data referring to the kinetics of histamine/anti-histamine antagonism (Charniere Theory) was especially dear to Rocha e Silva. It is characterized by simplicity and ingenuity. Inexplicably, neither this theory nor the related "rate theory", advanced by W.D.M. Paton to explain agonist-receptor interaction in kinetic terms, have received their deserving attention. Yet, together with Ariens' modification of Clark's occupation theory they stand as mathematical pillars of molecular pharmacology.

Rocha e Silva often requested the collaboration of laboratory colleagues for his writing. Many of us owe much of our international recognition to the generous stimulation and encouragement to publish research results in internationally accepted periodicals. Table I presents a list, certainly incomplete, of those who should be considered to have been influenced, direct or indirectly, in their scientific careers by Mauricio. They make up two groups: the first interacted with him at the Biological Institute of São Paulo; the second shared his scientific work or teaching at the Department of Pharmacology of the School of Medicine of Ribeirão Preto. Exceptions are myself and C.R. Diniz, who worked with him both in São Paulo and Ribeirão Preto.

Two enduring scientific societies were conceived and founded by Rocha e Silva, in collaboration with other senior scientists active in Brazil. The Brazilian Society for the Advancement of Science (SBPC), in 1948, and the Society of Pharmacology and Experimental Therapeutics (SBFTE), in 1966. Both have given opportunities to young

Table I

SOME SCIENTISTS OF MAURICIO ROCHA E SILVA'S CIRCLE:

A) At The Biological Institute in São Paulo (1937-1957)

Silvia O. Andrade	Eline and Jose Prado de Carvalho
Wilson T. Beraldo	Mauricio Rocha e Silva Junior
Carlos R. Diniz	Adolfo Max Rothschild
Saul Shenberg	Ulla Hamberg
Olga and Sebastião B. Henriques	Elisabeth Holzhacker
Adolfo Martins Penha	

B) At The Medical School of Ribeirão Preto (1958-1980)

Alexandre Pinto Corrado	Frederico G. Graef
Armando Otavio Ramos	Irene R. Pelá
Abilio Antonio	Fernando M.A. Correia
Itamar Vugman	Antonio C.M. Camargo
Carlos Ribeiro Diniz	Antonio R. Martins
Ivan F. Carvalho	Marina L. Reis
Adolfo Max Rothschild	Ivone B. Queiroz
Sergio H. Ferreira	Lyoko O. Yoshigai
João Garcia Leme	Ana M. Oliveira
Elfriedes S. Shapoval	Flavio Fernandes

scientists during yearly meetings; their importance is well-described by W.T. Beraldo and S.B. Henriques on pgs. 134 and 7 of this volume. An event representing a maximal organizational effort of Rocha e Silva was the III International Congress of Pharmacology held in 1966 in São Paulo. Carried out under circumstances financially much more precarious than they would have been today, the Congress was a resounding success attaining the same level as preceeding IUPHAR Congresses at Stockholm and Prague and succeeding ones in Basel, San Francisco, Helsinki and Paris. I, having organized meetings in Brazil, can only offer enthusiastic homage to the resolution of Rocha e Silva to launch a big International Congress in our country 25 years ago.

Last, but not least, a very important aspect of Rocha e Silva: His writings on the meaning of Science for man both as a unique and irreplaceable being – as he himself was – and as a member of humanity, a conglomerate much larger than the sum of its parts. Larger because contributing towards it were the gifted minds of Leonardo da Vinci, Johann Wolfgang von Goethe, Friedrich Hegel, Mauricio Rocha e Silva and Noam Chomsky, to cite but a few. Chomsky, the linguist, creator of the theory of generative grammar of not only words, but especially of their deeper meaning in psychological terms, was greatly admired by Rocha e Silva, who contrasted him with Skinner, a behaviourist. Chomsky, by indissolubly tying the universe's creative arts evolved through millennia of mythology to the scientific language of the twentieth century and Jungian symbology, deeply satisfied Rocha e Silva's idea of himself as a scientist and thinker. In "The Rational Frontiers of Science" he expands this view. Excerpts from a highly praising critique of this book(1) are reproduced below:

"Mauricio Rocha e Silva is a Brazilian pharmacologist who, in "The Rational Frontiers of Science," has written a very instructive book of scientific explanation, wise, warm, and wide-ranging. I do not know for sure whether a school of Latin American scientific philosophers is rising to help inject a rational humanism into this technological age. I suspect there is, if the work of the Chilean physiologist-philosopher Humberto Maturana is any indication. But I do know that when one reads Latin American literature, the result almost always is surprise at the many levels of meaning and perception with which novelists like Jorge Luis Borges and Gabriel Marquez dazzle the senses.

So, too, with Silva. But the process is a subtle one. Silva introduces a dance of ideas that follow a not-easy-to-track stream of thought but take the reader along an intricate excursion from linguistics and dialects to enzymology and the Bohr electron. *The lovely aspect of this book*, to me, anyway, *is Silva's attempt to explain science to itself* so that it can better lead the way toward solving the challenges faced by a postindustrial world. This is a world where mankind will have to fashion technology to be more in tune with the laws of nature and of humanism. Silva's book deals directly with such issues and for that reason is exciting. "The philosophies of all times", he writes, "have been marked by the opposition between abstract and concrete, analytic and synthetic, soul and body, conscious and unconscious, essence and phenomena, form and matter, finite and infinite, freedom and necessity, possible and real, theory and practice. Mankind continues to struggle between two poles that could be expressed in terms of another opposition: tragedy and comedy, the first resulting from a subjective interpretation of different ideologies, and the second in the Balzacian sense of *Human Comedy*, as a novelist's description of the common man who places in science his hopes for liberation". What Silva is saying is that it is worth searching through such fields as mythology, linguistics, depth psychology, development of the wave-particle theory of the electron, Hegelian and Marxist philosophy, and political theory for approaches to broadening the base of creativity in science. Why? Because science offers a way out of the debilitating effects of technology while needing some new perceptions about itself. His book is mainly a series of reflections on the underlying basis for creativity in science, an extension of the debate over whether science grows mainly through observation of phenomena or out of perceptions that already exist in the mind. What he asks implicitly, then, is to what degree thought and inner impressions shape science and vice-versa. He delves into these issues because problems beset the world. Most of these problems stem from the misuse of technology. A more rational way of approaching technology is needed, and Silva explores whether the source of that rationality can come from science through a better understanding of what science does, how it works, and how it can be taken to its next order of relevance.

All in all, "The Rational Frontiers of Science" is both an entertainment and an exploration. Rocha e Silva is representative of the Latin American approach to scientific investigation of the scientific age. *His is a thoroughly human approach to the problems posed by the reality of the irrational, and he remains true to the ideals of scientific integrity.* Marxist, Hegelian, linguistic, and psychological scholars may find plenty to argue about with Silva, but they can hardly fault his sincere attempt to broaden the meaning and purpose of science."

I wish to close this homage to Mauricio Rocha e Silva, man and scientist on both a sad and a cheerful note. Sad: much of the bitterness and the withdrawal into himself of Rocha e Silva after his compulsory retirement from the professorship which a mind as active as his could not accept, resulted from a sensation of abandonment and lack of understanding of his still brilliant intellect by his colleagues at Ribeirão Preto. How much he welcomed and relished the friendship and warmth of members of this group was confirmed by his satisfied look at the "merengão" anniversary party on September 19th of each year. Many of us here, who are also preparing their departure from professional life, may now perhaps understand the intellectual solitude which can afflict men of genius in the evening of their lives. And now, a cheerful ending note: a testimony of Rocha e Silva's sense of humor expressed by his representation of a being he much admired and who inspired his own life: Albert Einstein, depicted with the wit and charm of Mauricio's pictorial work of later years (Fig. 1).

Reference

1. Lepkowski, W., Chem. Eng. News, Sept. 27, 35-36 (1982).

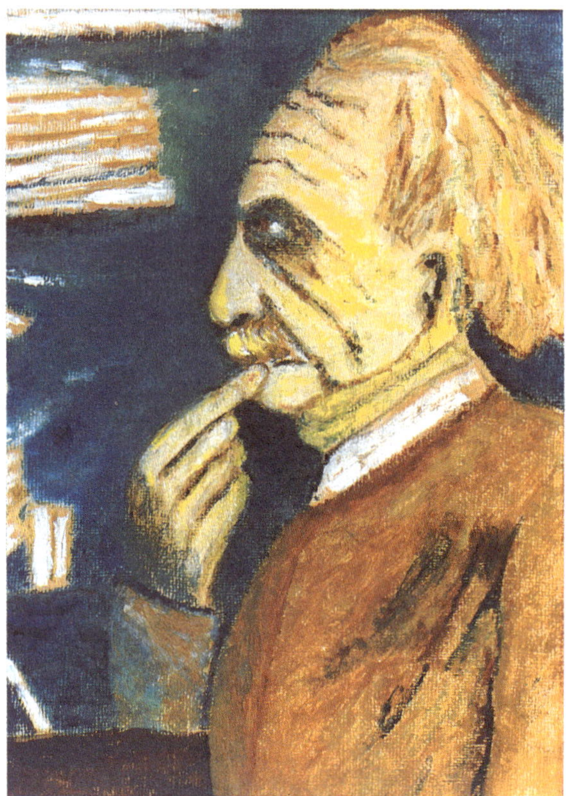

Fig. 1. Albert Einstein, depicted with the wit and charm of Mauricio's pictorial work of later years.

AAS 36
Contributions to
Autacoid Pharmacology

THE SCIENTIFIC THINKING OF PROFESSOR MAURICIO ROCHA E SILVA

S.B. Henriques

Laboratory of Molecular Biology, Instituto Butantan, 05504 São Paulo, SP, Brazil

In this talk, two aspects of the thinking of Rocha e Silva will be focussed upon. In the first two sections, this lecturer shall endeavour to show that Rocha e Silva's scientific thought is thoroughly evidenced by a description of the role he has played as an absolutely tireless fighter to change the situation of underdevelopment of scientific research in Brazil. In the latter sections – 3 and 4 – this speaker will try to show (a) the positions taken by Rocha e Silva in relation to the role played by the Greeks of the Classic Epoch in the development of World Science, and (b) of the attitude taken by Rocha e Silva towards Science in the Modern age.

1. The Situation of the Brazilian Universities Until the Middle of the Century

In the third decade of this century, the few "Universities" of the country were in reality, aggregates of professional Schools of Law, Medicine, Engineering, Pharmacy and Dentistry, bureaucratically administered by a decorative figure named the Rector. Professors of basic subjects were never research workers but, lawyers, medical professionals, engineers, pharmacists, or odontologists, who, with well-known exceptions, used their Departments only as places for undergraduate teaching, rendering them incapable of serving as centres of research at the post-graduate level.

In 1934, Dr. Armando de Salles Oliveira, Governor of the State of São Paulo, modified this situation. He set up the College of Philosophy, Sciences and Letters, aggregating new institutes to the existing professional faculties, to constitute the University of São Paulo. This initiative marked the beginning of research at the new University. Its departments of Physics, Chemistry, Mineralogy, Geology, General Biology, Genetics, Zoology and Botany, were charged with the double role of teaching undergraduates and of initiating graduate students in research[(1)].

2. Research in Brazil

Until the early fifties all significant research produced in the country, came from state institutes (Agronomico de Campinas, Oswaldo Cruz, Adolpho Lutz, Butantan, Biologico, Ezequiel Dias). Hence the phrase attributed in the thirties to Professor Rocha Lima: "In Brazil, those who want to dedicate themselves to research, must flee the Universities".

The scientific institutes maintained by the State had as their main tasks the solution of technical questions in Public Health, Agronomy, Phythopathology, Animal Husbandry, Soil Technology, Hydrography, etc., all concerns of the State. Two reasons caused these institutes to nevertheless carry weight in basic scientific research: the unsatisfactory situation of the Universities and the fact that these Institutes had clear-minded Directors who utilized their power to (a) promote real scientific research and (b) to endeavour, within the aims of the institutions they directed, to find the best solutions for the technical problems faced.

Conditions of technical underdevelopment, however, often rendered scientific communities unable to exert an influence powerful enough to make Administrators find the most intelligent solution when a new director of a scientific institution was to be appointed. The most devastating error happened in 1947 at the Butantan Institute. The new director, considered scientific research a job for the University, the role of the Butantan Institute being to produce arms to defend Public Health by preparing sera, vaccines and chemotherapeutic agents. Putting this into practice, he transferred to other state organizations all those who refused to abandon their research to put themselves at his disposal to solve any technical problem coming up. As a consequence, about ten research workers were suddenly transferred from the Institute, mostly to the School of Medicine of the University of São Paulo whose Director was not even consulted beforehand. He had great trouble accommodating such a sudden addition to his staff[(2)].

3. The Foundation of the Brazilian Society for the Progress of Science

The calamity affecting the Butantan Institute, by stressing the need for an organism responsible for the defense of Brazilian scientific institutions, gave Mauricio Rocha e Silva the opportunity to show that, besides being an internationally known research worker, he was also capable of applying a large part of his enormous energy to the interests of scientific work in his country. In 1948, associating himself with well-known Brazilian scientists (Rocha Lima, Miguel Ozorio de Almeida, José Reis, Paulo Sawaya, Otto Bier, José Ribeiro do Valle, Anisio Teixeira, J. Baeta Viana, André Dreyfuss, José Leite Lopes, Marcelo Damy de Souza Santos, Carlos Chagas Filho, and others) he set up the Brazilian Society for the Progress of Science (SBPC).

The SBPC has had very successful Annual Meetings since its foundation especially important for young research workers, who are entitled to a single presentation, strictly limited in time, of their experimental results. SBPC meetings are held in different regions of the country each year. In part, they are dedicated to discussions of local problems, chaired by guests invited ahead of time and known to have a considerable understanding of such problems. Thus, those living in the region where the meeting is being held, have an opportunity to become conscious and to think about its problems.

In the 42 years of its existence (the first SBPC annual meeting occurred in July, 1948), no July has passed without an annual SBPC meeting – even in the worst years of the "*Redeeming Revolution*". Rocha e Silva was always the most influential personality of the SBPC. One can say that even when his health became a source of concern for his friends, whenever a crisis threatened the SBPC, Rocha e Silva dedicated great energy to help the Society to overcome it. Thus, the influence exerted by Rocha e Silva in the development of Brazilian Science is the most eloquent illustration of the depth of his scientific thinking.

4. Rocha e Silva: Greek Science and Philosophy

As is well known, scientific activity may have one of two aims: experiment for applications, an activity usually called technology or applied science, or experiment and observe to acquire knowledge, an activity commonly, but improperly, called pure science. The difference between the two is not absolute, because "pure" acquisition of knowledge will always find, in the short or in the long run, somebody with the technological capacity to make the new knowledge useful to the community[3]. Historically, experiment for applications seems to have preceded the performance of experiments to acquire knowledge. Thus the Sumerians knew and utilized metals, Babylonians could foresee eclipses and the Egyptians were able to foresee the Nile floods. Nobody can surely affirm however, that such applications were not preceded by the acquisition of "pure" knowledge. Nobody can deny that owing to their wonderful accomplishments between the sixth Century, B.C. and fourth Century, A.D. when the Alexandria Museum was destroyed by fanatic Christians, the Greeks were pioneers in both systematic scientific investigation and philosophical meditation. During those ten centuries, Greek scientific production occurred in all fields of the material world (both physical and biological).

As an illustration, one should perhaps start by mentioning Heraclitus (sixth century B.C.), who stated that it was impossible for one to bathe twice in the same water of the same river: in a way, this is an anticipation of the modern concept that Nature is in a state of perpetual change. The list which follows is a very small reminder of the magnificent contribution of the "Golden Age" of Classical Greece to knowledge of Nature: Pythagoras (fifth century B.C.), a great mathematician and astronomer considered to be the founder of Acoustics; Leucippus (about 490 B.C.) and Democritus (about 460 B.C.) precursors of Atomic Theory, which is incompatible with the idea that Nature abhors a vacuum, a prejudice which lasted for 20 centuries; Euclid (third century B.C.), who developed Geometry to the point that his demonstrations are still used for teaching in our present-day schools. Archimedes (287-212 B.C.) the founder of hydrostatics.

5. The Negative Role Played by Aristotle in European Scientific Development

Aristotle was undoubtedly the Greek philosopher-scientist who most influenced European thinking for 20 centuries. This was due in the first place, because Aristotelism became the official philosophy of the Roman Empire, then the greatest military, political and economic power of the world; secondly, because under Emperor Constantinus (280-337 A.D.) this powerful empire adopted the Christian faith as its official religion; and thirdly, because writings of Aristotle did not contradict the set of dogmas of Christian Theology. With the collapse of the Western part of the Empire, history in that part of Europe went through a period of confusion during the Middle Ages, from which it started to emerge only at the end of the first third of the second millennium. To a large measure this was so because during all that period, Aristotelian philosophy in western Europe became a dogma, modified only in details by the Catholic theologians St. Augustine (354-1274), St. Thomas Aquinas (1224-1274), William Ockham (1280-1349), and others. As a consequence, errors contained in the Aristotelian dogma braked scientific progress of Europe. Such stagnation of knowledge led Roger Bacon (1210-1293) – the great paladin of experimentation as the only way to test validity of a theory – to exclaim, relatively to errors contained in Aristotle's writings:" I should like to burn them all, since their reading increases ignorance and causes a loss of time"(3). It is well-known that the long European medieval night only started slowly to light up with the return of the crusaders, a few of which were influenced by the Arabic philosophers, who although Aristotelians themselves, were not affected by Christian prejudices. Thereby becoming, at that time, the "vanguard" of philosophy and science.

6. The Thinking of Rocha e Silva on Modern Science

The notorious mistakes of Aristotle do not decrease his enormous importance as a pioneer of science and philosophy; if the Greeks gave a most remarkable contribution to the philosophic and scientific progress of humanity, this is due to the fact that they – and this most justly include Aristotle – were able to postulate extraordinary generalizations which became, in modified from, embodied in modern science. Still, one most admit with Heisenberg(4): "The enormous difference between present-day science and Greek philosophy, consists precisely in the empirical attitude of modern science..."

The expression "empiricism" is sometime utilized in the sense of obtaining information with the aid of "experience"; – and here one must stress that there is a difference between "experience" and "experiment". While the first is obtained at random, the latter is performed after a complete analysis of the phenomenon to be studied. This bad interpretation of the term empiricism still occurred in the United States in the fifties. When visiting Chicago this lecturer heard a professor explain that he wanted to measure electrical potential of the knee joint, with a potentiometer he had built himself. When asked what kind of results he expected to obtain, he retorted: "That is for experience to answer". Real knowledge cannot increase from such "experience" and, obviously this is not the type of empiricism that Heisenberg(3) had in mind. In homage to Rocha e Silva, one must mention that when planning an experiment to solve a given question, depending upon the phenomenon to be studied, he left the question to be discussed in depth by the experimenter and colleagues. It has been stated that the level of scientific production of countries of the third world is low because of experiments performed without proper discussion of the aspects to be studied, or often even without any discussion at all. This has been contrasted with the opinion that in France, physicists take 10% of their time in performing experiments, but 90% of it in discussing on how to perform them. The books by Rocha e Silva[3,4] are a precious source of his views about physics, physical-chemistry, biology, linguistics and sciences of the mind. Bernal[5], has dealt, also in a very knowledgeable form, with a similar subject.

7. On Some Disagreement with Rocha e Silva

It has always been a source of pride for me to have been honoured with the friendship of Mauricio Rocha e Silva and to have had the opportunity of having long, frequent debates with him. Sometimes these ended in complete disagreement – more often than not, when dealing with one or another aspect of Marxism. One source of disagreement was Rocha e Silva's comments (1976b): "Engels practically ruined his philosophy... pretending to extend Hegelian philosophy to natural phenomena...". Rocha e Silva apparently associated this phrase with the well-known errors committed by Lysenko in regards to wheat genetics. Since in my view these errors were based on demagogic and sectarian "Marxist" arguments, they should not be accepted as proof that Marxist philosophy cannot be extended to natural phenomena. In fact, one generalization made by Engels was to apply to nature the Marxist "law" of transformation of quantity into quality, obtained from the analysis of society. In favor of this generalization, Engels cited the case of the chemical elements, of the properties of the series of organic compounds, of the many species of living organism, and others.

To end, this author expresses his undying admiration for Rocha e Silva and his thanks to Professors Wilson Teixeira Beraldo and Adolfo Max Rothschild for the invitation to talk about the scientific thinking of the man to whom homage is rendered in this series of talks dedicated to his eightieth birthday.

References

1. Henriques, S.B., The Butantan Institute – An essay on the need for reformulation of our scientific Institutes (in Portuguese), Cienc. Cult. 35, 153-157 (1982).

2. Henriques, S.B., The stability of professors and the University's autonomy (in Portuguese), Cienc. Cult. 33, 3-8 (1980).

3. Rocha e Silva, M., The evolution of scientific thinking (in Portuguese). Hucitec Editora, São Paulo, Brazil 1976a.

4. Rocha e Silva, M., Pure science and applied science (in Portuguese). Hucitec Editora, São Paulo, Brazil 1976b.

5. Bernal, J.D., Science in History. Penguin Books, Ltd., Harmondworth, Middleser, England 1969.

The author expresses his thanks to Dr. Hanna Rothschild, for lending him the books of Rocha e Silva, quoted.

AAS 36
Contributions to
Autacoid Pharmacology

MAURICIO, A FRIENDSHIP AT ALL TIMES

H. Moussatché

FIOCRUZ, Rio de Janeiro, RJ, Brazil

I do not know precisely when I first met Mauricio. In searching through an already foggy memory of a distant past, I sometimes feel that it was yesterday, that our friendship had no starting day, that it was of all times. There are, it is true, well-defined facts in my memory: our first contacts in the second year of our medical course; to be precise, during the final moments of Physiology classes by professor Alvaro Ozorio de Almeida.

After several years of absence, Alvaro Ozorio had begun again in 1929 to teach the first year of the Physiology course then given to second and third year medical students of the School of Medicine of the University of Rio de Janeiro. His lectures required basic knowledge uncommon in most students, demanding from Ozorio de Almeida a frequent reassessment of the level of understanding of his lectures and frequent reinforcement of knowledge to understand basic concepts of Physiology. I do not wish however to refer any more to these classes; it was the "other lecture", which Almeida gave to a small group of students who looked him up after the main lecture, to question, to converse, for a period long enough to impress in all the personality traits of a researcher, which arose in a few, a very few, the wish to follow his example; among these, was Mauricio. I never asked to what extent such conversations and lectures influenced Mauricio's professional decisions.

Our almost daily companionship was kept up until the end of the medical course. The early thirties were a period of great revolutionary and electoral agitation. Classes and scheduled student shifts in the clinics were disturbed. Exams were passed by governmental decree. One day, on our way to the Medical School in a streetcar, I asked Mauricio whether he knew a gentleman sitting a little in front of us. He did not. It was our professor of Pharmacology. On one occasion, jokingly or not, Mauricio commented that, had he gone to Pharmacology lectures, he would never had become a pharmacologist. I myself attended only one of his lectures. Our professor was an admirer of language but not a pharmacologist. It was a rule rather than an exception then, that teachers of basic sciences in our School were not professionals in the fields they lectured on. Another reason for our low attendance of formal lectures but of frequent meetings in cafe and bookstores was the urge to discuss local and world politics, especially the possible consequences, to science and culture, of the rise to power of Hitler. Not rarely, our meetings ended in Mauricio's home, at a most pleasant spot on the Largo (square) of the Boticário (Apothecary) in Rio which, if memory does not betray me, has been chartered to the city by the government. Our chats often lasted for hours; in the Cafe Odeon, it was not unusual for the waiter to suggestively come and clear our table on which innumerable cups of coffee had been consumed, but little expense incurred. It was there however, that I became impressed by the already extensive literary and scientific background of Mauricio, especially in mathematics, a rare fact among medical students. Although my own training in mathematics was not deep, I could grasp the reach of his knowledge in tensorial calculus and other fundamental changes taking place in classical physics and mathematics. His continued interest in these fields made him often choose a physico-mathematical approach to problems in Pharmacology. When once asked whether in his search for the philosophical basis of science he had found Plato, he answered that not Plato, but Pythagoras and his school, looking for the equation behind the phenomenon, were what interested him most. In his last years he devoted much energy working on theoretical physics concerning electron jumps in hydrogenoid atoms and a relativistic approach in his studies on red shifted hydrogen spectral bands.

While still a medical student, he wrote a series of literary essays, published in 1934 after completion of his medical training. "Bonecos (Dolls) of Porcelana (Chinaware)" consists of nine essays, in two parts: eight in the first, under the collective aegis of "Everybody's and Nobody's Soul" and in the second part, a longer essay named "Picture of an Intelligent Girl". In the first tale, "The Merchant of Souls" he describes a writer in a corner of a large ferryboat, furtively watching other passengers talking or whispering to each other. A young couple in particular, the girl of shining and fixed eyes, the young man, apparently trembling under the impact of some deep, delicate, intimate feeling, attracted his attention. Getting closer, the writer still fails to gather their exchanged words of tenderness and rapture. The boat arrives at its destiny but the young man, imprudently steps aside, and falls into the sea. The girl in a cry of anguish terrible to hear, screams "My brother ... save him ... save him ..."; but the writer, carried by the crowd, disappears with an empty spirit and a pained feeling in his soul.

In this, as well in the other tales touching mostly on themes familiar to the writer, the excessive use of certain adjectives, reveals the beginner. However, in the second part of the book, one notes the improved style and depth of thematic focussing. "Picture of an Intelligent Girl" describes the changing spirits of a young woman, according to the development of a Symphony or a Concerto: Allegro, Andante, Presto and Prestissimo. Susan, intelligent, non conformist, excitedly curious, meets Richard, young but serene and mature. Impressed by his words and vision of the world, her hypnosis however, does not last long. She notices the antagonism and wants to free herself. In growing desperation she faces Richard's serene and understanding attitude by shouting at him: "Go, go away. I am a woman like the others, wanting to live. I don't want to see you anymore". And she flees by a rear window. The crescendo of Susan's despair, as described by Mauricio, deserves reading.

In his sixth medical year, Mauricio spent a short period of apprenticeship in Miguel Ozorio de Almeida's laboratory at the Osvaldo Cruz Institute. On finishing his course he accepted an invitation by André Dreyfuss to become an Assistant in Biology at the Faculty of Sciences of The University of São Paulo; in 1932 he started work at the Institute of Biology of São Paulo where in 1942 he was made head of the Department of Biochemistry and Pharmacodynamics. The years at the Institute of Biology (1937-1957) were the decisive period of Rocha e Silva's total dedication to scientific research. His frequent trips to the United States and Europe, his humanistic background, his excellent writing capacity in Portuguese helped him to excel also in English which was required for the writing of his publications, and became a second mother tongue to him.

It is not my purpose to review the extensive production of Rocha e Silva's forty years of scientific activity. W.T. Beraldo has done this in his talk to the Brazilian Academy of Sciences, of which Mauricio was also a member, giving special relevance to the discovery of bradykinin as well as to Rocha e Silva's other initiatives. These include the founding of the Brazilian Society for the Advancement of Science and of the great laboratory of Pharmacology at the School of Medicine of Ribeirão Preto, where a cluster of disciples of international projection in the physiological sciences was formed.

Mauricio was one the greatest men of science of Brazil. If science was his profession, his restless spirit, already outlined in his youth, led him to read and to think about other themes close to or far from Pharmacology, Physiology or Biochemistry. His already firm basis in scientific and literary knowledge allowed him upon graduating, to broaden his education in other areas, solidifying concepts, and correlating view-points.

This resulted in a series of books published as contributions to the philosophy of science between 1965 and 1982: "The Logic of Invention", "Science and Humanism", "The Evolution of Scientific Thought", "Pure Science-Applied Science", "The Cartesian Myth" and "The Rational Frontiers of Science". All of them constitute mostly fluent, pleasant reading arousing the reader's curiosity, not rarely his amusement and occasionally, his surprise with the apparent irreverent reference to someone the world had become used to refer to in most respectful terms. As an example, in "The Logic of Invention", analysing humanity as a whole he concludes: "As is well-known, only rarely, very rarely, do extraordinary men arise in Science as well as in Art. It may therefore be concluded, that such exceptional beings no longer belong to the human species; a new species is evolving from the present *Homo sapiens*, in the same way that the human species appeared, when there were only anthropoids, as a mutation, equivalent to an Einstein among anthropoids: the Einstein-anthropoid. Obviously this still simian anthropoid would not "in a state of intellectual exaltation" discover the equation relating matter and energy. Furthermore, the Manhattan project, would be entirely useless in the jungle". But what results from the appearance of the Einstein-anthropoid? It would permit anthropoids to profit from his inventions or creations to conquer the "small difference" between the anthropoid and *Homo sapiens*. Mauricio further concludes that this new anthropoid would have to be a female, which he describes as a "magnificent specimen of the human species, with a hairless breast, brown, silky hair and a smile capable of filling his not so favoured companions with envy, love or hate". Furthermore, this anthropoid would be a woman because as a man, he would hardly have resisted the competition by other, probably stronger males. Undoubtedly this essay holds a fair share of imagination and irony. But it would be equally valid to take it as a parable in the same manner as Rocha e Silva took the saying of Heraclitus that fire is the primeval substance, not as a mythological entity, but as "something concrete, obviously the cause of the transformation of the world in which he lived". In his book, Mauricio approached a varied array of themes: Darwin's evolutionary theory, Heraclitus' eternal return to the being and-not being, Descartes' dualism of spirit and matter, Hegelian and Marxist dialectics, Chomsky's Piagetean or Cartesian linguistics, always discoursing with the lucidity and elegance which we commemorate today when Mauricio Rocha e Silva would have become eighty years old.

AAS 36
Contributions to
Autacoid Pharmacology

MAURÍCIO ROCHA E SILVA'S CONTRIBUTION TO THE TRAINING OF NEW SCIENTISTS

F.G. Graeff

Laboratory of Psychobiology, School of Philosophy, Sciences and Letters of Ribeirão Preto, University of São Paulo, 14049, Ribeirão Preto, SP, Brazil.

When Maurício Rocha e Silva started his scientific career during the late thirties, experimental research in Brazil was the occupation of a selected few, and in spite of an exponential growth over the last fifty years, it still lies well below saturation level.

As a consequence, the contribution of Brazilian scientists should not be measured exclusively in terms of published work, but also by the seeds dropped in research soil in terms of new laboratories, research institutions and scientific societies founded and, above all, by the number and quality of new researchers trained.

In the last sense, Rocha e Silva's contribution was very important, since most of his former students are presently engaged in laboratory work and some of them rank among the leaders of pharmacological research in Brazil.

Why certain scientists like Rocha e Silva are able to detect and foster the development of young talents into creative and independent researchers is easier to acknowledge than to explain. Nevertheless, having personally experienced his influence both during my Ph.D. training and over nearly twenty years while working at the Department of Pharmacology of the Ribeirão Preto Medical School, University of São Paulo, I feel entitled to make a qualified guess at the main factors in Rocha e Silva's teaching ways that made him a successful breeder of new scientists.

First of all, it was the plain fact that he himself was a creative scientist of high stature – One cannot give what one does not have! More than simply a dedicated researcher Rocha e Silva was a "philosopher" in the genuine sense of the word; that is, he cherished knowledge in its broadest sense. His intellectual interests ranged from the biological sciences to liberal arts, especially painting and music, as well as philosophy, epistemology in particular. He was also especially fond of mathematics, physics and chemistry, was an amateur astronomer and gave some thought to psychology. Such Da Vincian intellectual life certainly exerted a powerful attraction on young inquisitive minds. In addition, Rocha e Silva enjoyed discussing his latest ideas with young people and feeling the resonance of his endeavours in their spirits. This fact may have helped him to detect, before any material proof was produced, creative talents that later became his students and collaborators.

Witnessing Rocha e Silva's workings in actual research was another source of deep-seated lessons for us. He was justly proud of having achieved international recognition for his work, in spite of the comparatively meager material resources and poor cultural environment that were available to him. This was achieved, I believe, through a combination of intellectual boldness, sharp intuition and wit. Rocha e Silva was brave enough to face relevant issues of both theoretical importance and potential for practical application. He followed his own ideas, guided by the intrinsic logic of his subject matter and by a piercing intuition. Once, while visiting our Department, a British pharmacologist, Desirée Armstrong, came right to the point with her view on Rocha e Silva's scientific strategy: "He does not do much, but he does the right things".

Rocha e Silva assembled a team of motivated students and collaborators that reached the "critical mass" necessary for performing competitive research. We worked with genuine enthusiasm and dedication, and often discussed freely the wildest research ideas, some of which later proved fertile. The ludical character of scientific research was in the air, spurring creative thought and action. However, it would be misleading to convey only this Edenic scenery. All of us have our Jungian "shadow" and Rocha e Silva was no exception. He was not always an affable person, although he could be charming when he wanted to be. His emotional reactions were quite unpredictable, and aggressive and unpleasant interactions often occurred, generating an atmosphere ladden with mistrust and persecutory feelings among the members of the group,that was short of unbearable. Like an immature parent, Rocha e Silva felt insecure about the growth of his "children" and at a certain stage clashes were inevitable. Interestingly enough, for those of his students who were strong enough to withstand his overwhelming personality, such incidents fostered early independence. It may have worked as an unintended school for leadership.

Despite the above shortcomings, those of us who learned from Rocha e Silva felt a powerful drive to emulate his example, within the limitations of our capabilities and with the different shades of our personalities. Like him, we feel the urge to help other young talented people grow as much as they can into independent and mature research workers. Hopefully this multiplicative process will result in a sizeable contribution to Brazilian pharmacology.

AAS 36
Contributions to
Autacoid Pharmacology

THIRTY YEARS AS A LABORATORY TECHNICIAN UNDER PROF. MAURICIO ROCHA E SILVA

D.S. Reis
Retired Laboratory Technician

Department of Pharmacology, School of Medicine of Ribeirão Preto, University of São Paulo, 14049 Ribeirão Preto, SP, Brazil

It is a reason of great pride for me to represent my colleague technicians and employees of the Department of Pharmacology, on this day honouring the memory of Professor Rocha e Silva. It was difficult to decide to accept the responsibility of presenting a convincing testimony of the affection and admiration which all employees of the Department of Pharmacology of the School of Medicine of Ribeirão Preto felt for Professor Rocha e Silva. All of us fondly recall how that austere countenance of an apparently severe and wary man of few words during working hours, hid a highly sensitive person, always preoccupied with human problems in general and especially with those of laboratory technicians; to us, he always lent a receptive ear. There were several instances in which he openly took our side against administrative officials of the School of Medicine and even the University of São Paulo. He always appreciated and encouraged our profession, fully understanding the importance of the laboratory technician's work as a complement to university teaching and research; among the many teachers and researchers whom I knew, only rarely did I meet anyone so ready to invest time and effort in the promotion of the technical career. Talking little, always between the reading of one or another article, his utterances were nevertheless always to the point, often humorous, sometimes even salty, adding zest to otherwise arid dialogues. He taught us to laugh and live, but also to love research work. The dedication and enthusiasm with which he performed his experiments were responsible for the interest in research not only of his co-workers, but also of his technical assistants. Countless were the occasions on which several of us would stay in the laboratory much beyond regular working hours, proving that technicians when made to feel their contribution is being appreciated gladly reciprocate initiatives to work. I also wish to testify about the professor's enthusiasm in setting up new techniques with his at the time, still young laboratory technicians. He stimulated us not only to learn, but also to be able to teach what we learned to undergraduate and graduate students in Pharmacology, as many of us still do.

I thank the organizers of this Symposium on behalf of my colleagues and of myself, for this opportunity to honour the memory of Professor Rocha e Silva.

AAS 36
Contributions to
Autacoid Pharmacology

RECENT OBSERVATIONS ON MECHANISMS OF STORAGE AND RELEASE OF MAST CELL HISTAMINE. APPLICABILITY TO OTHER BIOGENIC AMINES

B. Uvnäs

Department of Pharmacology, Karolinska Institutet, Stockholm, Sweden

Abstract

A new theory on non-degranulating release of histamine is presented.

Histamine is a very active biogenic amine localized to cells in almost all tissues of the body; in the mast cells of the interstitial tissues, in the basophils of the blood and in the enterochromaffin-like cells of the intestine. During the last years more evidence has appeared to indicate that histamine is also a nervous transmitter to be found in many neurons of the brain. In the cells and presumably also in the neurons, histamine is localized to granules from which it is released on activation of the storage cells. Due to its high biological activity, the release of histamine leads to pronounced effects in the body involving contractions of the smooth muscles of the lungs and in the circulatory systems, thereby causing symptoms characteristic of asthma and other allergic reactions.

Since histamine probably also plays functional although not yet identified roles in various bodily systems, it is of importance to know the mechanism by which it is released. Most studies on the storage and release of histamine have been performed on mast cells, especially mast cells isolated from the rat peritoneal fluid, since these cells are relatively easy to isolate. I will therefore confine my presentation today to studies of the release of histamine from rat mast cells.

The isolated mast cell from the rat peritoneal cavity is a spherical body with an average diameter of about 10 μ. Each cell contains about 1000 – 1200 granules with a diameter of about 0.5 μ. Since the histamine content of rat peritoneal mast cells has been estimated to about 15–30 μg per million cells, the concentration of histamine in the granule should, if being in solution, be about 0.7 mM. When a mast cells is challenged with histamine releasing agents, degranulation is a common response; in other words, the granules are expelled from the cell. According to current teaching, degranulation is a prerequisite for histamine release from a mast cell. Histamine should be released from the granules when they become exposed to the extracellular cations. We have since many years studied the properties of mast cell granules from the rat and found that these particles have the properties of a weak cation exchanger resin. The matrix of a mast cell granule consists mainly of two components, a strongly acid polymer (heparin) and a strongly basic protein. These two components occur in the rat mast cell granule as a water-insoluble complex. To this complex histamine is assumed to be ionically linked, to carboxyl end terminals in the protein part of the complex[1]. The mechanism of release should therefore be as illustrated in Fig. 1. When the granules are expelled into the extracellular space, their exposure to sodium ions in the extracellular fluid will result in a complete immediate release of the histamine by $Na^+ \rightleftharpoons HA^+$ ion exchange. However, I will now be heretic enough to propose another release mechanism withouth degranulation as the initial process.

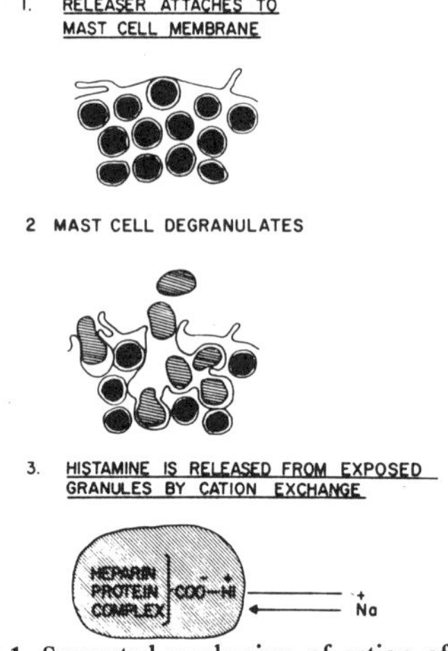

Fig. 1. Suggested mechanism of action of degranulating agents (from Handbook in Experimental Pharmacology 1978).

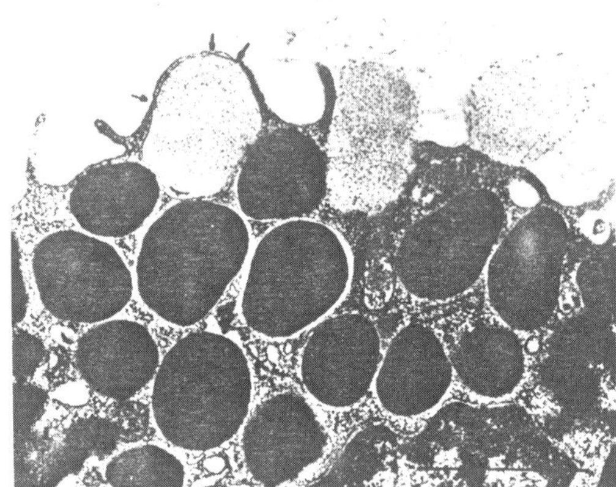

Fig. 2. Electron microscopic picture of begining degranulation of a mast cell exposed to compound 48/80 (from Handbook in Experimental Pharmacology 1978).

Look at the electron microscopic picture of a degranulating cell (Fig. 2). You can see three translucent granules; the two to the right are on their way out of the cell and have no membrane. The third, the left one, has also lost its electron density but is still shielded from the extracellular space by a membrane. In other words, since reduced electron density means loss of histamine, histamine can evidently be lost even before the granule has left the cell. In case the histamine loss is due to ion exchange there are two alternatives, either that cations have entered the granule from the outside or the other possibility, that cations from inside the cell have penetrated into the granule. To study these possibilities we have during the last years focused our interest on the kinetics of histamine release from granules and mast cells.

A release from a cation exchanger satisfies special cation exchange equations. The Rothmund-Kornfeld equation is well known and is a slight modification of the mass action law. The release of histamine from mast cell granules satisfies this equation[1]. But we also found that under our experimental conditions where we perfused the mast cell granules, the release also fitted two other equations based either on the occurrence of free histamine or the retainment of stored histamine in the mast cell granules during the release process (Fig. 3).

IONICALLY BOUND STORE

Ion exchange equations

F = released histamine (conc.)

a) $$F = F_0 e^{-k_F \sqrt{\Sigma ml}}$$

or the straight line:

$$\ln F = \ln F_0 - k_F \sqrt{\Sigma ml}$$

B = amount of bound releasable histamine in store

b) $$B = B_0 e^{-k_B \sqrt{\Sigma ml}} \qquad B_0 = B_{max}$$

or the straight line:

$$\ln B = \ln B_0 - k_B \sqrt{\Sigma ml}$$

Fig. 3. Kinetic equations valid for release of ionically bound cations in weak cation exchanger.

In our experiments we superfused mast cell granules, or mast cells, placed on a semipermeable filter in a special pump device[2]. Superfusion of granules with various salt solutions under isoosmotic conditions caused a release of histamine and this histamine release satisfied the characteristic ion exchange equations mentioned above, confirming that mast cell granules behave like cation exchanger materials. One day we decided to superfuse mast cells, not granules but intact mast cells, and found then to our surprise that histamine was released. Since histamine was released when we perfused the mast cells with various isotonic salt solutions including isotonic sodium chloride, we thought from the beginning that the histamine release was due to cation exchange between sodium and histamine in the mast cells. However, when we then observed that perfusion with isotonic deionized sucrose also led to a histamine release we had to change our mind. Especially since the histamine release also under these conditions satisfied the ion exchange equations. The sucrose did not contain any cations and the responsible cations had therefore to come from the mast cells, the best candidates then being potassium ions. We had in previous studies on granules found that sodium and potassium ions were equipotent in their ability to release histamine. We decided to measure simultaneously the outflow of histamine and potassium and we found not only a simultaneous release of potassium and histamine (Fig. 4a) but also an equimolar efflux of these substances (Fig. 4b). Both histamine and potassium contents vary considerably between mast cell batches the histamine content throughout being 3-4 times higher than the potassium content (Table 1).

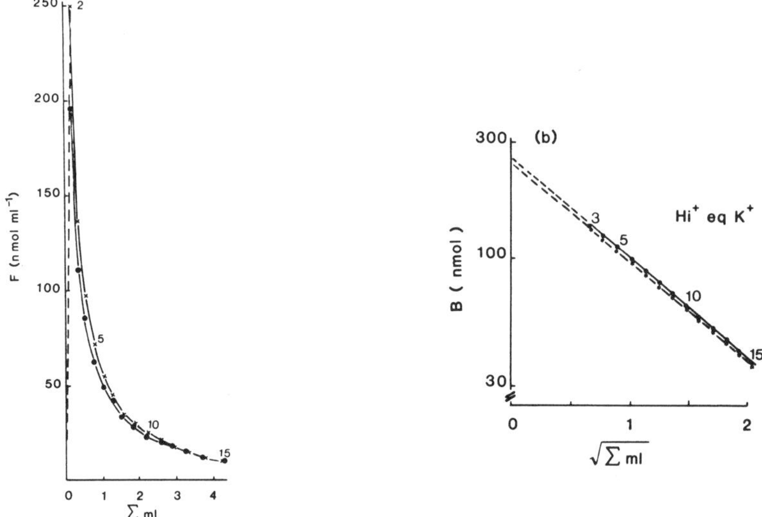

Fig. 4. Concomitant equimolar release of histamine and potassium on superfusion of mast cells with deionized isotonic sucrose solution (0.32 M, $7<pH<7.6$, 25°C, 0.2 ml min^{-1}). (a) Concentration of histamine and potassium versus cumulated effluent volume. (b) Release values for both histamine and potassium satisfy the ion exchange equation $\log B = K\sqrt{(\Sigma \text{ ml})} + \log B_{max}$. Histamine (× — ×). Potassium (• — •). (From Acta Physiol. Scand. 1989, 136: 309-320).

Table 1. Total content of histamine and potassium in 10^6 mast cells.

Exp Nº	Histamine nmol 10^6 cells	Potassium nmol 10^6 cells	Molar ratio Hi^+/K^+ cells
113	261.7	47.0	5.6
114	310.0	41.6	7.5
116	328.9	59.4	5.5
117	227.5	52.1	4.4
118	193.4	45.4	4.3
119	242.8	52.4	4.6
120	442.1	86.9	5.1
121	290.3	56.6	5.1
122	246.5	51.0	4.8
124	342.0	65.9	5.2
125	235.5	48.0	4.9
126	243.4	55.8	4.4
127	348.1	62.1	5.6
129	338.8	81.2	4.2
131	218.9	46.7	4.7
134	280.6	57.7	4.9
135	302.1	62.4	4.8
136	242.0	52.3	4.6
139	278.6	49.5	5.6
142	366.2	55.7	6.6
	Σ 5739.4	Σ 1129.7	Σ 102.4
	x = 287.0 ± 60.77	x = 56.5 ± 11.32	x = 5.1 ± 0.80
	(± 13.59)	(± 2.53)	(± 0.18)

x values are means ± SD (or ± SEM) for 20 experiments

A ratio of 1:1 between the histamine and potassium effluxes indicated therefore a dependence of histamine release on potassium release, suggesting that not all histamine should be released from the mast cell. In fact, Fig. 5 illustrates what happens when the cells are superfused. There is a continuous efflux of potassium and histamine but when the cytoplasmic potassium store is emptied (in the figure when the potassium curve hits the ordinate), the histamine release stops in spite of the fact that only 15% of the histamine store of the cells is released. In other words, the amount of histamine release depends on the amount of potassium available for the release process and not on the total histamine store.

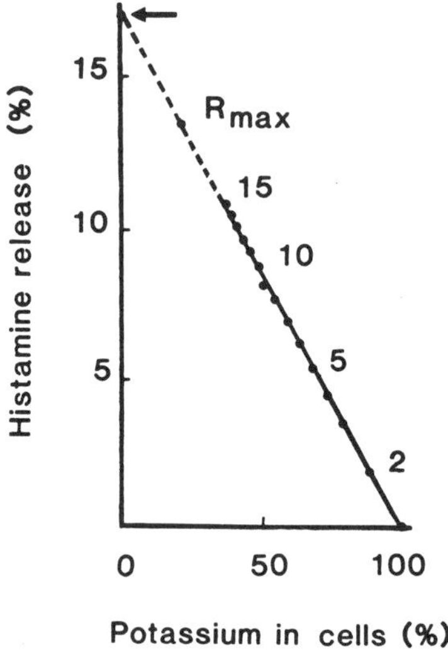

Fig. 5. Percentage release of histamine and depletion of potassium store on superfusion of mast cells with isotonic sucrose solution ($7<pH<7.6$, 25°C, 0.2 ml min^{-1}). Note that the intersection with the ordinata (arrow) corresponds exactly to the percentage ratio K^+/Hi^+ in the cells. Total K^+ (234 nmoles) × 100/total Hi^+ (1364 nmoles) = 17%. (From Acta Physiol. Scand. 1989, 136: 309-320).

The importance of potassium for the release of histamine might be an experimental curiosity occurring only in our artificial system, superfusion of the mast cell. However, when mast cells superfused with sucrose, in other words without any extracellular cations present, were exposed to compound 48/80, the histamine release was also here accompanied by an almost equimolar efflux of potassium, suggesting a similar dependence of the histamine release induced by compound 48/80 on potassium efflux as was the case with the superfused mast cells described above (to be published). My hypothesis is therefore, as illustrated in the schematic figure (Fig. 6) that when mast cells are superfused or challenged with compound 48/80 an internal flux of cytoplasmic potassium is initiated to pass across the histamine-containing granules. Histamine is released as reflected by the equimolar outpouring of histamine and potassium. In this situation degranulation is not obligatory. However, when the cells are challenged more intensely the potassium flux becomes so violent that also granules are expelled. In case this expulsion process is intense and rapid enough and the expelled granules still contain histamine this will immediately be released by ion exchange, primarily with sodium ions in the extracellular fluid. It should be mentioned that the idea of a histamine release from

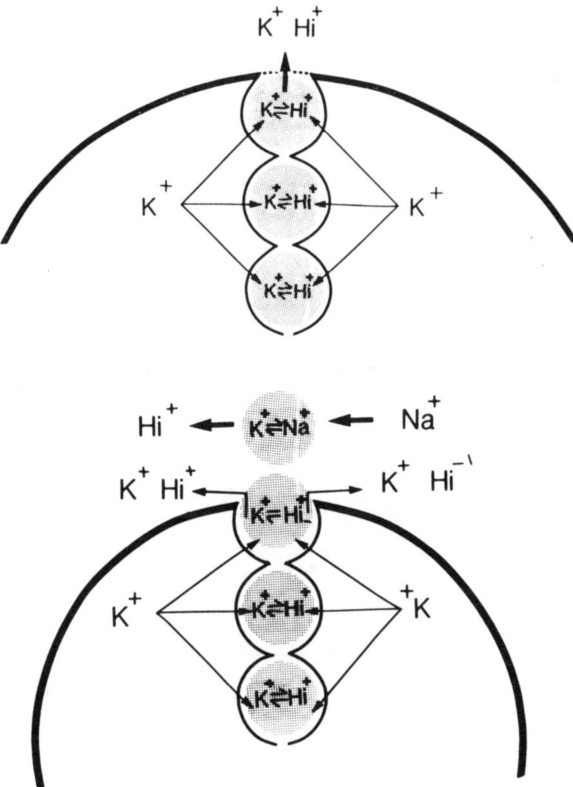

Fig. 6. Release of histamine from mast cells by intra- and extracellular ion exchange. (a) *Non-exocytotic phase*. Granules are exposed to a flux of cytoplasmic K^+ ions resulting in intracellular exchange $K^+ \rightleftharpoons Hi^+$. Released histamine and potassium pass out through membrane-bridged pores at the cell surface. Molar ratio of released K^+ to $Hi^+ = 1$. (b) *Exocytotic (degranulation) phase*. On more forceful response granules are dragged along with the potassium flux. Granules appearing extracellularly loose their remaining histamine by ion exchange with extracellular Na^+ ions ($Na^+ \rightleftharpoons Hi^+$). Molar ratio of released K^+ to $Hi^+ < 1$. (From Acta Physiol. Scand. 1989, 136: 309-320).

mast cells without concomitant degranulation is not new. The idea was presented for instance by Smith[3]. He describes histamine release into the cavity of the rat without concomitant degranulation of mast cells challenged with the granulating agents protamine and toluidine blue. His observation is evidently since long forgotten.

The next question arose. Why do mast cells release histamine on superfusion? One alternative could be that the superfusion disturbed some balance between the intra-and-extracellular compartments. Since histamine release appeared also on perfusion with salt solutions containing all physiologically occurring ions, one reason for the histamine release could be removal of an inhibitory factor. Histamine being considered a possible candidate we added histamine to the superfusion fluid. An inhibition was observed to occur with histamine concentrations within the μmolar range, ED_{50} being around 25 μM (Fig. 7). Interestingly enough, the remaining histamine release still occurred according to

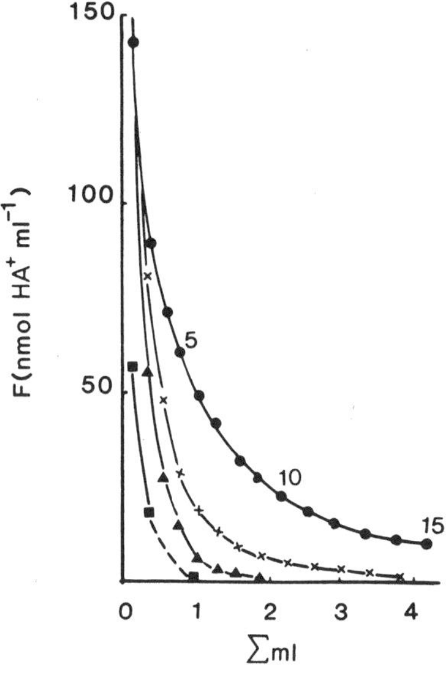

Fig. 7. Inhibition of histamine release from superfused mast cells by addition of histamine to the superfusion fluid (isoosmotic deionized sucrose 0.32 M, 0.2 ml min^{-1}, pH around 7, room temperature). • No external histamine, × 25 μM external histamine, ▲ 50 μM external histamine, ▪ 100 μM external histamine in superfusion medium. Note that added histamine is expressed in μ-molar concentrations but release of histamine in nmoles ml^{-1}.

ion exchange. The ratio between the released potassium and histamine diminished, approaching zero values (Fig. 8). In other words, the potassium efflux continued but was evidently diverted from the granules to leave the cell by some other route. In fact, the release of "excess" potassium outflow changed from being the result of an ion exchange

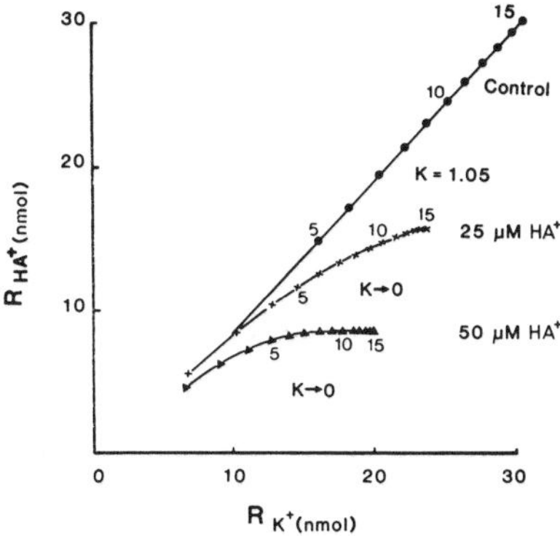

Fig. 8. Superfusion of mast cells with isoosmotic sucrose. Decline of potassium/histamine rations in eluates approaching zero on addition of histamine. In other words, histamine release goes towards total inhbition, while the efflux of potassium remains.

process to being a diffusion process obeying first order equation. Time does not allow me to go into this interesting phenomenon but it can be seen from Fig. 9 how the relationship between the histamine release and the external histamine concentration changes.

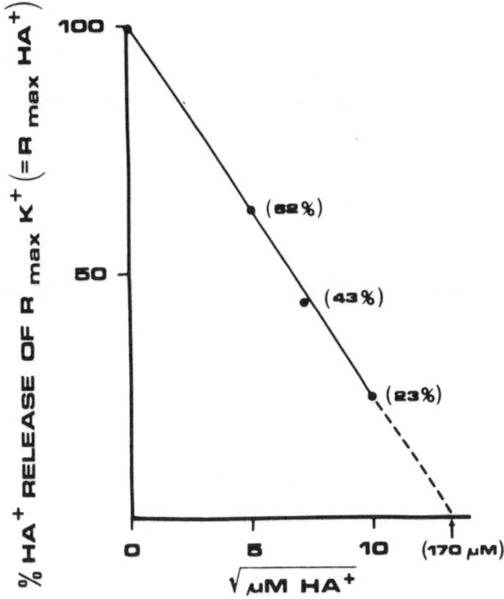

Fig. 9. Superfused mast cells. Sucrose 0.32 M. Linear relationship between release of histamine (in per cent of control) and square root values of external histamine concentrations. Release is expressed as R_{max}.

The more histamine in the external fluid the less histamine release on superfusion. Extrapolated values towards the intersection with the abscissa suggest that at an external concentration of about 170 μM histamine the histamine release approaches zero values. This is a very interesting curve, because it suggests that the functional histamine release from the mast cell in vivo may be counterbalanced by the extracellular histamine concentration. It is known that mast cells show a spontaneous histamine release which might then be checked by the extracellular histamine concentrations. In the rat peritoneal fluid we determined the histamine concentration in pleural and abdominal cavities to be around 30–40 μM. In other words, concentrations which should suffice to have inhibitory influences on the histamine release from the mast cells.

The ion exchange properties of mast cell granules prompted us to study the properties of catecholamine containing granules from adrenals(4). It turned out that the chromaffin granule material behaved just as the mast cell granules do, as cation exchange materials. The superfusion of the granules caused a release of catecholamines satisfying the cation exchange equations. With the mast cell studies in mind we also studied the release of catecholamines from living cells. In cats the splanchnic nerves were stimulated and the catecholamine release determined(5). The release turned out to satisfy the same cation exchange equations found valid for granules in vitro. The idea that nerve impulses induce a catecholamine release on cation exchange basis was strengthened by the observation that when splanchnic nerve stimulation was stopped during the estimated height of the catecholamine release the kinetics of the release immediately changed from satisfying an ion exchange equation to satisfying an equation of first order, suggesting the continuous release of catecholamines to come from a free depot formed during the nerve stimulation. Identical results were obtained with acetylcholine as the catecholamine releasing agent.

We have in previous experiments observed that granule materials from various peripheral and central neurons also behave like cation exchange particles and the release of catecholamines and other amines from superfused granule materials satisfies ion exchange equations. These observations are of interest in connection with the current exocytosis theory, according to which transmitter amines, as also the catecholamines from the adrenal gland, are released by evacuation of catecholamine-containing vesicles. In other words, transmitter amines should be released in quanta corresponding to the contents of vesicles. The minimal quantum that can be released according to this exocytosis theory is the content of one vesicle. However, there are many quantitative discrepancies between the exocytosis theory and several experimental observations. At adrenergic nerve terminals in cat or rat there are for example about 50 varicosities in each terminal; each varicosity contains about 1,000 vesicles and each vesicle 10–15,000 noradrenaline molecules[6]. It can be calculated that if the nerve impulse activates only one vesicle at each varicosity, the released quanta of catecholamines should result in extremely high concentrations of the transmitter amine in a narrow junctional space. Folkow and his group[7] as well as others have experimentally calculated the amount of noradrenaline released on sympathetic nerve stimulation and found that each nerve impulse should release only 300–400 molecules per varicosity, in other words, only a fraction of the contents of a vesicle. It has previously been difficult to understand how a fractional release of a vesicle content can occur, but in case the storage and release of amines is dependent on cation exchange, then it will be possible to explain the transmitter amine release not as due to a total evacuation of a vesicle but to a fractional release from perhaps numerous vesicles, the size of the released quanta being dependent not any more on the total content of amine in the vesicle but on the size of the ion flux, possibly potassium flux, initiated by the nerve impulse. If the ion exchange theory will be verified to play a role in the release of catecholamines and transmitter amines, many new questions will be opened for discussion both in neurophysiology and neuropharmacology.

References

1. Uvnäs, B., The mechanism of histamine release from mast cells, In: Handbook of Experimental Pharmacology, vol. XVIII/2, pp. 75-92 (Eds. G.V.R. Born, O. Eichler, A. Farah, H. Herben and A.D. Welsh). Springer-Verlag, Berlin, Heidelberg, New York 1978.

2. Uvnäs, B., C.-H. Aborg, L. Lyssarides and L.-G. Danielsson, Intracellular ion exchange between cytoplasmic potassium and granule histamine, an integrated link in the histamine release machinery of mast cells, Acta Physiol. Scand. 136, 309-320 (1989).

3. Smith, D.E., Nature of the secretory activity of the mast cell, Am. J. Physiol. 193(3), 573-575 (1958).

4. Uvnäs, B. and C.-H. Aborg, In vitro studies on a two-pool storage of adrenaline and noradrenaline in granule material from bovine adrenal medulla, Acta Physiol. Scand. 109, 345-354 (1980).

5. Uvnäs, B., C.-H. Aborg and M. Goiny, The kinetics of adrenal catecholamine secretion elicited by splanchnic nerve stimulation or by Ach is consistent with non-exocytotic, multivesicular release on cation exchange basis, Acta Physiol. Scand. 123, 249-259 (1985).

6. Dahlström, A., J. Häggendal and T. Hökfelt, The noradrenaline content of the nerve terminal varicosities of sympathetic adrenergic neurons in the rat, Acta Physiol. Scand. 67, 289-294 (1966).

7. Folkow, B., F. Häggendal and B. Lisander, Extent of release and elimination of noradrenaline at peripheral adrenergic nerve terminals, Acta Physiol. Scand. Suppl. 307 (1967).

AAS 36
Contributions to
Autacoid Pharmacology

HISTAMINE AND ANTIHISTAMINES IN ANAESTHESIA AND SURGERY: FROM EXPERIMENTAL PHARMACOLOGY TO CLINICAL DECISION MAKING

W. Lorenz

Institute of Theoretical Surgery, Centre of Operative Medicine I, Phillipps - University Marburg, Baldingerstrasse, W-3550 Marburg, FRG

Abstract

The problem of whether antihistamines (histamine H_1+H_2-antagonists) should be administered prophylactically before surgical interventions rose after animal experiments with hypnotics, opioids, muscle relaxants and plasma substitutes. It could, however, not be solved by classical biomedical research, but needed a heuristic problem-solving strategy. This strategy was formalized and in this way changed into a scientific structure by the thinking-aloud technique and the building of a decision tree with 9 nodes and various study designs to answer questions at particular decision nodes. The first question, whether the incidence of the reactions was high, was answered by several controlled clinical trials. The second question of life-threatening degrees of severity in single cases, was answered by a drug surveillance study. The third question, of whether severe incidents could always be avoided was answered by medical audit. The same was the case if death had to be considered as the final therapeutic failure. The fifth question was, "are the risks of histamine release comparable to other risks in the perioperative period?" They were - if thromboembolism, infection and stress ulcers were considered. The sixth and seventh questions referred to an experimentally and clinically effective prophylaxis. They were answered by animal and clinical studies with histamine antagonists, mainly with dimetindene and cimetidine. Undesired, adverse reactions to prophylaxis are rare since the drugs are given only once. Prophylaxis was calculated to be fairly cost-effective. Problem-solving strategies are very helpful in transferring facts and conclusions from experimental basic research to clinical decision making. This was convincingly demonstrated in antihistamine prophylaxis in anaesthesia and surgery.

Introduction

In the environment of experimental pharmacology as an important part of basic science in medicine, preoperative preparation of a surgical patient is in a state of nearly unbelievable pharmacological chaos (Fig. 1). Within about 40 min up to 15 drugs are administered into a "poor" single patient – all well-conceived to improve his vital safety, homeostatic stability and physiological and psychological comfort[1,2]. However, all these drugs and measures including intubation, gastric tube insertion and patient positioning, also produce side-effects. One of these is histamine release, serious enough to be prevented in its biological effects by a cost-effective prophylaxis with histamine H_1-+H_2-receptor antagonists[3,4]. However, the road from experimental pharmacology to clinical decision making is more arduous than expected from the promising results of animal experimentation and controlled clinical trials[1,4].

The role of experimental pharmacology in the concept of antihistamine prophylaxis in anaesthesia and surgery

How did this concept arise? It started clearly with reductionistic experimental pharmacology[5]. All components of induction of anaesthesia were first studied in animals. It is the sincere intention of this issue of Agents and Actions to celebrate the work of Rocha e Silva and his collaborators in London and Ribeirão Preto because they have, by extensive animal investigation, prepared the way for meaningful clinical decision making, several decades later.

The induction of anaesthesia starts with the giving of a small dose of the muscle relaxant alcuronium chloride (Fig. 1) to avoid postoperative muscular pain. The muscle relaxant d-tubocurarine was investigated many years ago for its histamine-releasing side-effects in the classical article of Rocha e Silva and Schild[6] Fig. 2 of this presentation shows histamine release as a very explosive event occurring mostly during the first 5 min following injection of the relaxant. This holds true also in man, as later clinical studies have shown[7]. However, experiments in animals were used to predict the activity of the most potent muscle relaxants having low histamine-releasing capacity (Table 1). The index of autonomic margin of safety as a measure of increased neuromuscular blocking potency, but reduced histamine-releasing activity for each drug was developed in cats[9] and is now generally accepted for the assessment of drugs newly released into the pharmaceutical market.

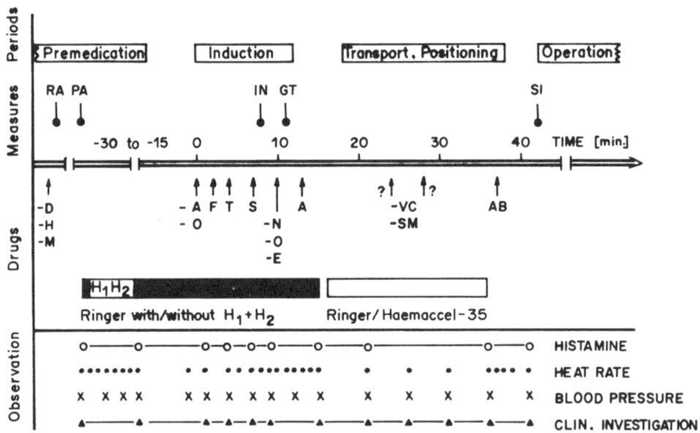

Fig. 1. Schematic description of the treatment and investigations in a single anaesthetized patient in the study (Mainz-Marburg trial). D = diazepan; H = heparin; M = miscellaneous; RA = randomization; PA = peripheral access; A = alcuronium; O = oxygen; F = fentanyl; T = thiopental; S = suxamethonium; N = nitrous oxide; E = enflurane; IN = intubation; GT = gastric tube; VC = vasoconstrictors; SM = stabilization medications; AB = Antibiotics; SI = skin incision. For further conditions of the trial see Lorenz *et al.*[(1)].

Table 1. Index of autonomic margin of safety for neuromuscular blocking drugs in cats.

Drug	Cat $\frac{ED_{50} \text{ (HR)}}{ED_{95} \text{ NMB)}}$	Man Plasma histamine (% of control) AT ED_{95} (NMB)
dTC	1.14	318%
BW785U	6.0	260%
BW444U	15.7	134%
Atracurium	>16	77%

From Moss et al., Klin. Wochenschrift (8)

– The second drug in the induction of anaesthesia (Fig. 1) is fentanyl, an opioid analgesic drug. The symptoms of histamine release by morphine were first described by the first investigator of morphine in an experiment on himself Friedrich Wilhelm

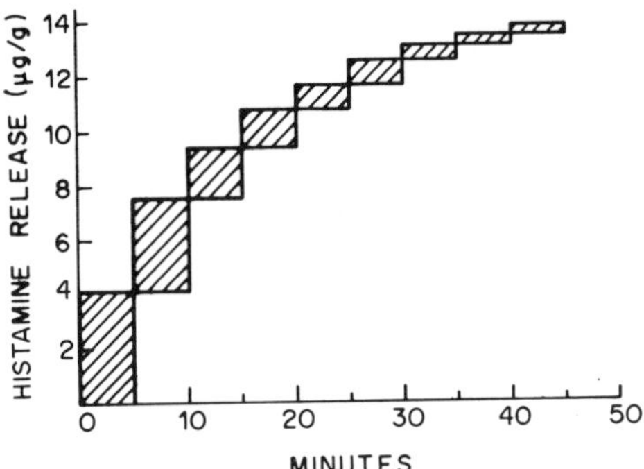

Fig. 2. Total histamine released from a rat diaphragm left during successive periods of 5 min in solutions of d-tubocurarine (1:1000), in Tyrode solution. From Rocha e Silva and Schild[6].

Sertürner from Einbeck close to Hannover in 1817: erythema, nausea and general weakness, probably due to hypotension[10]. Histamine release by opioids in experimental pharmacology was first described by Feldberg and Paton[11] (Fig. 3), who found again, that histamine release after morphine was an explosive event as demonstrated by Schachter[12] for pethidine, a synthetical opioid product of the Hoechst Company (Fig. 4). Most of the histamine released appeared in the first 5–10 min in the bathing fluid of cat's skin which was *fortunately* the particular isolated tissue investigated. Not all mast cells react to opioids with the same potency as do skin mast cells[13,14].

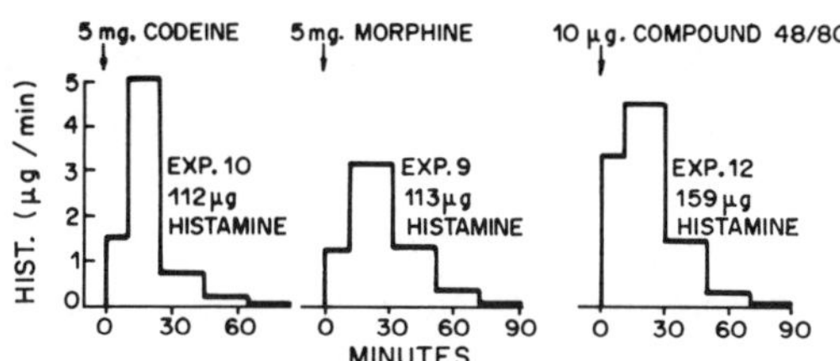

Fig. 3. Histamine output from perfused cat's skin by 5 mg codeine, 5 mg morphine and 10 μg compound 48/80. The numbers of the experiments refer to those of Table 5. From Feldberg and Paton[11].

– The third drug in the induction of anaesthesia was thiopentone (Fig. 1), the barbiturate hypnotic agent so frequently shown to release histamine in man[15-17]. In

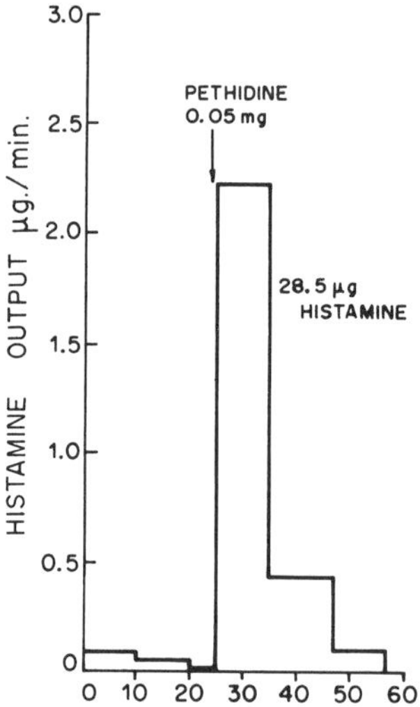

Fig. 4. Histamine release from cat skin by the opioid analgesic drug pethidine. From Schachter[12].

experimental pharmacology there is as yet no model for clinical histamine release; in isolated human skin mast cells, histamine release by this world-wide distributed drug was shown[18]. Other hypnotic agents such as propanidid, althesin and propofol, shown to release histamine[15-17,19,20], have a problem in common. They are all dissolved in cremophor E1, a derivative of fatty acids and a wetting agent, shown to be effective on its own in dogs, as a very potent histamine releaser[21,22]. As Fig. 5 demonstrates, arterial blood pressure fell dramatically after injection of small doses of cremophor E1. It was the delayed blood pressure response classically described by Paton[23]. Histamine release was identified by measuring blood histamine concentrations in several circulatory areas of the dog[24]. In addition, antihistamines prevented hypotension[5]. The results of this study indicated that histamine was liberated both from the periphery of the body (skin) and from the gastrointestinal tract: blood levels were higher in the portal vein than in the hepatic vein and in the abdominal aorta. This finding was most remarkable[26,27] since it was the first example in the literature describing histamine release from the mucosal mast cell[28,29]. Cremophor E1 is a solubilizer used not only for various hypnotic drugs, but also for a series of other compounds used in the induction of anaesthesia (Table 2). Its place, therefore, is well established in pharmacology, but it has created clinical problems in transplantation surgery as the solubilizer of cyclosporin A.

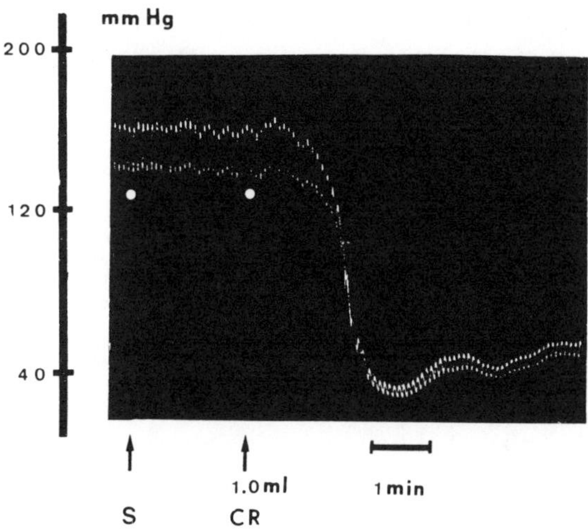

Fig. 5. Blood pressure response in a dog following administration of the solubilizer, cremophor El. Ordinate: arterial blood pressure in mm Hg. Abcissa: time in mins. S. = Saline, CR = cremophor El (1 ml/dog; weight of the animal 14 Kg).

Table 2. Drugs "dissolved" in cremophor E1 for parenteral administration.

<u>Anaesthetics</u>	<u>Antibiotics</u>
- Diprivan	- penicillins
- (Propanidid - Epontol^{R})	- sulphonamides
- (Althesin^{R})	
	<u>Vitamins</u>
	- Vitamin A, D, E
<u>Steroid Hormones</u>	
- derivatives of oestrogen	<u>Immunosuppressants</u>
- derivatives of cortisone	- Cyclosporin A

After the muscle relaxants, analgesics and hypnotics, plasma substitutes are the fourth drugs given in order to prevent or treat hypotension, relative hypovolaemia and other cardiovascular disturbances of the surgical patient (Fig. 1). Again, this problem was carefully investigated in animal experiments (Fig. 6). In agreement with the human situation, the most potent histamine releaser was Haemaccel – in its now outdated

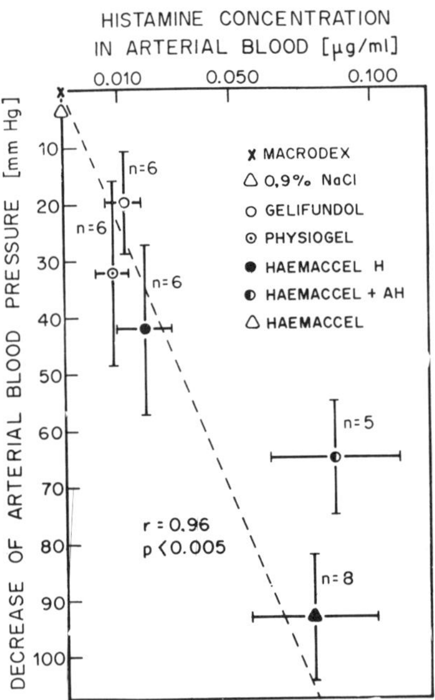

Fig. 6. Correlation between maximal increase of histamine concentration in the arterial blood and maximum fall of the arterial blood pressure in dogs undergoing isovolemic hemodilution by means of different plasma substitutes. The data from animals pretreated with the antihistaminic Neclastinum (0.1 mg/Kg), (Haemaccel + AH) were not included for the calculation of the regression line. From Messmer *et al.*[30].

formulation[31]. Its side effect, eliciting adverse anaphylactoid reactions was blocked by histamine antagonists – the earliest finding of a successful antihistamine prophylaxis, in 1970[30]. This problem was further investigated using H_2-blockers[32] and compound 48/80 at doses which produced plasma histamine levels as high as those occurring in really severe anaphylactoid clinical reactions in man[3,33] (Fig. 7). A dose of only 50 µg/kg compound 48/80 was necessary – dissolved in 500 ml Ringer solution imitating gelatin or other histamine-releasing plasma substitutes[34] – to increase plasma histamine levels up to an average of 70 ng/ml. As in human anaesthesia with doses of drugs commonly used[3], large

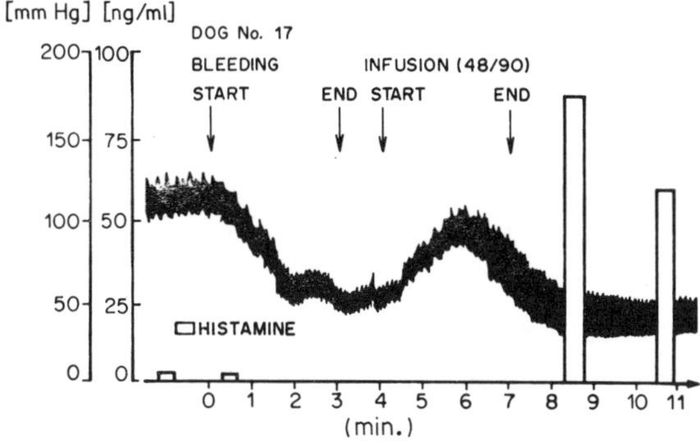

Fig. 7. Blood pressure and arterial plasma histamine in a dog after bleeding 1/3 of its blood volume and immediate replacement by Ringer solution containing 50 μg/Kg 48/80 (normovolaemic haemodilution). As premedication saline instead of antihistamines or corticosteroids was given. Histamine in ng/ml, blood pressure in mm Hg.

Table 3. Prophylaxis of life-threatening pseudoallergic reactions to 48/80 in dogs by histamine receptor blockade or methylprednisolone.

Prophylaxis	Hypotension (mm Hg, $\tilde{x}$)	Histamine release (ng/ml, $\tilde{x}$)
Saline	60	52
H_1	28	32
$H_1 + H_2$	0	11
MP 3	63	32
MP 15	88	90

H_1 = 0.5 mg/kg i.v. dimethindene, H_2 = 5 mg/kg i.v. cimetidine, MP = 3 or 15 mg/kg i.v. methylprednisolone. Randomized study, n = 12/group. From Dietz et al. (33)

variations were observed with this dog model and recently also with pigs. The results on Table 3 were obtained applying several prophylactic measures. In this randomized controlled trial in dogs, saline served as control. The H_1-receptor antagonist dimethindene with a pA_2-value of 9[35] similar to that of mepyramine, was partly effective; the combination of dimethindene with the H_2-receptor antagonist cimetidine fully inhibited the pharmacological effect of 48/80; it also effectively reduced histamine release. The corticosteroid methylprednisolone was not effective at all in a conventional dose[36]; it did worse in the high dose commonly used in traumatic and septic shock[37-39]. These findings strongly recommend H_1-+H_2-prophylaxis in anaesthesia and surgery.

The gap between concepts developped in experimental pharmacology and clinical decision making

Why was the histamine H_1-+H_2-prophylaxis not in every-day use in anaesthesia and surgery? As a clinical chemist and biochemical pharmacologist, the author of this review had to learn his lesson when, about 20 years ago he moved from basic to clinical research in a Department of Theoretical Surgery and, in a team of basic scientists, anaesthetists and surgeons, tried to convince a clinical environment[(40)] to use H_1-+H_2-blockade.

– Problem Nº 1 was *incidence*. Several groups reported, after more than 20 controlled clinical trials with single drugs, a high incidence[(4)]; the majority of the clinicians, even after hundreds of talks and two dozen symposia, books and articles[(4)], was however not convinced that this occurred during clinical routine[(1,4,41)].

– The second problem was *severity*. Hundreds of case reports were collected in reviews about life-threatening allergic and pseudoallergic reactions[(42-44)]. The calculated incidence was similar to that of thromboembolism, pulmonary infection in surgery and stress ulceration - but: the majority of clinicians was not convinced that this was dangerous enough to use prophylactic intervention[(45)].

– Problem Nº 3 was *effectiveness*. Although effectiveness was demonstrated in controlled clinical trials[(4)] and in a field study[(46)], the majority of clinicians was not convinced that such a prophylaxis had any significant effect on the postoperative outcome[(1)].

Heuristic problem-solving strategy to overcome the gap between basic science and clinical medicine: example of H_1- + H_2-prophylaxis

Three different strategies were conceived and applied to overcome a situation frustrating for supporters and of potential risks and costs in health for millions of patients undergoing surgery every year.

– A *controlled clinical trial* was carefully conceived over a period of about three years; the protocol was published in 1988[(1)]. In addition, a discussion forum was built with known pro and contra experts putting forward their arguments against the concept and methodologies of this trial[(45)]. Experts included surgeons, anaesthetists, pharmacologists and immunologists. The trial started in December 1988 and has now enrolled 200 of 240 planned patients.

– A careful *causality analysis* was performed for typical situations in anaesthesia and surgery in which histamine release was frequently demonstrated[(47)]. Koch-

Dale criteria, Hill-criteria, a multivariate model with several types of determinants, calculation of conditional probabilities and a causal network were taken into account. This analysis was published in a book series[48] whose first two volumes on Histamine had been edited by Mauricio Rocha e Silva[49,50]: the Handbook of Experimental Pharmacology.

– However, during the performance of the first two strategies, rejection of the H_1-+H_2-prophylaxis by anaesthetists posed questions and lead to statements against the use of such a premedication; they could not be contradicted by the result of a controlled clinical trial only. This dilemma led to the application of a third strategy developed by information scientists and medical decision makers. It has been denominated a *problem-solving strategy*[51]. One of its methods is the thinking-aloud technique[52]. Experts in the field with contradicting opinions were asked to pose their arguments, explanations, and especially decisions, in a lively discussion. This discussion was taped and analysed. Decisions proposed in this dialogue were formally structured in a so called *heuristic decision tree* (Fig. 8). Decisions were presented as answers to the questions using results of available *differents types* of experimental and clinical studies. They ended in an acceptance of the H_1-+H_2-prophylaxis. Using this strategy both supporters and rejectors of premedication were forced to argue rationally, formally and systematically and hence more scientifically in face of this complex problem.

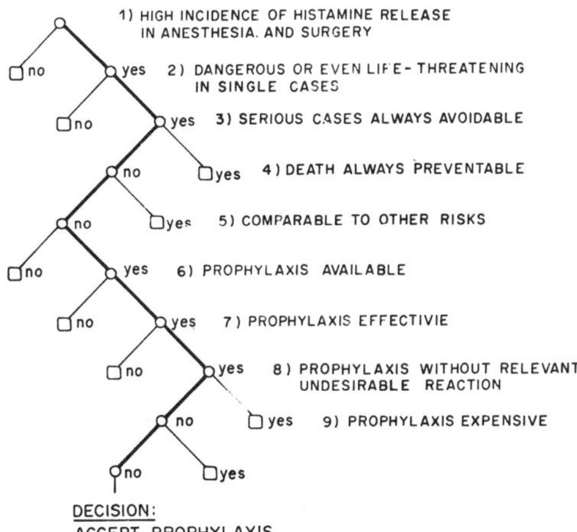

Fig. 8. Decision tree for heuristic decision-making developed by the "think-aloud techinique" with three experts. It includes nine hierarchically ordered decision nodes at which questions had to be answered. Data from different types of clinical studies (controlled trials, epidemiological surveys,postmarketing surveillance and cost-effectiveness analysis) were used in creating this tree. The final decision was acceptance of the prophylaxis. From Lorenz *et al.*[4].

The *first of 9 questions* was that on high incidence. Its answer was given in a controlled clinical trial in 600 orthopaedic patients[(53)], using outdated, classical Haemaccel with an excess of cross-linking hexamethylene diisocyanate[(54)]. 30 out of 600 patients, showed a systemic anaphylactoid reaction which in 3, was life-threatening. The incidence of reactions including those with only skin manifestations, was 30 per cent. Individual values are shown on Figs. 9 and 10.

However, the rejectors of the H_1-+H_2-prophylaxis may oppose: if the outdated Haemaccel was replaced by a new, less toxic drug formulation, the problem would be solved by the so called treatment paradox and no H_1-+H_2-prophylaxis would be needed. Yet, the many drug combinations used in anaesthesia (Fig. 1) keep the incidence high. The present status of the Mainz-Marburg trial[(1)], in 200 patients is: 85% of the patients show at least one episode of histamine release reaction to one of the many drugs given. 4 life-threatening reactions were observed, of which only 1, associated with skin reactions, could not be diagnosed as a histamine release reaction had not plasma histamine been determined. The incidence of histamine release reactions of various grades of severity, in anaesthesia and surgery is still *at least* 20–30%.

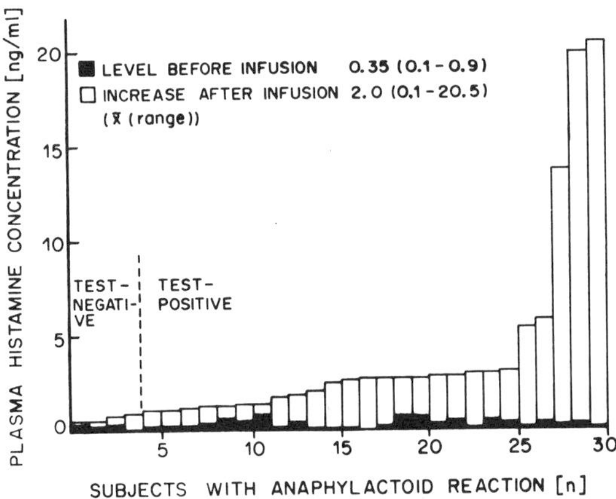

Fig. 9. Plasma histamine levels before and after infusion of Haemaccel in patients with systemic pseudoallergic reactions. Single values from each of the patients. Dotted line = cut-off point for a plasma histamine level > 1 ng/ml. From Lorenz *et al.*[(53)].

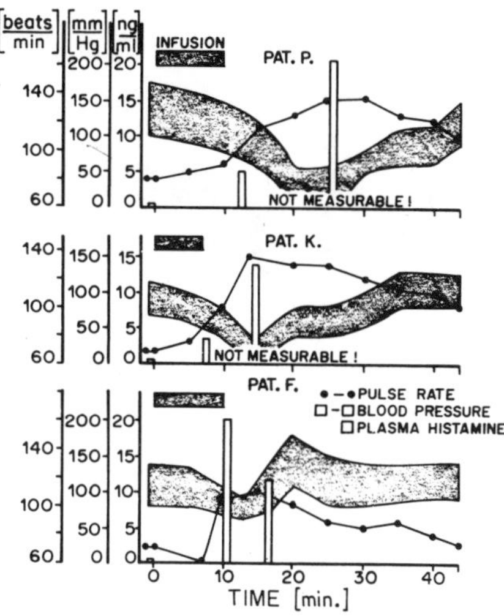

Fig. 10. Life-threatening anaphylactoid reactions to polygeline in a clinical trial with orthopedic patients. Single values from each of the patients. From Lorenz *et al.*[53].

The *second question* in the decision tree is that on dangerous or life-threatening severity in single cases. Case reports can answer this question[42-49,56,57]. Deliberately, the chosen one, deals with a drug which never seems to be outdated: human albumin (Fig. 11). The patient with oesophageal cancer suffered from ventricular fibrillation and therefore circulatory arrest. His plasma histamine level was 110 ng/ml, the highest value we ever measured over a period of 20 years in more than 24,000 estimates. It did not return to normal levels even 8 hours after the incident. He was admitted to the intensive care unit[55].

The *third question* is whether serious incidents are avoidable. Clinicians argue that the development of shock, of circulatory breakdown, of cardiac or respiratory arrest have to be considered as bad clinical practice. It was urgently demanded by them to improve medical care and to introduce more effective medical audit, rather than to introduce a new prophylaxis. The answer to this question is given by incidents occurring during clinical trials with well-trained anaesthetists who were aware of the possibility of a life-threatening reaction in every case of the study (Hawthorne effect). Hundreds of cases collected from various parts of England[56,58,59] indicate that medical practice is not better than what can be observed in a nation-wide surveillance system.

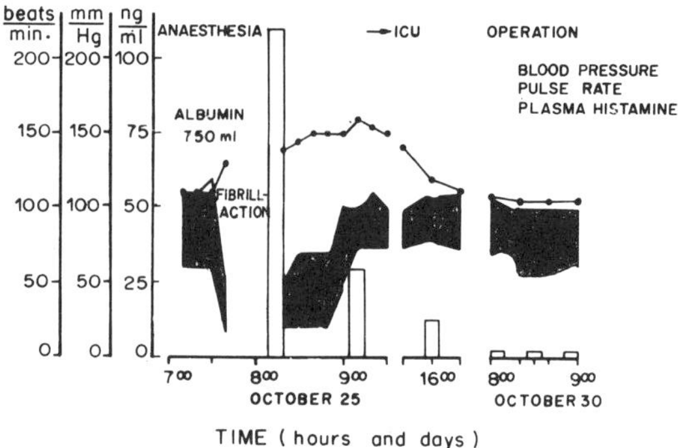

Fig. 11. Histamine release by human albumin. Plasma histamine levels, blood pressure, and heart rate from a patient with esophageal carcinoma. From Doenicke and Lorenz(55).

This problem is proposed even more seriously by the *fourth question:* Is death always preventable? The first answer to this are the reports about patients in the author's own experience: An urological patient received 20 ml of dextran. The patient died within a few min - despite emergency treatment(34). So did 30 other patients reported to the committee for safety of drugs in West Germany during one year(60). Again, the treatment paradox argues: give him low-molecular weight dextran as a hapten! So we proceed to the second patient: An 82 years old female received bone cement for an artificial hip replacement. She died within a few min(55). Some clinicians may argue: was it only histamine? But this is not a problem if we accept causality as a contributory determinant(61), as impressively demonstrated by a field study with chymopapain (Table 4). Although histamine release to this drug, used to dissolve an incarcerated intervertebral disc, is considered a true anaphylactic reaction releasing a whole battery of mediators other than histamine, the H_1- + H_2-prophylaxis reduced death rate by a factor of 20–60.

The second answer to the fourth question has nothing to do with biomedical research, but with the problem of distinguishing between efficiency and effectiveness of a medical technology(62). Effectiveness is the success of a treatment under optimum conditions (e.g. a randomized trial), whereas efficiency is the success under routine clinical conditions.

Effectiveness is always better than efficiency in technology assessment. It cannot be achieved in routine. It is remarkable that those arguing against H_1- + H_2-prophylaxis under conditions of routine anaesthesia, immediately switch to clinical trials, when arguing against a change in their daily practice. This inconsistency can be supported by animal experiments (Table 5). A healthy animal may not be dying from histamine release. However, bleeding and substitution of blood lost by a plasma substitute, produces death even at low plasma histamine levels.

Table 4. Incidence of anaphylactic reactions to chymopapain in a field study in USA.

Events	period 1 - (1982)	period 2 $H_1 + H_2$ (1983)	period 3 $H_1 + H_2$ (1984)
- operated (n)	1585	16 177	28 736
- reactants (n,%)	13 (0.82)	126 (0.78)	126 (0.44)
- death (n)	2	2	1
- mortality (%)	0.13	0.006	0.002

From Moss *et al.*(46).

Table 5. Plasma histamine levels and incidence of death before the end of the experiment following bleeding and volume substitution by a plasma substitute releasing histamine. (Ringer's solution with compound 48/80 imitating a histamine-releasing plasma expander such as human albumin or polygeline).

Dose of compound 48/80	1 mg/kg[a]	1 mg/kg[b]	0.3 mg/kg[b]	0[b]
Blood loss before releaser (ml)	5	500	150	500
Time of administration (min)	0.5	3	3	3
Plasma histamine level (ng/ml)	855 (305–2520)	510 (0–1100)	94 (0–1120)	0.3 (0.1–1.3)
Incidence of death during experiment	0/8	5/8	1/8	0/8

From Lorenz *et al.*(47).

Drug surveillance studies by industrial companies all over the world reveal that anaesthesiological and surgical practice is associated with death rates which should not, but do, occur. The most convincing example is that of the British CEPOD study (Table 6). It demonstrates human failure as part of clinical routine. Prophylaxis helps to overcome this imperfection.

The *fifth question* is: "are risks of histamine release comparable to other risks in the perioperative period?" The answer is "yes" if thromboembolism, surgical infection and stress ulcers are considered as conditions for which a medical prophylaxis is fairly well accepted (Table 7). Clinically less important endpoints of these complications are very common; severe events are less frequent - common practice continues to accept this for decision making.

Table 6. Confidential enquiry into perioperative deaths (CEPOD).

- criteria -
- Appropriateness of the operation. - Appropriateness of the preoperative preparation. - Appropriateness of the grade and special interests of the surgeon. - Soundness of the organization. - Equipment failure - Adverse drug reaction. - Human failure: lack of knowledge failure to apply knowledge lack of experience lack of care inadequate supervision fatigue physical or mental imparement other.

Pollock, Evans, Surgical audit[(63)].

The *sixth question* is that calling for effective prophylaxis. It has already been answered by the randomized study in dogs using H_1-receptor antagonists, H_1- + H_2-receptor antagonists and corticosteroids (Fig. 3).

The *seventh question*, on effectiveness in clinical conditions, can only be answered positively by a series of controlled clinical trials[(4)]. All phases of anaesthesia

Table 7. Classes of severity and incidence of complications occurring in surgical conditions selected for prophylaxis.

Complications	Classes of severity and incidence (%) I	II	III
- Thrombo-embolism	Fibrin split products (10-100)	Deep vein thrombosis (1-10)	pulmonal embolism (0.01 - 1)
- Wound infection	anastomotic leakage (20-50)	pelvic abscess (1-5)	septic shock (0.1 - 0.5)
- Stress ulceration	endoscopic lesion (20-80)	clinically manifest bleeding (1-5)	haemorrhagic gastritis (0.05 - 0.2)
- Histamine release reactions	cutaneous (20-30)	systemic (1-5)	life-threatening (0.1 - 0.5)

From Lorenz *et al.*[64].

(Fig. 1) have been investigated with single drugs as histamine liberators. They include hypnotics, analgesics, muscle relaxants and plasma substitutes. This question is remarkably well-documented. Table 8 provides a few examples. The general scepticism is difficult to understand if the clinical success of the positive results of H_1-+H_2-prophylaxis in so many trials is considered. Undesirable side-effects of the H_1-+H_2-prophylaxis are minimal since the drugs are given only *once* before operation. Hence the *eighth question* is easily answered.

Is H_1-+H_2-prophylaxis cost-effective, is the *final question* reached in the decision tree. It can only be answered by a formal cost-effectiveness study[65] not yet performed. However it can be calculated that one day in an intensive care unit costs about 2000 DM; 1 package of the prophylastic treatment costs about 10 DM; hence, 200 patients can be treated with the antihistamines at a price equal to one life-threatening reaction, not considering the anxiety and discomfort the patient suffers from such a reaction. Since the incidence of life-threatening reactions in the Mainz-Marburg study was about 4 in 200 or 1 in 50, the prophylaxis is cost effective if it prevents only 1 of the reactions in 200 patients. Hence the H_1-+H_2-prophylaxis is cost-effective and preferable to present-day wait-and-see strategy.

Table 8. Clinical trials investigating the effectiveness of a combined prophylaxis witgh H_1- and H_2-receptor antagonists to prevent adverse pseudoallergic/allergic reactions.

Drug, Severity of Reactions, Number of Patients, Antihistamines Used	Result	Author and Reference Number
	Induction of anesthesia and preparation of the surgical patient	
Morphine (1 mg/kg), grade 2 40 patients, cardiac bypass surgery diphenhydramine 1 mg/kg cimetidine 4 mg/kg	Cardiac index (CI) unchanged, diastolic blood pressure (DP) slightly reduced (7 torr) $H_1 + H_2$. CI increased, DP reduced by ca. 26 torr saline, $p < 0.05$	Philbin et al.[91]
Propanidid, grade 1 + 2 32 volunteers dimetindene 0.1 mg/kg + cimetidine 10 mg/kg	4/16 with flush $H_1 + H_2$ 11/16 flush saline tachycardia significantly reduced in $H_1 + H_2$ group $p < 0.02$	Lorenz et al.[21]
Suxamethonium, grade 1 + 2 60 surgical patients (20 saline, 20 H_1, 20 $H_1 + H_2$) general surgery promethazine 0.5 mg/kg (i.m.) + cimetidine 400 mg (i.m.)	1/20 had increased HR > 9 beats/min ($H_1 + H_2$) 9/20 (saline), 6/20 (H_1) $p < 0.01$ $H_1 + H_2$ v. saline	Tryba et al.[95]
d-Tubocurarine, grade 2 + 3 24 patients (placebo, H_1, H_2, $H_1 + H_2$), cardiac surgery chlorpheniramine 0.1 mg/kg cimetidine 4 mg/kg	$H_1 + H_2$ reduced decrease in SVR caused by tubocurarine $p < 0.05$	Inada et al.[12]
Atracurium, grade 1 + 2 40 patients, general surgery dimetindene 0.1 mg/kg ranitidine 1.25 mg/kg	0/20 histamine release reactions $H_1 + H_2$ 10/20 reactions saline $p < 0.01$	Doenicke et al.[10]
Polygeline, grade 1 + 2 50 volunteers dimetindene 0.1 mg/kg + cimetidine 5 mg/kg	0/25 reactions $H_1 + H_2$ 9/25 reactions saline $p < 0.01$	Schöning et al.[96]
Polygeline, grade 1 300 patients, orthopedic surgery dimetindene 0.1 mg/kg or chlorpheniramine 0.3 mg/kg + cimetidine 5 mg/kg	4/150 reactions $H_1 + H_2$ 27/150 reactions saline $p < 0.005$	Schöning et al.[96]
	Intraoperative measures and drug delivery	
DSA, Ultravist, grade 1–3 200 patients, radiodiagnostics dimetindene 0.1 mg/kg + cimetidine 5 mg/kg	1/100 mild reaction $H_1 + H_2$ 5/100 reactions saline $p < 0.05$	Beyer et al.[97]
Urography, Telebrix, grade 1 + 2 500 patients, urology dimetindene 0.1 mg/kg + cimetidine 5 mg/kg	16/300 reactions $H_1 + H_2$ 76/200 reactions saline less severe reactions with $H_1 + H_2$	Tauber et al.[98]
Urography, amidotrizoate, grade 1 + 2 196 patients $H_1 + H_2$, 194 patients saline, urology clemastine 0.03 mg/kg + cimetidine 5 mg/kg	1% incidence with $H_1 + H_2$ 4.6% incidence saline $p < 0.05$	Ring et al.[99]
Palacos implantation, grade 1–3 20 patients, emergency surgery clemastine 4 mg + cimetidine 400 mg	Changes in systolic blood pressure (SP) and DP and number of therapeutic interventions reduced with $H_1 + H_2$ $p < 0.01$ (BP), $p < 0.05$ (interventions)	Tryba et al.[72]

Trials listed in the sequence of their common use in anesthesia and surgery. DSA = digital subtraction angiography; SVR = systemic vascular resistance; Ultravist^R = Iopromide; Telebrix^R = Ioxithalamate. From Lorenz et al. (4). The reference numbers refer to the original paper.

Conclusion

Society has recognized that basic science does not exist for its own sake but is related to social aims especially in the case of a science of action like medicine. Pharmacology was never a discipline of pure interest such as anatomy, but always a science of living individuals; not of corpses. Likewise, Rocha e Silva was always a man of action, and not only of contemplation. This article, which may be read both as a review and a hypothesis contains an answer to his first book on Histamine (Fig. 12): after 35 years we are struggling in the cause for histamine – but we believe that we are closer than ever to a decision.

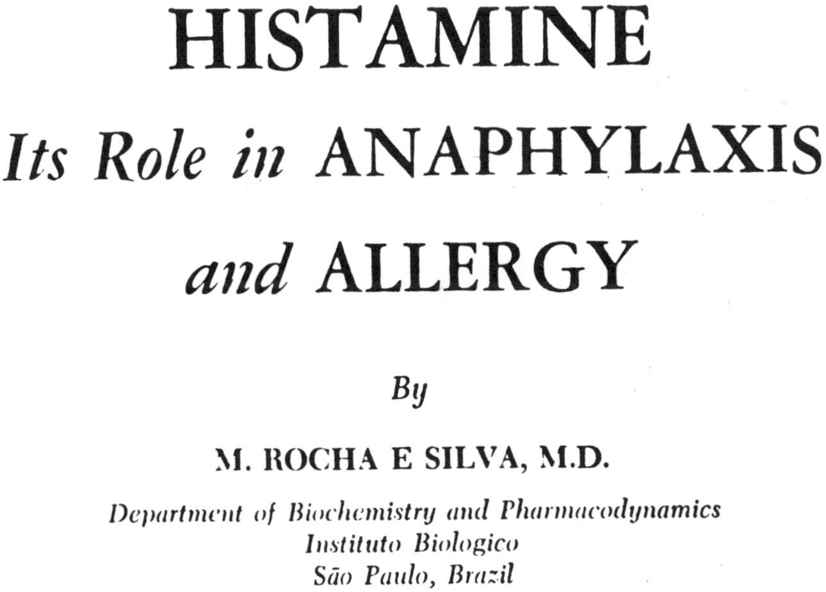

HISTAMINE

Its Role in ANAPHYLAXIS

and ALLERGY

By

M. ROCHA E SILVA, M.D.

Department of Biochemistry and Pharmacodynamics
Instituto Biologico
São Paulo, Brazil

Fig. 12. Photography of the first important book on histamine in allergic and pseudoallergic reactions – published by Rocha e Silva in 1955, Charles C. Thomas, Springfield, Illinois[66].

Acknowledgement: This article was supported by a grant from the Deutsche Forschungsgemeinschaft (Lo 199/16-1).

References

1. Lorenz, W., W. Dick, T. Junginger, C. Ohmann, M. Ennis, H. Immich, B. McPeek, W. Dietz and D. Weber, Members of the Trial Group Mainz/Marburg, Induction of anaesthesia and perioperative risk: Influence of antihistamine H_1-+H_2-prophylaxis and volume substitution with Haemaccel-35 on cardiovascular and respiratory disturbances and histamine release - Protocol of a controlled clinical trial, Theor. Surg. 3, 55-77 (1988).

2. Suttmann, H., A. Doenicke, W. Lorenz, M. Ennis, O.A. Müller, R. Dorow and M. Ackenheil, Is perioperative stress a real surgical phenomenon, of merely a drug-induced effect?, Theor. Surg. 1, 119-135 (1986).

3. Lorenz, W. and A. Doenicke, H_1-+H_2-blockade: a prophylactic principle in anaesthesia and surgery against histamine-release responses of any degree of severity, New Engl. Reg. Allergy Proc., Part I: 6, 37-57 (1985), Part II: 6, 174-194 (1985).

4. Lorenz, W., M. Ennis, A. Doenicke and W. Dick, Perioperative uses of histamine antagonists, J. Clin. Anesth. 2, 345-360 (1990).

5. Lorenz, W., M. Thermann, H. Hamelmann, A. Schmal, D. Maroske, H.-J. Reimann, J. Kusche, F. Schingale, P. Dormann and P. Keck, Influence of H_1-+H_2-receptor antagonists on the effects of histamine in the circulatory system and on plasma histamine levels, In: Int. Symposium on Histamine H_2-Receptor Antagonists, pp. 151-168 (Eds. C.J. Wood and M.A. Simkins). Deltakos, London 1973.

6. Rocha e Silva, M. and H.O. Schild, The release of histamine by d-tubocurarine from the isolated diaphragm of the rat, J. Physiol. 109, 448-458 (1949).

7. Moss, J., C.E. Rosow, J.J. Savarese, D.M. Philbin and K.J. Kniffen, Role of histamine in the hypotensive action of d-tubocurarine in humans, Anesthesiology 55, 19-25 (1981).

8. Moss, J., D.M. Philbin, C.E. Rosow, S.J. Basta, C. Gelb and J.J. Savarese, Histamine release by neuromuscular blocking agents in man, Klin. Wochenschr. 60, 891-895 (1982).

9. Savarese, J.J., The autonomic margins of safety of metocurine and d-tubocurarine in the cat, Anesthesiology 50, 40-46 (1979).

10. Sertürner, F.W.A., Über das Morphium, eine neue salzfähige Grundlage, und die Mekonsäure als Hauptbestandteil des Opiums, Annalen der Physik 55, 56 (1817).

11. Feldberg, W. and W.D.M. Paton, Release of histamine from skin and muscle in the cat by opium alkaloids and other histamine liberators, J. Physiol. 114, 490-509 (1951).

12. Schachter, M., The release of histamine by pethidine, atropine, quinine, and other drugs, Brit. J. Pharmacol. 7, 646-654 (1952).

13. Benyon, R.C., The human skin mast cell, Clin. Exp. Allergy 19, 375-387 (1989).

14. Ennis, M., C. Schneider, E. Nehring and W. Lorenz, Histamine release induced by opioid analgesics: a comparative study using porcine mast cells, Agents Actions (in press).

15. Doenicke, A. and W. Lorenz, Histaminfreisetzung und anaphylaktische Reaktionen bei Narkosen. Biochemische und Klinische Aspekte, Anaesthesist 19, 413-417 (1970).

16. Lorenz, W., A. Doenicke, R. Meyer, H.-J. Reimann, J. Kusche, H. Barth, H. Geesing, M. Hutzel and B. Weissenbacher, Histamine release in man by propanidid and thiopentone: Pharmacological effects and clinical consequences, Brit. J. Anaesth. 44, 355-369 (1972).

17. Lorenz,W., A. Doenicke, R. Meyer, H.-J. Reimann, J. Kusche, H. Barth, H. Geesing, M. Hutzel and B. Weissenbacher, An improved method for the determination of histamine release in man: Its application in studies with propanidid and thiopentone, Europ. J. Pharmacol. 19, 180-190 (1972).

18. Hirshman, C.A., R.A. Edelstein, J.M. Ebertz and J.M. Hanifin, Thiobarbiturate-induced histamine release in human skin mast cells, Anesthesiology 63, 353-356 (1985).

19. Doenicke, A., W. Lorenz, R. Beigl, H. Bezecny, G. Uhlig, L. Kalmar, B. Praetorius and G. Mann, Histamine release after intravenous application of short-acting hypnotics: a comparison of etomidate, althesin (CT 1341) and propanidid, Brit. J. Anaesth. 45, 1097-1104 (1973).

20. Doenicke, A., W. Lorenz, D. Stanworth, T. Duda and J.B. Glenn, Effects of propofol (Diprivan) on histamine release immunoglobulin levels and activation of complement in healthy volunteers, Postgraduate Medical Journal 61, 15-20 (1985).

21. Lorenz, W., H.-J. Reimann, A. Schmal, P. Dormann, B. Schwartz and E. Neugebauer, Histamine release in dogs by cremophor El and its derivatives: oxethylated oleic acid is the most effective constituent, Agents Actions 7, 63-67 (1977).

22. Lorenz, W., A. Schmal, H. Schult, S. Lang, C. Ohmann, D. Weber, B. Kapp, L. Lüben and A. Doenicke, Histamine release and hypotensive reactions in dogs by solubilizing agents and fatty acids: analysis of various components in cremophor El and development of a compound with reduced toxicity, Agents Actions 12, 64-80 (1982).

23. Paton, W.D.M., Histamine release by compounds of simple chemical structure, Pharm. Rev. 9, 269-328 (1957).

24. Lorenz, W., M. Thermann, K. Messmer, A. Schmal, P. Dormann, J. Kusche, H. Barth, R. Tauber, M. Hutzel, G. Mann and R. Uhlig, Evaluation of histamine elimination curves in plasma and whole blood of several circulatory regions: a method for studying kinetics of histamine release in the whole animal, Agents Actions 4, 336-356 (1974).

25. Lorenz, W., Histamine release in man, Agents Actions 5, 402-416 (1975).

26. Lorenz, W., A. Doenicke, B. Schöning and E. Neugebauer, The role of histamine in adverse reactions to intravenous agents, In: Adverse Reactions of Anaesthetic Drugs, pp. 169-238 (Ed. A. Thornton). Elsevier North-Holland Biomedical Press 1981.

27. Lorenz, W., J.V. Parkin, H. Rohde, H. Barth, H. Troidl, K. Thon, E. Hinterlang, D. Weber, R. Albrecht and H.D. Röher, Histamine in gastric secretory disorders: the relevance of the mucosal histamine content and the origin of histamine in gastric aspirate, In: Gastric Secretion, Basic and Clinical Aspects, pp. 29-51 (Eds. St. J. Konturek and W. Domschke). Georg Thieme Verlag, Stuttgart 1981.

28. Enerbäck, L., Mast cells in rat gastrointestinal mucosa. 1. Effects of Fixation, Acta path. et microbiol. scandinav. 66, 289-302 (1966);
Enerbäck, L., Mast cells in rat gastrointestinal mucosa. 2. Dye-binding and melachromatic properties, Acta path. et microbiol. scandinav. 66, 303-312 (1966);
Enerbäck, L., Mast cells in rat gastrointestinal mucosa. 3. Reactivity towards compound 48/80, Acta path. et microbiol. scandinav. 66, 313-322 (1966);
Enerbäck, L., Mast cells in rat gastrointestinal mucosa. 4. Monoamine storing capacity, Acta path. et microbiol. scandinav. 67, 365-379 (1966).

29. Lorenz, W., A. Schauer, St. Halbach, R. Calvoer and E. Werle, Biochemical and histochemical studies on the distribution of histamine in the digestive tract of man, dog, and other mammals, Naunyn-Schmiedebergs Arch. Pharmak. 265, 81-100 (1969).

30. Messmer, K., W. Lorenz, L. Sunder-Plassmann, W. Klövekorn and M. Hutzel, Histamine release as cause of acute hypotension following rapid colloid infusion, Naunyn-Schmiedebergs Arch. Pharmak. 267, 433-445 (1970).

31. Lorenz, W., A. Doenicke, B. Schöning, H. Karges, A. Schmal, Incidence and mechanisms of adverse reactions to polypeptides in man and dog, In: Joint WHO/IABS Symposium on the Standardization of Albumin, Plasma Substitutes and Plasmapheresis, Geneva 1980, Develop. biol. Standard Vol. 48, pp. 207-234 (Ed. W. Hennessen). Karger Verlag 1981.

32. Black, J.W., W.A.M. Duncan, C.J. Durant, C.R. Ganellin and E.M. Parsons, Definition and antagonism of histamine H_2-receptors, Nature 236, 385-390 (1972).

33. Dietz, W., H. Lennartz, I. Köpf, A. Schmal, U. Kaiser and W. Lorenz, Lebensbedrohliche anaphylaktoide Reaktionen im perioperativen Zeitraum: Blockade durch Histamin H_1-+H_2-Antagonisten oder Methylprednisolon?, Langenbecks Arch. Chir., Suppl. Chir. Forum 333-337 (1987).

34. Lorenz, W., A. Doenicke, K. Messmer, H.-J. Reimann, M. Thermann, W. Lahn, J. Berr, A. Schmal, P. Dormann, P. Regenfuss and H. Hamelmann, Histamine release in human subjects by modified gelatin (Haemaccel[R]) and dextran: an explanation for anaphylactoid reactions observed under clinical conditions?, Brit. J. Anaesth. 48, 151-165 (1976).

35. Reinhardt, D. and U. Borchard, H_1-receptor antagonists: comparative pharmacology and clinical use, Klin. Wochenschr. 60, 983-990 (1982).

36. Tryba, M., Therapie allergischer Reaktionen, Ergebnisse einer interdisziplinären Konsensuskonferenz (in press).

37. Neugebauer, E., A. Dietrich, B. Bouillon, W. Lorenz, A. Lechleuthner and H. Troidl, Steroids in trauma patients - right or wrong?, Theor. Surg. 5, 44-53 (1990).

38. The Veterans Administration Systemic Sepsis Cooperative Study Group, Effect of high-dose glucocorticoid therapy on mortality in patients with clinical signs of systemic sepsis, N. Engl. J. Med. 317, 659-665 (1987).

39. Bone, R.C., C.J. Fisher, T.P. Clemmer *et al.*, A controlled clinical trial of high-dose methylprednisolone in the treatment of severe sepsis and septic shock, N. Engl. J. Med. 317, 653-658 (1987).

40. McPeek, D., Formal and informal strategies in clinical decision making - the role of order in the information environment, Theor. Surg. (in press).

41. W. Lorenz and A. Doenicke, Anaphylactoid reactions and histamine release by barbiturate induction agents: clinical relevance and pathomechanisms, Anesthesiology 63, 351-352 (1985).

42. Ahnefeld, F.W., A. Doenicke and W. Lorenz, Histamine and Antihistamines in Anaesthesia and Surgery, Klin. Wochenschr. Vol. 60, pp. 1-1062. Springer-Verlag, Berlin-Heidelberg-New York 1982.

43. Laxenaire, M.-C., Prevention des reactions anaphylactoides peranesthesiques, Ann. Fr. Anesth. Reanim. Vol. 4, pp. 1-244, Masson, Paris 1985.

44. Laxenaire, M.C. and D.A. Moneret-Vautrin, Le Risque Allergique en Anesthesie-reanimation, pp. 1-154. Masson, Paris 1990.

45. Hobsley, M., J. Moss, S.S. Gross, R.S.J. Clarke, M. Fisher and J. Watkins, Discussions about a protocol of a controlled clinical trial: induction of anaesthesia and perioperative risk, Theor. Surg. 3, 132-151 (1988).

46. Moss, J., M.F. Roizen, E.J. Nordby, R. Thisted, J.L. Apfelbaum and D.J. McDermott, Decreased incidence and mortality of anaphylaxis to chymopapain, Anesth. Analg. 64, 1197-1201 (1985).

47. Lorenz, W., W. Dietz, M. Ennis, B. Stinner and A. Doenicke, Histamine in anaesthesia and Surgery: causality analysis, In: Handbook of Experimental Pharmacology Vol. 97, pp. 385-439 (Ed. B. Uvnäs). Springer-Verlag, Berlin-Heidelberg-New York 1991.

48. Uvnäs, B., Handbook of Experimental Pharmacology, Vol. 97, pp. 1-841, Springer-Verlag, Berlin-Heidelberg-New York 1991.

49. Rocha e Silva, M., Histamine and Anti-Histaminics. Part 1. Histamine. Its Chemistry, Metabolism and Pharmacological Actions. Handbook of Experimental Pharmacology, Vol. 18, pp. 1-991, Springer-Verlag, Berlin-Heidelberg-New York 1966.

50. Rocha e Silva, M., Histamine II and Anti-Histaminics. Chemistry, Metabolism and Physiological and Pharmacological Actions, Handbook of Experimental Pharmacology, Vol. 18, pp. 1-700, Springer-Verlag, Berlin-Heidelberg-New York 1978.

51. Elstein, A.S., L.S. Shulman and S.A. Spralka, Medical problem solving: an analysis of clinical reasoning, pp. 64-121, Harvard University Press, Cambridge 1978.

52. Stinner, B., W. Dietz, W. Lorenz and M. Rothmund, "Think aloud technique" für dichotome Entscheidungsprozesse: ein neues Studiendesign für umstrittene Prophylaxiemaßnahmen zur Reduzierung des perioperativen Risikos, Langenbecks Arch. Chir. Suppl. Chir. Forum 171-176 (1990).

53. Lorenz, W., A. Doenicke, B. Schöning, C. Ohmann, B. Grote and E. Neugebauer, Definition and classification of the histamine-release response to drugs in anaesthesia and surgery: studies in the conscious human subject, Klin. Wochenschr. 60, 896-913 (1982).

54. Lorenz, W., A. Doenicke, B. Schöning, J. Mamorski, D. Weber, E. Hinterlang, B. Schwartz and E. Neugebauer, H_1-+H_2-receptor antagonists for premedication in anaesthesia and surgery: a critical view based on randomized clinical trials with Haemaccel and various antiallergic drugs, Agents Actions 10, 114-124 (1980).

55. Doenicke, A., M. Ennis and W. Lorenz, Histamine release in anaesthesia and surgery: a systematic approach to risk in the perioperative period, In: Anaphylactoid Reactions in Anaesthesia (Ed. D.J. Sage), International Anesthesiology Clinics 23, 41-66 (1985).

56. Watkins, J. and C.J. Levy, Guide to Immediate Anaesthetic Reactions, pp. 1-128, Butterworths, London 1988.

57. Fisher, M.McD., Adverse Reactions. Clinics in Anaesthesiology, Vol. 2, pp. 1-697, W.B. Saunders Company, London 1984.

58. Watkins, J., Adverse anaesthetic reactions, Anaesthesia 40, 797-800 (1985).

59. Watkins, J., Second report from an anaesthetic reactions advisory service, Anaesthesia 44, 157-159 (1989).

60. Kimbel, K.H., Spontanerfassung unerwünschter Arzneimittelwirkungen, Münch. med. Wschr., 119, 841-844 (1977).

61. Lorenz, W., H.D. Röher, A. Doenicke and C. Ohmann, Histamine release in anaesthesia and surgery: a new method to evaluate its clinical significance with several types of causal relationship, Clin. Anaesthesiol. 2, 403-426 (1984).

62. Lorenz, W. and M. Rothmund, Grundlagen der Technologiebewertung in der chirurgischen Diagnostik, Langenbecks Arch. Chir. Suppl. II, 369-376 (1988).

63. A. Pollock and M. Evans, Surgical Audit. Confidential enquiry into perioperative deaths, pp. 83-88. Butterworth, London 1989.

64. Lorenz, W., H. Sitter, B. Stinner, D. Duda, B. Kapp, B. Gstrein, W. Dietz, A. Doenicke and W. Dick, Controlled clinical trials and cross-sectional studies with plasma histamine measurements and histamine receptor antagonists: solving the problem of preoperative H_1- + H_2-prophylaxis by asking new questions?, In: New Perspectives in Histamine Research, pp. 197-230 (Eds. H. Timmermann and H. v.d. Goot) Birkhäuser Verlag, Basel 1991.

65. Sitter, H., W. Lorenz and M. Rothmund, Measuring effectiveness and costs in surgery - 10th Meeting of the Permanent Working Party on Clinical Studies (CAS) of the German Surgical Society, 9-11 November 1989 in Marburg, FRG, Theor. Surg. 5, 211-213 (1990).

66. Rocha e Silva, M., Histamine. Its Role in Anaphylaxis and Allergy, pp. 1-249, Charles C. Thomas Publisher, Springfield, Illinois 1955.

AAS 36
Contributions to
Autacoid Pharmacology

MICROORGANISMS AND MEDIATOR RELEASE: NEW ASPECTS IN AIRWAY DISEASES

S. Norn

Department of Pharmacology, University of Copenhagen, Juliane Maries Vej 20, 2100, Copenhagen 0, Denmark

It has been shown that infections in the respiratory tract can provoke or exacerbate attacks of bronchial asthma[(1-8)]. Viral infections are a major cause of exacerbations of asthma in children, but the association is less clear in adult asthmatics. Although the role of bacteria are still obscure due to difficulties in obtaining microbiological evidence of invasion of bacteria or their soluble products, many physicians propose that bacterial respiratory infections (except for sinusitis) are not important to the provocation of asthma. However, they might play a role in chronic obstructive pulmonary disease and the endotoxins might be responsible for the symptoms, including subjective breathing difficulties in humidifier disease[(9,10)] and for the decrease in respiratory function in the byssinosis syndrome[(11-13)].

To date, a single, unifying mechanism has not been identified to explain how respiratory tract infections contribute to or cause airway diseases, but a number of important mechanisms have been suggested which include mediator release, IgE directed against bacteria or virus, bronchoconstriction, decreased β-adrenergic function, enhanced α-adrenergic response, a reversible damage of the airways epithelium and inflammation in the small airways with desquamation of destroyed epithelial cells (For references see 14,15).

Since recent advances in connection with mediator release caused or influenced by microorganisms and their soluble constituents seem to open new aspects pointing towards a relationship to asthma and other airway diseases, this paper will focus on microorganisms and mediator release.

Virus Enhances Basophil Histamine Release

Cellular studies on mediator release have mainly been performed on peripheral blood leukocytes to obtain information about the influence of virus on histamine release from basophil leukocytes. The first study was performed by Ida *et al.*[16] and included longterm experiments in which the leukocytes were incubated for 24 hours at 37°C in a 5% CO_2 atmosphere with herpes simplex virus, type 1, adenovirus type 1 or influenza A virus. The supernatant fluids were then assayed for their histamine content and showed no release of histamine with either live or inactivated viruses. That viruses *per se* did not release histamine from the basophilocyte was also observed by Busse *et al.*[17] and by Chonmaitree *et al.*[18] using infectious influenza A virus, respiratory syncytial virus (**RSV**) and rhinovirus. However, in higher concentrations **RSV**, parainfluenza type 3 virus and Sendai virus were found to trigger histamine release and the release was completed within 0.5 – 1 hour[19]. Another important effect was, however, found in the presence of lower concentrations of virus, i.e. virus increased the mediator release. Preincubation of the leukocytes with either herpes simplex virus type 1, adenovirus type 1 or influenza A virus followed by stimulation with anti-IgE enhanced IgE-mediated histamine release[16]. It was necessary to preincubate the cells with virus for at least 8 hours to obtain this effect, and it seemed that interferon production was responsible for the enhancement of the histamine release. Busse *et al.*[17] found a similar indirect effect of influenza A virus on the anti-IgE-induced basophil histamine release. However, virus, which causes no production of interferon, was also able to enhance the anti-IgE-induced histamine release, thus suggesting that other, unknown factors are responsible for the potentiating effect of virus[18].

In short-term experiments we examined a direct effect of influenza A virus on IgE-mediated histamine release from human basophil leukocytes. Peripheral blood leukocytes (containing approx. 2% basophilocytes) obtained from normal individuals by Ficoll-Hypaque gradient centrifugation were washed twice and suspended in glucose-free Tris-AMC containing 25 mM Tris at pH 7.6, 0.12 M NaCl, 5 mM KCl, 0.6 mM $CaCl_2$, 1.1 mM $MgCl_2$, and 0.3 mg of human serum albumin/ml[20]. IgE-mediated histamine release was obtained by incubating the cells for 40 min at 37°C with anti-IgE, and the release was determined spectrofluorometrically. To obtain a moderate release (< 25% of the total histamine content of the sample) the cells were stimulated with rabbit-antihuman IgE (Beringwerke AG, FRG) used in final concentrations from 4 to 40 IU/ml. When human influenza A virus (A/Caen/I/84 (H3N2)) was included in the samples the mediator release was enhanced by 60 to 200%, and the peak was obtained in low concentrations of the virus corresponding to the range of 10^{-3} to 1 ng viral protein per ml. (Fig. 1)[20]. Also

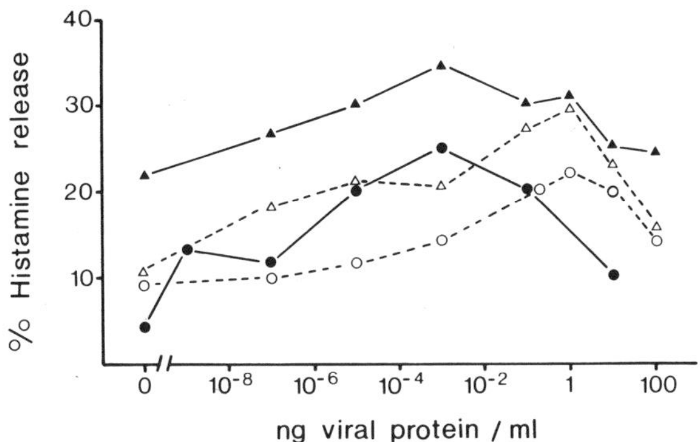

Fig. 1. Potentiation by influenza A virus of histamine release induced by anti-IgE in leukocyte suspensions from 4 normal individuals. Duplicate determinations. Note that the virus *per se* caused no release of histamine.

when histamine release was induced by specific allergens in cell suspensions from patients allergic to house dust mite, grass pollen, birch pollen or cat dander, inclusion of influenza A virus caused an enhanced mediator release which is shown in Fig. 2 and Table 1. The potentiating effect of virus was due to synergism, since virus did not release histamine per se, either in cell suspensions from normal individuals or in cell suspensions from the sensitized patients.

It seems doubtful whether a production of interferon could be responsible for the potentiating effect of virus in these short-term experiments, since a virus-induced production takes more time[16]. However, there are some indications that viral neuraminidase on the surface of the influenza A virus could be responsible for the potentiation of mediator release.

Firstly we examined the effect of a potent neuraminidase inhibitor, DDNANA (2–deoxy–2,3–dehydro–N–acetyl–neuraminic acid) which inhibits both viral neuraminidase, bacterial neuraminidases including *Vibrio cholerae* neuraminidase and mammalian neuraminidases[21].

This inhibitor was found to be a suitable tool for investigating the potentiating effect of the virus, as it did not interfere with the histamine release process induced by specific allergen or anti-IgE[20,22]. Fig. 3 shows experiments with cells from patients allergic to house dust mite or grass pollen, and it appears that the potentiation of histamine release by influenza A virus was completely abolished by the neuraminidase inhibitor[20]. *Secondly*, a purified neuraminidase preparation obtained from *Vibrio cholerae* was able to mimic the potentiating effect of influenza A virus and potentiation by the isolated neuraminidase was also abolished by DDNANA[20]. The potentiation and its abolition is

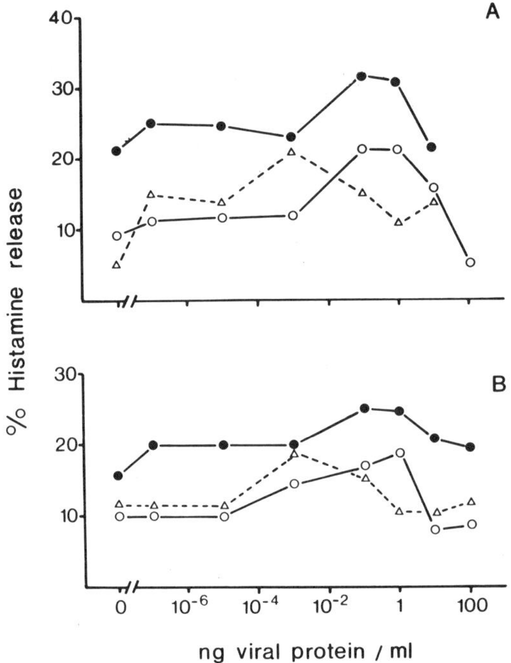

Fig. 2. Potentiation by influenza A virus of histamine release induced by specific allergens in leukocyte suspensions from 3 patients sensitized to house dust mite (A) and 3 patients sensitized to grass pollen (B). Duplicate determinations. Note that the virus *per se* caused no release of histamine.

Table 1. Potentiation by influenza A virus of histamine release induced by specific allergens in sensitized persons. The histamine release is given independent of the antigen and virus dilution in the experiments. Mean ± SEM is given.

Patients allergic to	№ of subjects tested	№ of responders	Histamine caused by allergen alone	Maximal histamine release caused by allergen + influenza A virus
House dust mite	5	4	14.4 (±2.7)	25.4 (± 1.9)
Grass pollen	7	5	10.8 (±1.6)	18.6 (± 1.5)
Birch pollen	2	2	9.5	19.0
Cat dander	3	2	12.0	20.3

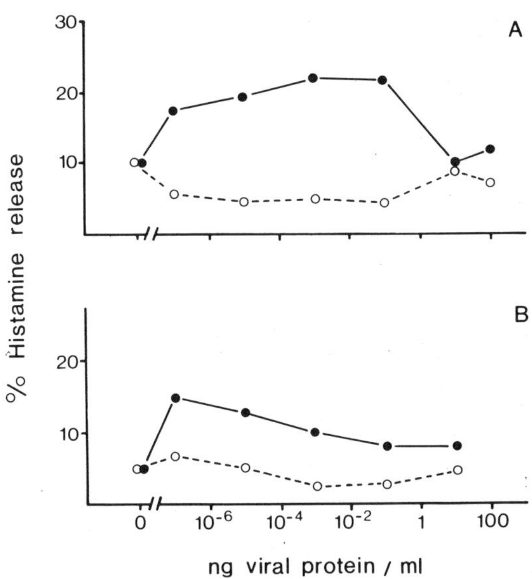

Fig. 3. Potentiation of histamine release by influenza A virus (•—•) and the complete abolishment by the neuraminidase inhibitor 2–deoxy–2,3–dehydro–N–acetylneuraminic acid (○ — ○). Cells from a patient sensitized to house dust mite (A) and to grass pollen (B). Duplicate determinations.

shown in Fig. 4 in connection with allergic histamine release. *Thirdly*, the effect of monoclonal antibodies directed against the viral neuraminidase (serotype N2) was studied in connection with the potentiation by influenza A virus of anti-IgE triggered histamine release, and this experiment also showed a complete abolition of potentiation[(23)]. All these findings indicate that the viral neuraminidase is responsible for the potentiating effect of the virus.

Since viral haemagglutinin is responsible for virus adsorption onto the cell surface[(24,25)] it seems possible that a binding of virus to the cell is necessary for the viral neuraminidase to cause potentiation of mediator release. Such a binding hypothesis was supported by the finding that monoclonal antibodies directed against the haemagglutinin (serotype H3) abolished the potentiating effect of influenza A virus[(23)].

Bacteria Trigger Histamine Release

The capability of bacteria to release histamine from human basophilocytes was examined in peripheral blood leukocytes using the method mentioned before. The studies include the most frequently encountered strains in the flora of the upper respiratory tract. Table 2 shows that both Gram-positive and Gram-negative bacteria cause basophil histamine release in leukocyte suspensions from normal individuals, children with intrinsic asthma, and allergic patients suffering from bronchial asthma and hay fever[26-29]. Recently, bacteria-induced histamine release has also been observed in human lung and tonsillar mast cells[30] and in nasal mucosa[31]. Furthermore, experiments with cells from human broncho-alveolar lavage (BAL) shows that *Staph. aureus* causes release of histamine from the superficially lying mast cells in the airway epithelium and that the bacterium stimulates the BAL-cells to generate leukotriene B_4 (Fig. 5)[32]. The mediator release caused by bacteria might be of importance for the exacerbation of bronchial asthma in respiratory tract infections, since histamine is assumed to increase the epithelial permeability with entrance of allergens and other insulting particles[33,34] and leukotriene B_4 to facilitate airway inflammation.

By examining the effect of *Staphylococcus aureus* (a protein A-deficient strain) we found that bacteria can trigger histamine release from basophils by two different mechanisms (Fig. 6), an immunological (IgE-dependent) and a non-immunological one[35,36]. The new mechanism might be of importance for our understanding of the role of bacteria in asthma and infectious diseases since a subject does not need to be sensitized to bacteria in order to induce histamine release. To differentiate between the two mechanisms the IgE molecules were removed from the cell surface of the basophils. This was done by brief exposure of the cells to pH 3.8, which dissociated IgE from the cells (Fig. 7)[37]. If bacteria cause histamine release in the intact cells but not in the nude cells stripped of IgE, the mechanism is IgE-dependent. On the other hand, a non-immunological mechanism is prevalent when intact and nude cells cause a similar release of histamine.

Fig. 8 shows the verification of IgE-mediated histamine release in cells from patients infected with and sensitized to bacteria; the non-immunological mechanism caused by bacteria with which the patient was not infected appears from fig. 9[36].

The non-immunological mechanism was found to operate in the major part of the persons tested. These subjects included allergic patients suffering from hay fever and asthma, children with intrinsic asthma and normal individuals[26,28,35,36]. Only in some cases an IgE-dependent mechanism was found, indicating that the person should be sensitized to the bacterium (antigen). However, it should be noted that only a limited

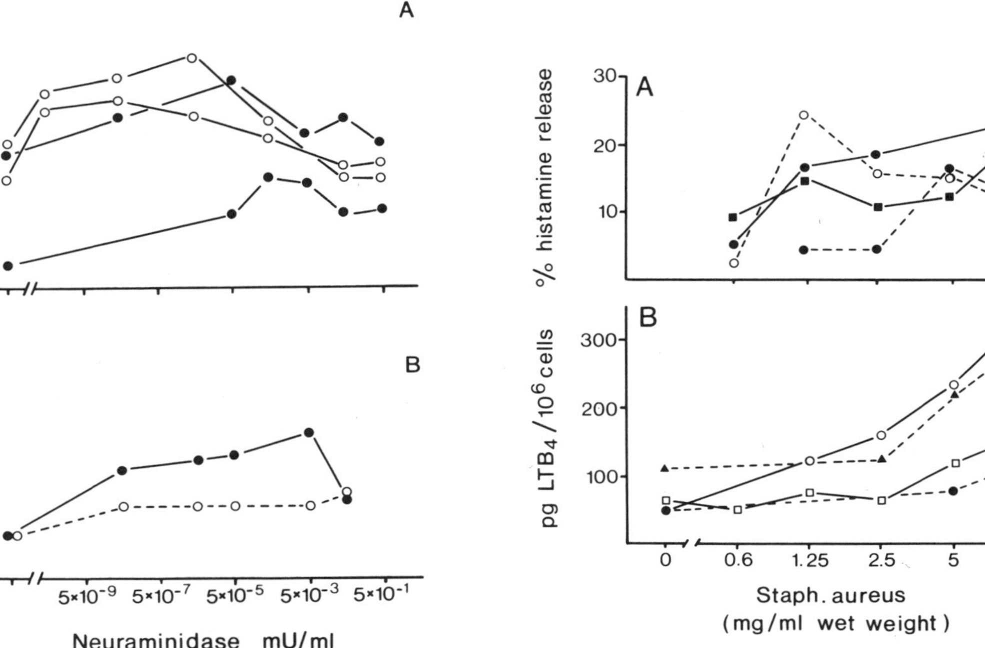

Fig. 4. Potentiation of histamine release by a purified neuraminidase (——) and the complete abolishment by the neuraminidase inhibitor 2-deoxy-2,3-dehydro-N-acetylneuraminic acid (– – –). Cells from patients sensitized to grass pollen (•) and to house dust mite (○). Duplicate determinations.

Fig. 5. Mediator release induced by *Staph. aureus* in BAL-cells from non-atopic subjects. (A) Histamine release and (B) LTB_4 production. Duplicate determinations.

Table 2. Bacteria causing histamine release in vitro from human basophil leukocytes.

Gram-positive		*Gram-negative*	
Aerococcus sp.	2	*Branhamella catarrhalis*	2
Corynebacterium sp.	2	*Enterobacter cloacae*	1
Group A and B *strept.*	1	*Escherichia coli*	1
Staph. aureus	1–2	*Haemophilus influenzac*	1–2
Staph. epidermidis	1	*Haemophilus parainfluenzae*	1–2
Strept. mitior	2	*Klebsiella oxytoca*	1
Strept. pneumoniae	1–2	*Klebsiella pneumoniae*	1
Strept. salivarius	2	*Neisseria pharyngis*	2
		Proteus mirabilis	1
		Proteus vulgaris	1

1: whole bacteria ; 2 : bacterial ultrasonicates.

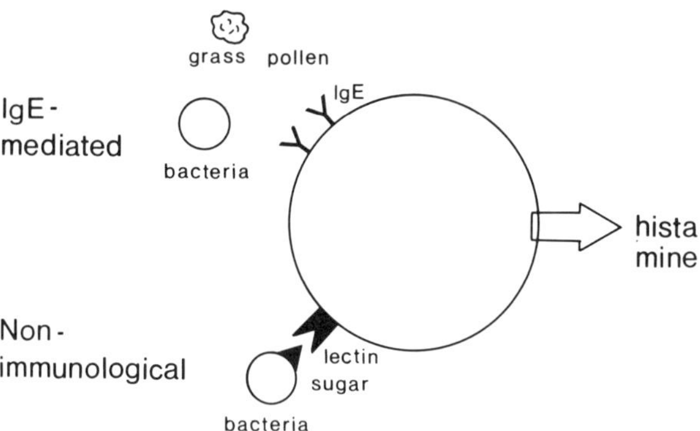

Fig. 6. Bacteria cause histamine release from basophils by two different mechanisms, an immunological and a non-immunological mechanism.

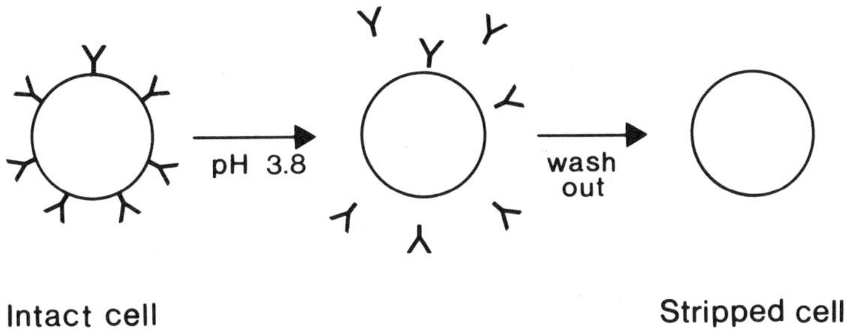

Fig. 7. IgE molecules are removed from the basophils by a brief exposure of the cells to pH 3.8 followed by wash out of dissociated IgE.

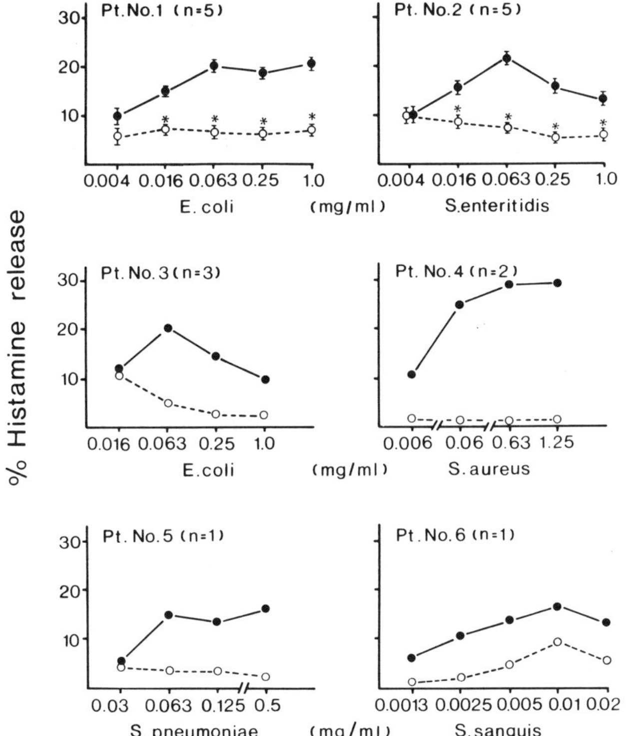

Fig. 8. Verification of IgE-mediated histamine release in cell suspensions from 6 patients infected with *E. coli*, *Salmonella enteritidis*, *Staph. aureus*, *Streptococcus pneumoniae* or *Streptococcus sanguis*. Intact cells (•—•) and cells deprived of IgE (o — o) were challenged with the patients own bacterium. Mean +/− SEM for n experiments in duplicate is given. *p<0.01 .

number of patients were tested and washed, whole bacteria were used; the effect of their toxins is now being investigated. The IgE-mediated histamine release from basophil leukocytes lasted from 2, to at least 8 weeks[36]. An IgE-dependent mechanism was demonstrated in 3 of 10 patients with intrinsic asthma, where *H. influenzae* and *Strep. pneumoniae* caused an IgE-mediated histamine release. Patiens with *E. coli* bacteriaemia and fever also showed an IgE-dependent histamine release by *E. coli*[28,36]. Other examples include 3 patients suffering from the syndrome of immune deficiency with hyper-IgE to their own *Staph. aureus* strain[35] and different categories of patients infected with various bacteria such as *Salmonella enteritidis* and *Streptococcus sanguis* (Fig. 8)[36].

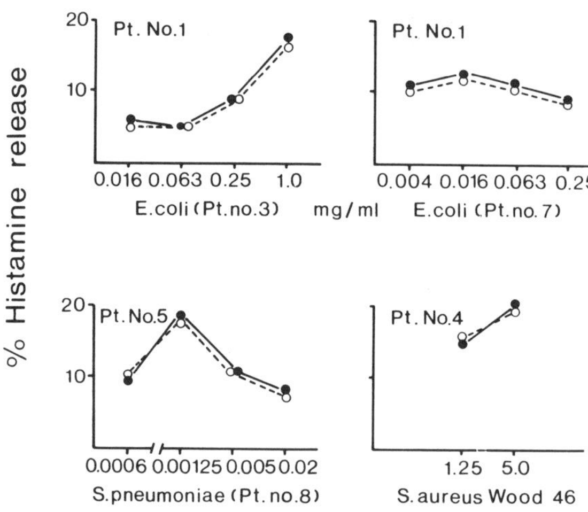

Fig. 9. Verification of non-immunological histamine release induced by bacteria strains to which the patients were not sensitized. Cells from patient no. 1, 4 and 5 were simulated with bacteria with which the patients were not infected. Intact cells (•—•) and cells deprived of IgE (o — o). Duplicate determinations.

We suspect that the non-immunological mechanism is a sugar-lectin mediated reaction. This means that sugars on the bacterial cell wall interact with lectins on the basophil cell membrane leading to histamine release (Fig. 6). Although a direct interaction between bacteria and the target cell has not been examined in connection with the basophilocyte, it was demonstrated for the mast cell using a 98% pure population of peritoneal mast cells from germ-free rats[35].

Both Gram-positive and Gram-negative bacteria contain peptidoglycan, and this bacterial cell wall component might be responsible for histamine release triggered by bacteria since in fact, isolated peptidoglycan releases histamine[26]. Peptidoglycan is composed of glycan strains of alternating, beta-(1,4)-glycosidically linked N acetyl glucosamine and N-acetylmuramic acid residues, which are cross-linked by peptide bridges[38]. If these long sugar chains interact with the basophil cell membrane, bacteria-induced histamine release should be inhibited by small fragments of the sugar chains or by the single sugars blocking the binding sites by competition. In fact both N-acetylglucosamine and N-acetylmuramic acid were found to inhibit *Staph. aureus*-induced histamine release[39]. Other indirect proofs for a sugar-lectin mediated reaction were the findings that lectin-binding sugars like α-methyl-D-mannoside and α-methyl-D-glucoside, inhibit bacteria-induced histamine release, in contrast to mediator release triggered by anti-IgE (Fig. 10)[35,40]. In agreement with this hypothesis, inhibition was also obtained when the cells were preincubated with the sugar, and unbound sugar was washed away from the cell surface before stimulation with *Staph. aureus*, whereas a similar pretreatment of the bacterium, before addition of the cells, did not result in decreased mediator release[40]. Furthermore, like bacteria, particle-bound sugars release histamine from the basophils, and this release was also abolished by specific sugars[40].

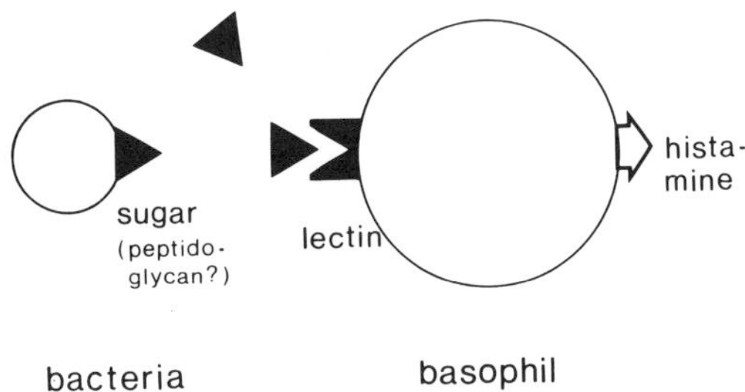

Fig. 10. Inhibition of bacteria-induced histamine release by lectin-binding sugars (Δ). An indirect proof of a sugar-lectin mediated reaction.

In connection with the hypothesis of sugar-lectin mediated reactions it should be mentioned that other mechanism might also co-operate in non-immunological mediator release, since lectin-binding sugars mostly caused only a partial inhibition of the bacteria-induced histamine release[30,40].

Bacteria and their Components Enhance Allergic Histamine Release

Bacteria and bacterial-constituents like endotoxins and peptidoglycan were found to enhance the allergic histamine release[28,41-43], an effect which might contribute to the exacerbation of airway diseases during infections. The in vitro experiments comprise cells obtained from house dust mite or grass pollen-allergic patients and cells from patients sensitized to bacteria (Table 3). A low histamine release was obtained when cells from mite-allergic patients were challenged with small amounts of specific antigen (Pharmalgen *Dermatophagoides pteronyssinus*). This was also the case by challenge with small amounts of bacteria (*Staph. aureus* or *E. coli*) to which the person was not sensitized. However, the combination of bacteria and specific antigen caused a high mediator release, exceeding the additive effect (synergism). Like bacteria, the bacterial cell wall component peptidoglycan markedly increased the release of histamine caused by specific antigen in cells from mite-allergic patients.

Table 3. Bacteria and their constituents enhance allergic histamine release in vitro, i.e. a synergistic effect is obtained by the combination of the allergic and the non-immunological reaction.

% Histamine release caused by			
patients	*Allergic reaction*	*Non-immunological reaction*	*combination of both*
Mite-sensitive	Mite 5 %	*S. aureus* 2%	58%
	Mite 4 %	*E. coli* 2%	22%
	Mite 7 %	Peptidoglycan 15%	45%
Grass-sensitive	Grass 17 %	*S. aureus* 16%	58%
	Grass 5 %	*K. oxytoca* 17%	39%
	Grass 5 %	Teichoic acid 3%	22%
	Grass 22 %	Endotoxin 2%	47%
Bacteria-sensitive	[1]*Pt. S. aureus* 5%	*S. aureus* 11%	37%
	[2]*S.pneumoniae* 11%	*S. aureus* 12%	42%
	[2]*S.pneumoniae* 15%	Endotoxin 2%	43%

[1] A *staph. aureus* strain isolated from the patient.

[2] A patient with intrinsic asthma.

Similar results were obtained in cells from grass pollen-allergic patients. The mediator release caused by grass pollen (Spectralgen 4-grass mix) was markedly enhanced by *Staph. aureus* or *K. oxytoca*, to which the person was not sensitized, and a similar synergistic effect was also found when the bacterium was replaced by endotoxins such as *E. coli*, *Salmonella* or *H. influenzae* LPS or by the bacterial cell wall component teichoic acid isolated from *Staph. aureus*.

Finally the table shows results obtained in cells from patients sensitized to bacteria. One patient was sensitized to his own *Staph. aureus* strain. A combination of this strain and another *Staph. aureus* strain, to which he was not sensitized, caused a similar synergistic effect. In analogy, a patient with intrinsic asthma who was sensitized to both *H. influenzae* and *Strept. pneumoniae* showed enhanced histamine release by the combination of one of these bacteria with either *Staph. aureus* (to which he was not sensitized) or endotoxin.

Virus Enhances Histamine Release Caused by Bacteria and Endotoxin

In mixed bacterial and viral infections an interaction might influence the mediator release. When such a interaction was examined in blood leukocytes, influenza A virus was found to enhance *Staph. aureus* induced histamine release[(44)]. The potentiating effect of the virus was caused by synergism, since virus itself did not induce mediator release. A similar enhancement was found in cells from normal individuals and from patients with intrinsic asthma. Although the trigger-mechanism was not examined in this study, it is most likely that the bacterium releases histamine from the basophilocyte by the non-immunological mechanism. However, recent findings show that the virus can enhance bacteria-induced histamine release caused both by the IgE-dependent mechanism and the non-immunological mechanism; this is in analogy with the enhancement of both anti-IgE- and calcium ionophore A23187-induced histamine release[(36,45)]. In these studies an IgE-mediated reaction was triggered by *Streptococcus pneumoniae*, *Staph. aureus*, *E. coli*, *Salmonella enteritidis* and *Streptococcus sanguis*, and non-immunological mediator release was caused by *Streptococcus pneumoniae*, *Staph. aureus* and *Salmonella enteritidis*, and overall the histamine release was enhanced by influenza A virus.

No direct release, or only a marginal release was obtained by endotoxins isolated from *E. coli* or *Salmonella bacteria* when examined in final concentrations from 1 pg to 100 μg/ml[(28)]. However, in the presence of serum, they trigger histamine release by complement activation, and this release is enhanced by influenza A virus[(22)]. Also here the potentiation by the virus seems to depend on the viral neuraminidase since the potentiation was abolished by DDNANA and mimicked by *V. cholerae* neuraminidase.

Mechanism of Potentiation

As mentioned, virus cause a synergistic enhancement of mediator release whether the release is triggered by IgE-dependent or non-immunological stimuli. This is also the case for bacteria and endotoxin where potentiation of the allergic reaction has been described (Table 3), and potentiation of a non-immunological reaction has been observed in experiments where histamine release was caused by calcium ionophore A23187(43).

A direct interaction between the microorganism or endotoxin and the target cell has not been demonstrated in connection with the potentiation. However, experiments with endotoxin suggest such an interaction(43). In these experiments the leukocytes were preincubated with *Salmonella typhimurium* LPS, then washed free of unbound endotoxin, and the cells were left for 30 min at 37°C before incubation with anti-IgE (37°C, 40 min). By this procedure a possible factor (f. inst. oxygen radicals) released from different types of cells is washed away. The potentiation did not differ from that obtained by the usual procedure by which the cells were stimulated at 37°C for 40 min with a mixture of anti-IgE and endotoxin (Fig. 11), indicating a direct interaction between LPS and basophilocyte.

It seems that carbohydrate residues in the microorganisms and endotoxins are responsible for the potentiation by interacting with binding sites on the basophil cell membrane. *Firstly*, the neuraminidase portion of influenza A virus contains carbohydrates such as galactose and N-acetyglucosamine(46). Endotoxins like *Salmonella typhimurium* LPS also contain these sugars(47); N-acetylglucosamine is found in the peptidoglycan structure of bacteria(38) and peptidoglycan isolated from *Staph. aureus* shows a potentiating effect(41). *Secondly*, the potentiation by influenza A virus, *Staph. aureus* and *Salmonella typhimurium* LPS is inhibited or abolished by low concentration (10^{-7} – 10^{-6} M) of the free sugars, galactose or N-acetylglucosamine(43,48,49). The inhibition was obtained whether the histamine release was triggered by an IgE-dependent (specific antigen or anti-IgE) or by a non-immunological (A23187) mechanism. Fig. 12 shows that in cells from patients allergic to house dust mite or birch pollen, the potentiation by bacteria or endotoxin of allergic mediator release was inhibited by galactose. The inhibitory effect seems to depend on a binding of the sugar to the cell membrane, since it persists after preincubation of the cells with galactose followed by wash-out of unbound sugar before the addition of anti-IgE plus

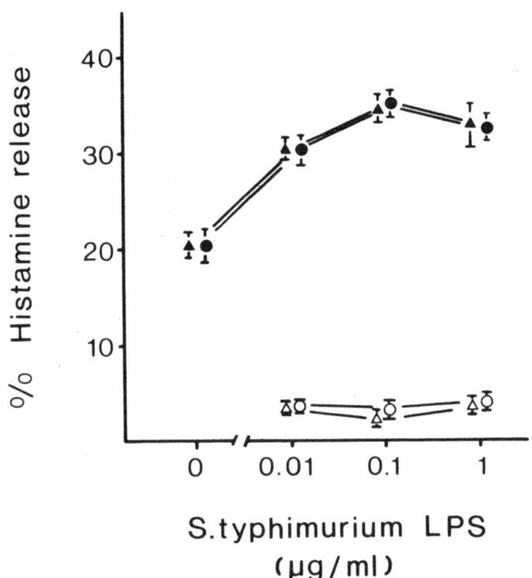

Fig. 11. Potentiation by *S. typhimurium* LPS of anti IgE induced histamine release. The cells were preincubated with LPS for 10 min, then washed and left for 30 min. at 37°C before incubation with anti-IgE (▲), or the cells were incubated with a mixture of LPS and anti-IgE (•). No significant release of histamine (<10%) was obtained when the cells treated by similiar procedures were incubated with LPS alone (open symbols).

virus (Fig. 13) or endotoxin(43,49). It is therefore possible that the microorganisms and endotoxins enhance the basophil cell response to IgE-dependent and non-immunological stimuli by such an interaction between microbial sugars and binding sites on the basophilocyte; this interaction seems to lead to a change in the subcellular handling of calcium rather than to its cellular influx(50).

Conclusion and Perspectives

Bacteria and bacterial constituents were found to cause release of histamine from human basophil leukocytes in vitro, and a similar release was also obtained from human lung and tonsillar mast cells and from mast cells in the airway epithelium obtained by broncho-alveolar lavage.

Mediator release caused by bacteria might be a pathogenic mechanism in airway diseases where a defect in the epithelium or failure of muco-ciliary clearence would promote invasion of bacteria or their soluble components. Another possibility is that they stimulate superficially lying mast cells in the airways epithelium (Fig. 14). Released

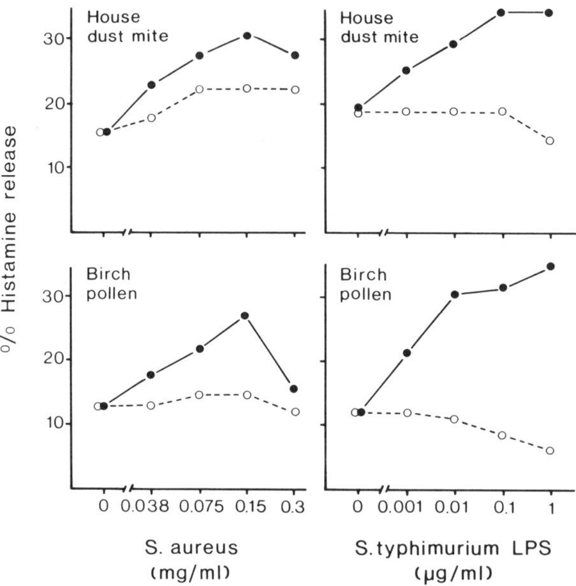

Fig. 12. Potentiation by *Staph. aureus* and *S. typhimurium* LPS of histamine release induced by specific allergens in leukocyte suspensions from patients sensitized to house dust mite or birch pollen. Potentiation (•) and its abolition (o) by galactose 10^{-6} M. Duplicate determinations. Note that *Staph. aureus* and *S. typhimurium* LPS did not release histamine *per se*.

histamine should then open the tight junctions in asthmatic patients (but not in normal individuals), where the number and the sensitivity of these cells are increased(51,52). The entrance of allergens, microorganisms and their soluble constituents would then lead to release of mediators and neurotransmitters and to accumulation of inflammatory cells responsible for the symptoms.

Two different mechanisms were found to operate in bacteria-induced histamine release, an immunological (IgE-dependent) and a non-immunological mechanism. The latter seems to be a sugar-lectin-mediated reaction, which means that to obtain a bacteria-induced histamine release, a person does not have to be sensitized to bacteria. Therefore this reaction cannot be disclosed by testing specific IgE to bacteria or their components.

Another important aspects is that virus, bacteria and their soluble components, endotoxins, peptidoglycan and teichoic acid enhance allergic mediator release by synergism. It is tempting to speculate that such an effect might play a role in infectious diseases and contribute to aggravate asthmatic attacks during respiratory tract infections.

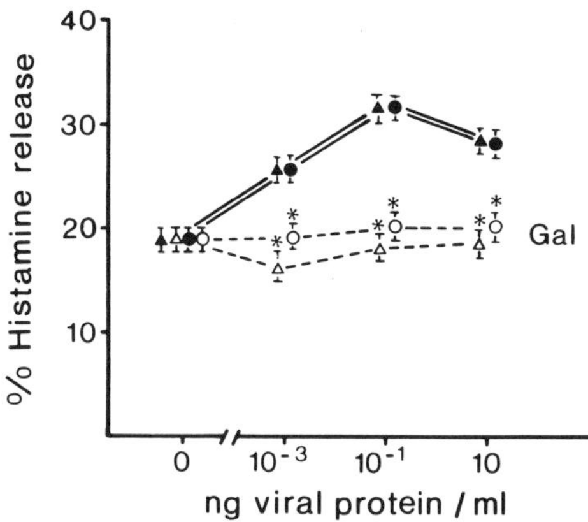

Fig. 13. Potentiation (closed symbols) by influenza A virus of anti-IgE induced histamine release and abolition (open symbols) of the potentiating effect by galactose (Gal) 10^{-6} M. The cells were preincubated with galactose (Δ) or buffer (▲) and then washed and incubated with anti-IgE and virus, or the cells were incubated with anti-IgE and virus in the presence (○) and absence (•) of galactose. Mean +/− SEM of 6 experiments in duplicate. *p<0.01.

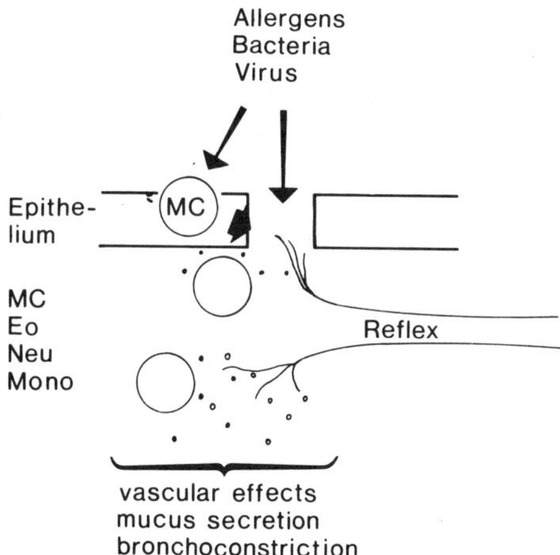

Fig. 14. Stimulation of epithelial mast cells (MC) might release significant amounts of histamine in asthmatic patients. Histamine opens the tight junctions leading to entrance of allergens and microorganisms, which trigger release of mediators and neurotransmitters responsible for the symptons.

The potentiating effect of the microorganisms and their constituents might depend on their carbohydrate chains interacting with binding sites on the cell membrane. Low concentrations of sugars such as galactose abolish the potentiation; this points to new medical aspects.

References

1. Busse, W.W., The relationship between viral infections and onset of allergic disease and asthma, Clin. Exp. Allergy 19, 1-9 (1989).

2. Horn, M.E.C., S.E. Reed and P. Taylor, Role of viruses and bacteria in acute wheezy bronchitis in childhood: a study of sputum, Arch. Dis. Child. 54, 587-589 (1979).

3. Hihi, E., T. Mokka, J. Nikoskelainen and P. Halonen, Association of viral and mucoplasma infections with exacerbations of asthma, Ann Allergy 33, 145-149 (1974).

4. Hudgel, D.W., L. Langstron Jr., J.C. Selner and K. McIntosh, Viral and bacterial infections in adults with chronic asthma, Am. Rev. Respir. Dis. 120, 393-397 (1979).

5. McIntosh, K., F.F. Elliot, L.S. Hoffman, T.G. Lybass, J.J. Eller, and V.A. Fulginiti, The association of viral and bacterial respiratory infections with exacerbations of wheezing in young asthmatic children, J. Pediatr. 82, 578-590 (1973).

6. Minor, T.E., E.C. Dick, J.W. Baker, J.J. Quellette, M. Cohen and C.E. Reed, Rhinovirus and influenza type A infections as precipitants of asthma, Am. Rev. Respir. Dis. 113, 149-153 (1976).

7. Minor, T.E., E.C. Dick, A.N. DeMeo, J.J. Quellette, M. Cohen and C.E. Reed, Viruses as precipitants of asthmatic attacks in children, JAMA 227, 292-298 (1974).

8. Welliver, R.C., Upper respiratory infections in asthma, J. Allergy Clin. Immunol. 72, 341-346 (1983).

9. Rylander, R. and P. Haglind, Airborne endotoxins and humidifier disease, Clin. Allergy 14, 109-112 (1984).

10. Rylander, R., P. Haglind, M. Lundholm, I. Mattsby, and K. Stenqvist, Humidifier fever and endotoxin exposure, Clin. Allergy 8, 511-516 (1978).

11. Castellan, R.M., S.A. Olenchock, K.B. Kinsley and J.L. Hankinson, Inhaled endotoxin and decreased spirometric values. An exposure-response relation for cotton dust. N. Engl. J. Med. 317, 605-610 (1987).

12. Kennedy, S.M., D.C. Christiani, E.A. Eisen, *et al.*, Cotton dust and endotoxin exposure-response relationships in cotton textile workers, Am. Rev. Respir. Dis. 135, 194-200 (1987).

13. Rylander, R., P. Haglind and M. Lundholm, Endotoxin in cotton dust and respiratory function decrement among cotton workers in an experimental cardroom, Am. Rev. Respir. Dis. 131, 209-213 (1985).

14. Norn, S., P. Stahl Skov and C. Jensen, C., Bacterial and viral infections in asthma, Allergy Today. vol. 1, nº 4, 37-39 (1985).

15. Busse, W.W., Infections, In: Asthma. Basic Mechanisms and Clinical Management, pp. 483-502 (Eds. P.J. Barnes, I.W. Rodger and N.C. Thompson). Academic Press, New York 1988.

16. Ida, S., J.J. Hooks, R.P. Siraganian, and A.L. Notkins, Enhancement of IgE-mediated histamine release from human basophils by viruses: Role of interferon, J. Exp. Med. 145, 892-906 (1977).

17. Busse, W.W., C.A. Swenson, E.G. Borden, M.W. Treuhaft and E.C. Dick, E.C., Effect of influenza A virus on leukocyte histamine release, J. Allergy Clin. Immunol. 71, 382-388 (1983).

18. Chonmaitree, T., M.A. Lett-Brown, Y. Tsong, A.S. Goldman and S. Baron, Role of interferon in leukocyte histamine release caused by common respiratory viruses, J. Infect. Dis. 157, 127-132 (1988).

19. Sanchez-Legrand, F. and T.F. Smith, Interaction of paramyxoviruses with human basophils and their effect on histamine release, J. Allergy Clin. Immunol. 84, 538-46 (1989).

20. Clementsen, P., C. Hannoun and S. Norn, Influenza A virus enhances allergic histamine release. Effect of neuraminidase, Allergy 44, 33-38 (1989).

21. Schauer, R. and A.P. Corfifeld, Sialidases and their inhibitors, In: Medicinal chemistry advances, pp. 423-434 (Eds. F.G. de Las Heras and S. Vega). Pergamon Press, Oxford 1981.

22. Clementsen, P., C.B. Jensen, C. Hannoun, M. Soborg and S. Norn, Influenza A virus potentiates basophil histamine release caused by endotoxin-induced complement activation, Allergy 43, 93-99 (1988).

23. Clementsen, P., A.R. Douglas, J.J. Skenel, C. Hannoun, N. Bach-Mortensen and S. Norn, Influenza A virus enhances IgE-mediated histamine release from human basophil leukocytes. Examination of the effect of viral neuraminidase and haemaglutinin, Agents Actions 27, 58-61 (1989).

24. Kingsburgy, D.W., Orthomyxo- and paramyxoviruses and their replication, In: Virology, pp. 1157-1178 (Ed. B.N. Fields). Raven Press, New York 1985.

25. Weis, W., J.H. Brown, S. Cusack, J.C. Paulson, J.J. Skehel and D.C. Wiley, Structure of the influenza virus haemagglutinin complexed with is receptor, sialic acid, Nature 333, 426-431 (1988).

26. Espersen, F., J.O. Jarlov, C. Jensen, P. Stahl Skov and S. Norn, S., Staphylococcus aureus peptidoglycan induces histamine release from basophil human leukocytes *in vitro*, Infect. Immun. 46, 710-714 (1984).

27. Koch, C., P. Andersen, J.B. Hertz, N. Hoiby, E. Kappelgaard, N.E. Moller, S. Norn, P. Pedersen, P. Stahl Skov and P. Tonnesen, Studies on hypersensitivity to bacterial antigens in intrinsic asthma, Allergy 37, 191-201 (1982).

28. Norn, S., L. Baek, C. Jensen, P. Stahl Skov, H. Permin, J.O. Jarlov and C. Koch, Influence of bacterial endotoxins on basophil histamine release. Potentiation of antigen- and bacteria-induced histamine release, Allergy 41, 125-130 (1986).

29. Norn, S., P. Stahl Skov, C. Jensen, F. Espsersen and J.O. Jarlov, Bacteria-induced histamine release. Examination of the bacterial cell wall components peptidoglycan, teichoid acid and protein A, Agents Actions 16, 273-276 (1985).

30. Church, M.K., S. Norn, G.J.K. Pao and S.T. Holgate, Non-IgE dependent bacteria-induced histamine release from human lung and tonsillar mast cells, Clin. Allergy 17, 341-353 (1987).

31. Baenkler, H.W., H. Hosemann and F. Dechant, Bacterial induced in vitro histamine release from nasal mucosa and polyps, Ann. Allergy 55, 240 (1985).

32. Clementsen, P., H. Bisgaard, M. Pedersen, H. Permin, E. Struve-Christensen, N. Milman, B. Nuchel-Petersen and S. Norn, *Staphylococcus aureus* and influenza A virus stimulate human bronchoalveolar cells to release histamine and leukotrienes, Agents Actions, vol. 27, 107-109 (1989).

33. Hogg, J.C., Bronchial mucosal permeability and its relationship to airways hyperreactivity, J. Allergy Clin. Immunol. 67, 421-425 (1981).

34. Norn, S and P. Clementsen, Bronchial asthma, Pathophysiological mechanisms and corticosteroids, Allergy 43, 401-405 (1988).

35. Jensen, C., S. Norn, P. Stahl Skov, F. Espersen, C. Koch and H. Permin, Bacterial histamine release by immunological and non-immunological lectin-mediated reactions. Allergy 39, 371-377 (1984).

36. Clementsen, P., M. Pedersen, H. Permin, F. Espersen and S. Norn, Influenza A virus potentiates bacteria-induced histamine release. Examination of normal individuals and patients allergic to bacteria, Allergy, in press.

37. Stahl Skov, P., H. Permin and H.J. Malling, Quantitative and qualitative estimations of IgE bound to basophil leukocytes from hay fever patients, Scand. J. Immunol. 6, 1021-1028 (1977).

38. Schleifer, K.H. and O. Kandler, Peptidoglycan types of bacterial cell walls and their taxonomic implications, Bacteriol. Rev. 36, 407-477 (1972).

39. Norn, S., P. Stahl Skov, C. Jensen, F. Espersen, T.C. Bog-Hanses, C. Koch and H. Permin, Lectin-mediated reactions in bacterial histamine release. A new mechanism in bronchial asthma, In: J.S. Schou, A. Geisler and S. Norn, Drug receptors and dynamic processes in cells, pp. 228-241. Munksgaard 1986.

40. Jensen, C., P. Stahl Skov, S. Norn, F. E{persen, T.C. Bog-Hansen and A. Lihme, Complexity of lectin-mediated reactions in bacteria-induced histamine release, Allergy 39, 451-456 (1984).

41. Norn, S., J.O. Jarlov, C.B. Jensen, P. Clementsen, B.T. Dahl, F. Espersen and P. Stahl Skov, Bacteria and their products peptidoglycan and teichoic acid potentiate antigen-induced histamine release in allergic patients, Agents Actions 20, 174-177 (1987).

42. Clementsen, P., N. Milman, M. Kilian, A. Fomsgaard, L. Baek and S. Norn, Endotoxin from *Haemophilus influenzae* enhances IgE-mediated and non-immunological histamine release, Allergy 45, 10-17 (1990).

43. Clementsen, P., S. Norn, K.S. Kristensen, N. Bach-Mortensen, C. Koch and H. Permin, Bacteria and endotoxin enhance basophil histamine release and the potentiation is abolished by carbohydrates, Allergy, in press.

44. Clementsen, P., C.B. Jensen, J.O. Jarlov, C. Hannoun, M. Soborg and S. Norn, Influenza A virus enhances *Staphylococcus aureus*-induced basophil histamine release in normal individuals and patients with intrinsic asthma, Allergy 44, 39-44 (1989).

45. Clementsen, P., M. Pedersen, H. Permin, F. Espersen, J.O. Jarlov and S. Norn, Virus enhances IgE- and non-IgE-dependent histamine release induced by bacteria and other stimulators, Agents Actions 30, 61-63 (1990).

46. Colman, P.M. and C.W. Ward, Structure and diversity of influenza virus neuraminidase, Current Topics Microbiol. Immunol. 114, 177-255 (1985).

47. Hitchcock, P.J., L. Leive, P.H. Makela, E.T. Rietschel, W. Strittmatter and Morrison, D.C., Lipopolysaccharide nomenclature – past, present and future, J. Bacteriol. 166, 699-705 (1986).

48. Norn, S., P. Clementsen, K.S. Kristensen, C. Hannoun and J.O. Jarlov, Carbohydrates inhibit the potentiating effect of bacteria, endotoxin and virus on basophil histamine release, Agents Actions 30, 53-56 (1990).

49. Clementsen, P., S. Norn, K.S. Kristensen and C. Hannoun, Influenza A virus enhances basophil histamine release and the enhancement is abolished by carbohydrates, Allergy, in press.

50. Clementsen, P., K.S. Kristensen and S. Norn, Virus, bacteria and LPS increase basophil cell response to histamine releasing stimulators and calcium. Examination of allergic and normal individuals, Allergy, in press.

51. Tomioka, M., S. Ida, Y. Shindoh, T. Ishihara and T. Takishima, Mast cells in bronchoalveolar lumen of patients with bronchial asthma, Am. Rev. Respir. Dis. 129, 1000-1005 (1984).

52. Flint, K.C., K.B.P. Leung, B.N. Budspith, J. Brostoff, F.L. Pearce, N. McI. Johnson, Bronchoalveolar mast cells in extrinsic asthma: A mechanism for the initiation of antigen specific bronchoconstriction, Br. Med. J. 291, 923-926 (1985).

AAS 36
Contributions to
Autacoid Pharmacology

PARASYMPATHETICALLY-MEDIATED SWELLING OF MAST CELL GRANULES DURING FEEDING

A.M. Rothschild, E.L.T. Gomes and M.A. Rossi*

Departments of Pharmacology and of Pathology*, School of Medicine of Ribeirão Preto, University of São Paulo, 14049 Ribeirão Preto, SP, Brazil

Abstract

Mesentery mast cells have been observed to swell and to spontaneously return to their original size following feeding of 12-h fasted rats. This effect may be controlled by parasympathetic efferent nerve impulses, since it is inhibited by atropine. It was reproduced *in vitro* in isolated rat peritoneal fluid mast cells exposed for 30s to $10^{-8} - 10^{-11}$M acetylcholine. When examined under the electron microscope, mast cell average granule diameters had increased by 29% ($p<0.001$) following treatment. Swollen granules did not leave (exocytose) acetylcholine-treated mast cells. They gradually and spontaneously returned to their original size. This recovery only differed from that occurring in the fed rat by its greater speed.

Introduction

Although I was a collaborator of Professor Maurício Rocha e Silva for a long time (1951-1966), the work dealt with in this article was no longer the product of our joint efforts. It actually represents the breaking of an old, established professional tie: Prof. Rocha e Silva, like so many histaminologists even up to this day was not enthusiastic about attributing actions to mast cells not connected with histamine release. Yet, starting with reports on the effects of epinephrine on mast cell morphology and enzymology (see review)[(1)], my experiments have drawn me more and more towards the conclusion that such cells are endowed with an exquisitely sensitive system of α-adrenergic[(2)] and cholinergic[(3)] receptors capable of setting off responses of as yet unclear functional significance, but certainly involving neither granule exocytosis nor the release of histamine[3]. Rapid, spontaneously reversible swelling of intracellular mast cell granules has so far been found to be the most conspicuous characteristic of these responses.

The finding that feeding rats after a fast caused them to present swelling of mast cells[4], encouraged further research on what had at first appeared a cytomorphological curiosity, but which gradually became a phenomenon imbued with a deeper physiological meaning. Results which have strengthened this conclusion, are presented below.

Material and Methods

Male, 180-250g, Wistar rats were used. All animals had undergone an overnight fast with access to water *ad libitum*. Fed animals were prepared by allowing them access to pelleted ration (Purina Chow), for 1 h, in a darkened room, between 8:00 and 10:00 A.M. Controls were kept fasted during this period. Mesenteric spreads were obtained from anesthetized, (Nembutal 80mg/kg, subcutaneously) freshly killed animals, by careful dissection following fixation and staining *in situ*[4]. For dimension (area) analysis, mast cell contours observed under the microscope at 630-fold magnification, were manually reproduced with a bright-point stylus on an electronic drawing board (digital tablet), connected to a microprocessor (Zeiss Morphomat), programmed to provide average cell areas ± standard errors of the mean[8]. One hundred randomly chosen mast cells were examined in each of three mesenteric fragments obtained from each animal. Mean mast cell area remained within 5 ± 5% of the mean area of 50 cells, when more than this number of cells were analyzed. This indicated that 100 cells adequately represent the total mast cell population of the tissue. Peritoneal fluid cells were harvested by lavage[4]. Following experimental treatment, specimens to be used for *electron microscopy* were rapidly cooled and centrifuged at 4°C for 5 min at 130g. After 10-15 min in the cold, pellets were fragmented and kept for 1 h at room temperature in 2.5% glutaraldehyde in 0.1 M, phosphate buffer, pH 7.3; they were dehydrated by acetone and included in Araldite. Semi-thin sections were prepared and pre-stained with a 1% toluidine blue, 1% Na borate water solution. After selection of sectors adequate for further processing, thin sections were prepared, stained for 20 min with 4% uranyl acetate in 50% ethanol, followed by another 20 min period in 0.3% lead citrate in 0.1N NaOH. After washing, first with NaOH, pH 12, then with bidistilled water, they were examined under the Zeiss 109 electron microscope, at 80 KV.

For *area measurements* mast cell suspensions were spread on a microscope slide; excess suspending fluid was evaporated under a stream of warm (35-45°C) air for 5 min. After fixation and staining with Giemsa fluid[(4)], cell areas were estimated by computerized morphometry.
Drugs. Acetylcholine (Ach), atropine and compound 48/80, Sigma, USA.

Results

Figure 1 shows changes in mast cells of the mesentery of rats sacrificed 60 min following feeding. Swelling without evidence of degranulation (b) contrasts with the picture of mast cell degranulation seen following compound 48/80 treatment (c). Two findings attribute a physiological meaning to mast cell changes evoked by feeding: first, full reversibility following a renewed fast (Fig. 2); second, inhibition by atropine (Fig. 2), suggesting involvement of muscarinic receptors, previously demonstrated in rat mast cells[(6,7)]. Earlier experiments[(3,5)], showing that intravenously injected parasympathomimetic drugs as well as stimulation of the abdominal branch of the vagus nerve mimic the effects of feeding on mast cells, further strengthened the belief that cholinergic receptors, stimulated during feeding, cause cell swelling. Further proof in favour of this conclusion is presented by results showing that low concentrations of acetylcholine also cause mast cells to swell *in vitro*. Since low doses of acetylcholine were partly destroyed by rat mesentery during incubation, rat peritoneal fluid mast cell-containing suspensions were used for these experiments. Figure 3 shows dose-dependent swelling of peritoneal mast cells incubated with 10^{-11} to 10^{-8} M acetylcholine for 5 min at 37°C. This response was extremely rapid and essentially complete within 30 sec. Return to the non-swollen state occurred between 10 and 20 min of incubation in spite of the presence of Ach in the incubation medium. Changes evoked by acetylcholine were blocked by 10^{-9} M atropine.

Figure 4 shows impressive ultrastructural differences between control mast cells (a), and mast cells exposed to 10^{-8}M acetylcholine for 30 sec (b). Marked swelling of granules, not accompanied by exocytosis or of rupture of the cell membrane, resulted from such treatment. Partial or total unfolding of membrane extensions (possibly a means of accommodating increased cell volume) was observed. A mast cell undergoing spontaneous reversal to the non-swollen condition is shown in panel 4c. This process apparently did not engage the whole mast cell at once; rather, it appeared as a progressing wave of shrinking granules and gradually returning folds of the cell membrane. Acetylcholine induced swelling differed from the unspecific swelling exhibited by mast cells exposed to moderate

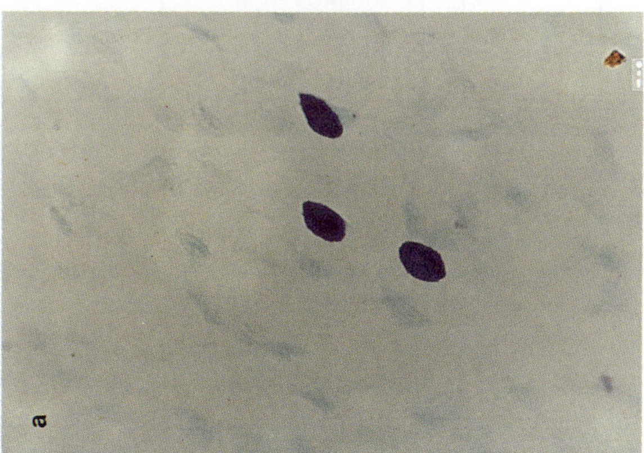

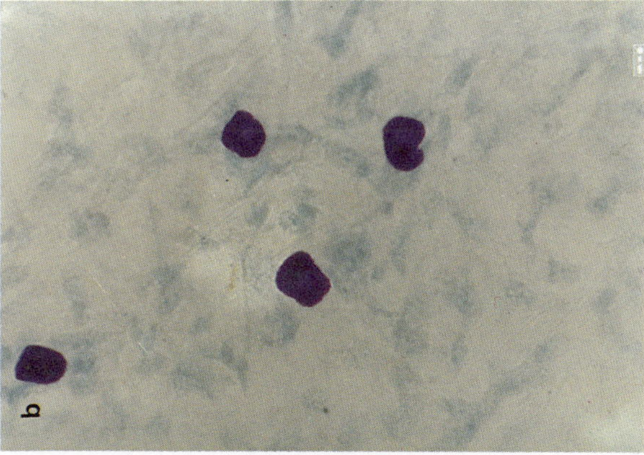

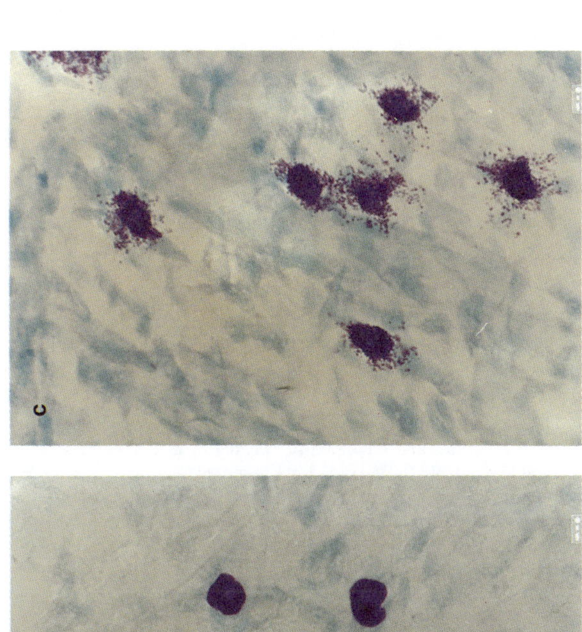

Fig. 1. Mast cell changes evoked in rat mesentery of a) fasted (12 h, water *ad libitum*), b) fed (1 h access to food after fast), and c) animals given an intravenous injection of 25 μg/kg of compound 48/80, 3 min prior to sacrifice. Note cell swelling in the absence of degranulation in cells of group b); conspicuous degranulation in group c).

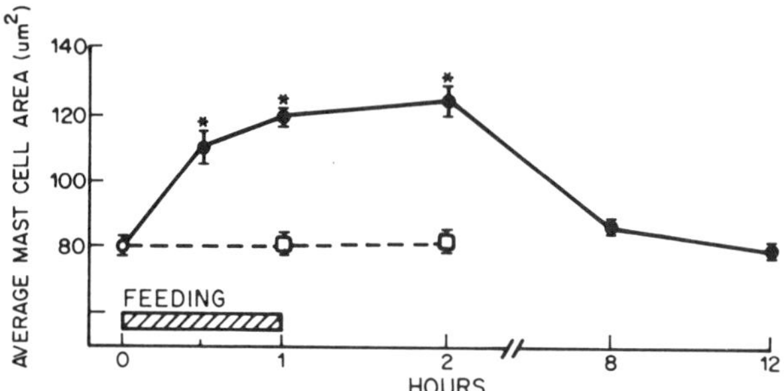

Fig. 2. Increase in mesenteric mast cell area following the act of feeding fasted rats; progressive spontaneous reversal during a renewed fast and inhibition of swelling by atropine. Rats were fasted for 12 h prior to being given access to food. ○, controls (fasted); •, Rats permited access to food for 1 h and sacrificed after different periods after this treatment; □ , rats fed 3 h following an intraperitoneal injection of 1 mg/kg atropine sulfate. Results are averages of 5 experiments. * Indicates a statistically significant ($p<0.05$, Student's *t*-test) effect of feeding. Mast cell areas were determined by computer-integrated cell morphometry at 630-fold magnification[2].

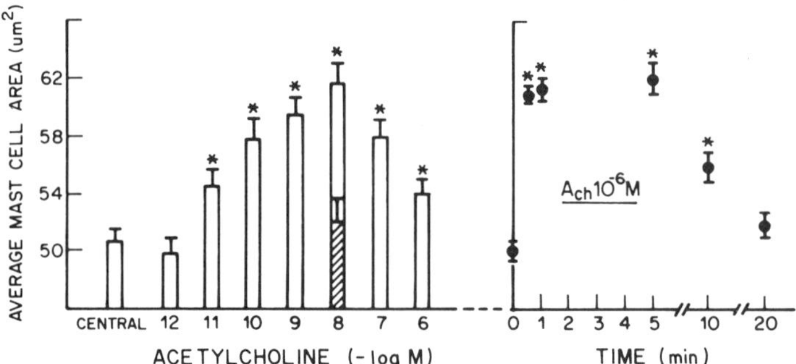

Fig. 3. Dependence on time, dose and absence of atropine of swelling evoked by acetylcholine (Ach) in rat peritoneal fluid mast cell suspensions *in vitro*. Results are averages of 5 experiments. Empty columns indicate average areas of mast cells incubated with Ach for 5 min at 37°C, in Krebs-Ringer phosphate buffer, pH 7.4. Hatched column refers to experiments conducted with cells pre-treated for 10 min with 10^{-9}M atropine. * Indicates a statistically significant effect of acetylcholine.

hyposmotic shock (Fig. 4d). In this case, 2 min after exposure to 2.5-fold diluted Krebs-Ringer buffer, the mast cell cytoplasmic matrix had undergone dilution evidenced by lessened electron density; retention of apparently unchanged, mostly non-swollen granules was observed.

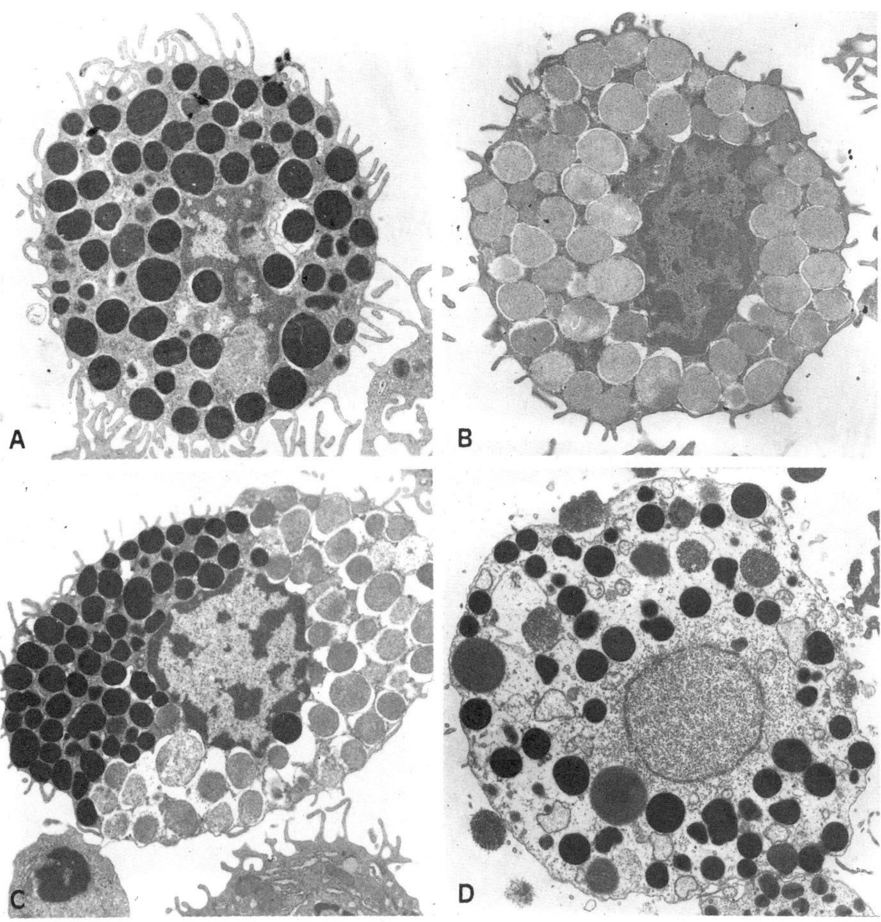

Fig. 4. Ultrastructural changes evoked in isolated rat peritoneal fluid mast cells by acetylcholine, observed under the electron microscope at 630–fold magnification. A) A control cell showing compact granules segregated within a well-defined cytoplasmic matrix. Projecting structures appear to be folded extensions of the cell membrane; B) following exposure to acetylcholine 10^{-8}M for 30 sec, granules appear swollen, less electron dense, but retained within the cell membrane; crowding by swollen granules does not seem to affect the cytoplasmic matrix; cell membrane extensions have become scarce and short; C) a mast cell, photographed 7.5 min following exposure to acetylcholine, is in the process of returning to its pretreatment appearance; note return of compact electron-dense granules and of membrane folded projections; D) a mast cell swollen in consequence to a 2 min exposure to a hyposmotic medium (2.5* diluted, i.e. 0.06 M Krebs-Ringer phosphate buffer, pH 7.4). Note rarefied appearance of the cell cytoplasm in contrast to compact aspect of some apparently unchanged granules. These unspecific changes are clearly different from those shown in panel B.

The frequency distribution of the diameters of control and acetylcholine-treated peritoneal fluid mast cells, respectively, is depicted in Fig. 5. Average diameters of granules of control cells were 0.48±0.13 μm and thus, significantly smaller than diameters of granules of Ach-treated cells which were 0.62 ± 0.15 μm (mean ± S.D.).

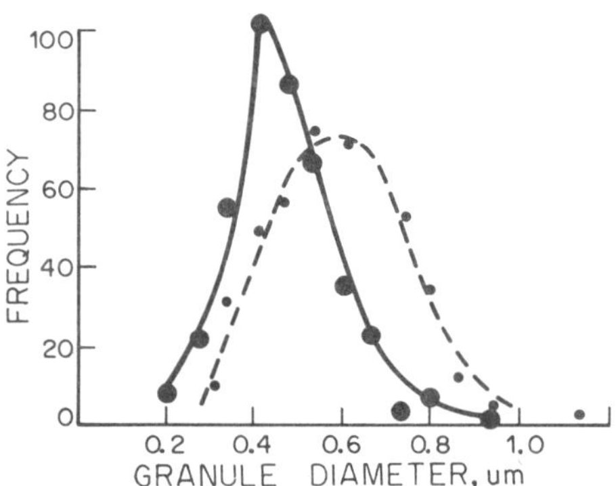

Fig. 5. Frequency distribution of the averages of the two major perpendicular diameters of granules contained in cross sections of respectively, control and acetylcholine-treated, aleatorily chosen, rat peritoneal fluid mast cells. Cell dimensions have been measured from photographs obtained under the electron microscope; they represent a total of approximately 400 granules each. Averaged diameters of the granule populations of control and treated cells, respectively, were statistically highly different ($p<0.001$ by Student's *t*-test).

Discussion

In spite of the extraordinary amount of information available concerning mast cell changes in disease, next to nothing is known about roles of such cells in normal physiology. Catecholamines, both *in vivo* and *in vitro*, physical exercise or exposure of rats to cold, have been shown to lead to spontaneously reversible changes in mast cell granule size(1). Observations showing that unfavourable environmental conditions like lack of glucose(2), low temperature(3) or low pH also evoke such changes suggested, at first, that mast cell granule swelling would be nothing more than the result of biochemical restrictions imposed by an unfavourable micro-environment. Further studies revealed however, that a physiologically all-important activity like the act of feeding caused the appearance of these very same changes in mast cells(4). They were reproduced by carbamylcholine, a parasympathomimetic drug. Atropinization prevented the effect of feeding on mast cells. This outcome was not due to an interference with the fasted animal's appetite (result not shown). Rather, it appeared to be the consequence of direct effects on muscarinic receptors controlling mast cell hydration, since carbamylcholine[3,5], as well as acetylcholine (present work), were capable of causing mast cell granule swelling *in vitro*. Mesentery mast cell granule swelling could be evoked by stimulation of the isolated abdominal vagus nerve, an effect again sensitive to inhibition by atropine[3]. The importance of vagal activity in the modulation of digestive activity is well-known. Although sympathetic innervation of the mesentery has been described[8], recent histochemical evidence has shown that parasympathetic fibers exist in this tissue[9]. A significant percentage of mesenteric cholinergic, possibly parasympathetic innervation, has been found in close proximity to mast cells[3]. Topographic support in favour of a functional relationship between mast cells and parasympathetic nerve fibers is provided by these results.

Reproduction of a cellular response by local application of its postulated mediator is one of the criteria suggesting physiological significance of an interaction between a neural pathway and its effector cell. The present report, by showing that minute amounts of acetylcholine applied to isolated rat peritoneal fluid mast cells cause cell swelling in a manner indistinguishable from that evoked by feeding or vagal stimulation, speaks in favour of an interpretation in physiological terms of this event.

Rat mast cells and circulatory basophils have been shown to mediate consumption of circulatory kininogen and release of kinin following carbamylcholine treatment[10], Feeding, vagal impulses and olfactory perception of food have been recently shown to evoke these very same effects in fasted rats[11]. A role of mast cells in post-prandial, putatively kinin-mediated vasodilatation in the mesenteric area is therefore suggested.

Acknowledgements

The authors are grateful to Prof. F.A. Amenta, Department of Neurological Science, University La Sapienza, Rome, for histochemical advice. Mrs. I.A.C Fortunato & Mrs. M.H. Nasi Gomes are thanked for technical assistance and the Fundação de Amparo à Pesquisa do Estado de São Paulo, Brazil, for financial support. Mrs. F.H. Ferreira provided expert typing.

References

1. Oliveira, M.P. and A.M. Rothschild, Effects of catecholamines on rat mesentery mast cells, Nature 218, 381-384 (1968).

2. Rothschild, A.M., E.L.T. Gomes and R.P. Gonçalves, Non-histamine releasing activities of mast cells, In: Adv. in Biosciences 33, pp. 57-68 (Ed. B. Uvnäs and K. Tasaka). Pergamon Press, Oxford 1982.

3. Rothschild, A.M., E.L.T. Tamburus and M.A. Rossi, Reversible mesenteric mast cell swelling caused by vagal stimulation or sham-feeding, Agents Actions 34, 295-301 (1991).

4. Tamburus, E.L. and A.M. Rothschild, Reversible swelling evoked by epinephrine, 8-bromo-cyclic 3', 5'-guanosine monophosphate and feeding in the mast cells of the rat, Biochem. Pharmac. 30, 469-479 (1981).

5. Rothschild, A.M. and E.L.T. Gomes, Atropine and hexamethonium-sensitive, Ca/KK-modulated, reversible swelling of mast cells in rat mesentery, due to feeding or exposure to carbachol, Agents Actions 25, 4-10 (1988).

6. Blandina, P., R. Fantozzi, P.F. Mannaioni and E. Masini, Characteristics of histamine release evoked by acetylcholine in isolated rat mast cells, J. Physiol. 301, 281-291 (1980).

7. Bani-Sacchi, T., M. Barattini, S. Bianchi, P. Bladina, S. Brunelleschi, R. Fantozzi, P.F. Mannaioni and E. Masini, The release of histamine by parasympathetic stimulation in guinea-pig auricle and rat ileum, J. Physiol. 371, 29-43 (1986).

8. Furness, J.B., Arrangement of blood vessels and their relation with adrenergic nerves in the rat mesentery, J. Anat. 115, 347-364 (1973).

9. Amenta, F., C. Cavallotti, E. Ceccarelli and F. Evangelisti, Cholinergic nerves in the rat mesentery, Acta. Histochem. 69, 125-131 (1981).

10. Rothschild, A.M. and A. Castania, Sensitivity to cyclic nucleotides and to aspirin of the kininogen-consuming system activated by adrenaline or carbamylcholine in rat blood, Agents Actions 8, 132-138 (1978).

11. Rothschild, A.M. and I.C. Fortunato, Changes in plasma kininogen evoked by feeding and related stimuli in the rat, this volume, pp. 230-237.

AAS 36
Contributions to
Autacoid Pharmacology

AGENTS THAT INHIBIT HISTAMINE RELEASE: A REVIEW

J.C. Gomes

Department of Pharmacology, Institute of Biosciences, Unesp, Botucatu, SP, Brazil

It is well known that histamine is found in high concentration in mast cell granules(1). The histamine content of these granules may be released to the extracellular space if an appropriate stimulus is provided(2). Besides histamine, other preformed active substances like enzymes, chemotatic factors and proteoglycans, as well as newly generated mediators like eicosanoids, platelet activating factor and adenosine are released during the secretion process of mast cells(3).

The activation of mast cell degranulation has been associated with a number of pathologic disorders, most frequently, diseases derived from the atopic state(4). It is now evident that mast cells are the primary effector cells in the early reaction in both allergic and non-allergic asthma(5,6), although some authors doubt that the late reaction of asthma is a mast cell dependent event(6). Other studies point towards basophils as cellular elements involved in the secondary phase of inflammation in allergic diseases(7). Secretion would depend on a histamine releasing factor, and on the presence of IgE on the basophil's surface(8). There is also evidence suggesting involvement of mast cells in some non-allergic inflammatory processes like arthritis(9). The pharmacological management of these diseases basically consists in the use of methylxantines, beta$_2$-adrenergic agonists, glucocorticoids, sodium cromoglycate-like drugs, anticholinergic and antihistaminic H_1 antagonists(10). Their therapeutic effects include bronchodilatation, receptor and physiological antagonism, prevention of inflammatory responses induced by secondary cells, and finally, inhibition of mast cell activation(11). This review is concerned with compounds having inhibitory action on mast cell activation, and their possible importance on the pathophysiology of mast cell-related diseases.

Sodium Cromoglycate and Nedocromil

Identified in 1965, sodium cromoglycate is known to inhibit antigen effects in sensitized tissue[12]. It was further shown to inhibit histamine release from mast cells in various locations and animal species including the rat.[13], mouse[14], monkey[15]. Although ineffective on human basophils[16], and on mucosal mast cell from the gut[17], it does inhibit histamine release induced by anti-human IgE in mast cells derived from human lung. It is more active against mast cells from bronchoalveolar lavage than against those obtained from human lung dispersed by collagenase[16]. The mechanism by which sodium cromoglycate exerts its inhibitory effect has been reviewed[18-20], and suggested to be a cell surface phenomenon. The acidic character of this drug makes it a highly ionized compound at physiological pH, and probably prevents it from crossing cell membranes by simple diffusion. Most likely, cromoglycate inhibits protein kinase C and the phosphorylation of a 78K protein. Protein kinase C represents a family of at least seven subspecies, four of them having molecular weights close to 78K[21]. Nedocromil is a sodium cromoglycate-like drug that has about the same effects as cromoglycate on the activation of mast cells. Nevertheless it has greater potency and efficacy in most sites assayed[22,23]. These drugs have a non-specific action; they also inhibit secretion by other inflammatory cells[22]. Thus inhibition of mast cell activity is probably not the only reason for the anti-allergic/antiinflammatory effects of cromoglycate-like drugs.

Antihistaminics H_1 Receptors Antagonists

Mota and Dias da Silva[24] were the first to describe the inhibition of histamine release from guinea-pig and rat mast cells by antihistaminic drugs. Further reports[25], have shown H_1 antagonists to inhibit histamine release from human basophils. Phenothiazine-analogues were the more potent members of this group. However, the concentration needed for an antihistaminic to exert its inhibitory effect on histamine release, is far higher than that required for it to inhibit H_1 receptors[26]. More recent antihistaminic drugs like ketotifen, terfenidine, ceterizine, azelastine and azatadine are most potent inhibitors of the histamine H_1 receptors; their inhibitory activity on the effects of mast cell stimulation, like that of the earlier antihistaminic drugs, also seems to be of low specificity[18,27,28].

Theophylline

High doses ($10^{-4} - 10^{-3}$ M), of this dimethylated xantine inhibit histamine release from human, basophil-containing leukocytes[29]. This effect was suggested to be due to the inhibition of phosphodiesterase, leading to the accumulation of cyclic 3', 5' -AMP. This hypothesis was strongly shaken by results showing that two methylxantines, isobuthylmethylxantine and theophylline increased cyclic 3', 5' -AMP in rat mast cells to the same level; however, only theophylline inhibited histamine release induced by antigen[30]. In lower doses, theophylline is a specific inhibitor of adenosine receptors[31]; when activated, such receptors potentiate histamine release from rat mast cells[32]. It was therefore suggested that theophylline's inhibitory action on mast cells was due to adenosine receptor blockade[33]. Neither theophylline-evoked increase of cyclic 3', 5' -AMP nor the antagonism of adenosine's effects on mast cells definitely explain the inhibition of histamine release by the xanthine. The effects of cyclic 3', 5' -AMP and adenosine on mast cell activation are, by themselves, a controversy. Besides potentiating it, adenosine, at low doses inhibits histamine release. This effect has been shown in rat peritoneal mast cells[34], and human basophils[35,36]. Adenosine inhibits adenylate cyclase activity by an A_1 type of action, or activates it by acting on A_2 receptors. These actions lead respectively, to decreases or increases in intracellular levels of cyclic 3', 5' -AMP[37]. Cyclic 3', 5' -AMP in it is turn, has been reported to inhibit histamine release from human lung and basophils[38], but, according to other reports, to potentiate it in human basophils[39], rat peritoneal mast cells[40], and guinea-pig heart[41].

Beta Adrenergic Agonists

Isoproterenol and epinephrine inhibit histamine release from human leukocytes. The mechanism of this effect was suggested to be activation of adenyl cyclase leading to increased conversion of adenosine triphosphate to cyclic AMP[29]. These findings were extended by Assem and Schild[42] who showed inhibition of histamine release in human chopped lung by sympathomimetic amines, and suggested this effect to be due to increased cyclic AMP levels resulting from the activation of $beta_2$ adrenergic receptors. Using radioligand assays and evaluation of the pattern of pharmacologic modulation of mediator release, the presence of such receptors was recently demonstrated on purified dog mastocytoma cells[43]. The inhibitory effect of $beta_2$ adrenergic agonists on histamine release seems to depend on the IgE mediated stimulus[44]. β-sympathomimetic amines show only a slight effect on compound 48/80-induced histamine release from dog mastocytoma cells[43]. Histamine release induced by concanavalin A in canine fundic mucosal mast cells is also inhibited by beta adrenergic agents[45]. It is known that concanavalin A induces histamine release by activating mast cells in a fashion very similar to that caused by IgE[2]. Much evidence relates beta adrenergic inhibition of histamine release to increased cell levels of cyclic AMP. Yet, as described for theophylline, this change causes a number of non-specific and variable effects on cell metabolic activity.

Calcium Channel Blockers

The dependence on calcium of mast cell secretion was first demonstrated by Mongar and Schild[46]. In 1977, the uptake of ^{45}Ca by rat mast cells stimulated with antigen, concanavalin A, dextran or ionophore A23187 was demonstrated. Inhibition of transmembrane calcium ion influx may be therapeutically beneficial in processes involving cell activation. Studies using the calcium channel blocker nifedipine, have shown that this compound could inhibit the increase in plasma histamine caused by exercise-induced asthma[48,49]. Calcium channel blockers have been shown to inhibit histamine release induced by immunological and non-immunological stimuli in rat peritoneal mast cells and in human basophils[50-52]. The inhibitory effect of calcium antagonists was however, considered not to be related to specific blockade of calcium channels because high doses were found to be necessary to inhibit histamine release *in vitro*[50]. Interestingly, calcium channel antagonists have been shown to inhibit the release and uptake of adenosine by human erythrocytes[53]. As previously discussed, this substance may play a role in mast cell histamine release.

Attempts to Find New Histamine Release Inhibitors

It has been widely demonstrated that mast cells from different sites exhibit marked morphological and functional heterogeneity[54-57]. In common with this, or perhaps due to it, histamine release inhibitors, besides low specificity, show variable effects on mast cells. The development of new and more specific inhibitors of histamine release would be a very valuable aid in studies on the pathophysiological role of mast cells in disease as well as in therapy. Not intending to discover a panacea, but believing in the possibility that such inhibitors might be found in plant extracts, we have been studying aqueous extracts of brazilian plants whose teas have been in popular use in allergic diseases. In preliminary trials, two plants have shown promise: *Hymenaea courbaril and Anchietea salutaris.*

The crude material obtained from aqueous extracts of stem and root bark of these species, inhibited histamine release caused by compound 48/80 or antigen from rat peritoneal cells, by 50%. Doses not higher than 10 microgram/ml, sufficed (Fig. 1). Since they refer to crude extracts, high potency of the active principles is to be expected upon further purification. Ten seconds of pre-incubation were enough for *A. salutaris* to inhibit histamine release induced by compound 48/80, by 30%; inhibition was maximal after 3 minutes (Fig. 1). Extracts of *A. salutaris* and *H. courbaril* also inhibited histamine release induced by *in vitro* anaphylaxis in the guinea-pig heart (Fig. 2). 30 microgram/ml of

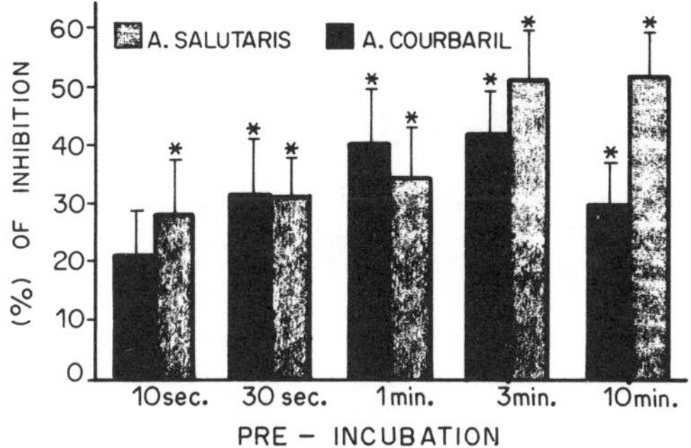

Fig. 1. Effects of pre-incubation with *H. courbaril* or *A. salutaris* (10 ug/ml) on histamine release induced by compound 48/80 (0.5 ug/ml) in rat peritoneal mast cells. Columns represent means of 10 experiments; vertical bars show S.E.M.. *Indicates significant differences of means (*t* test for paired samples).

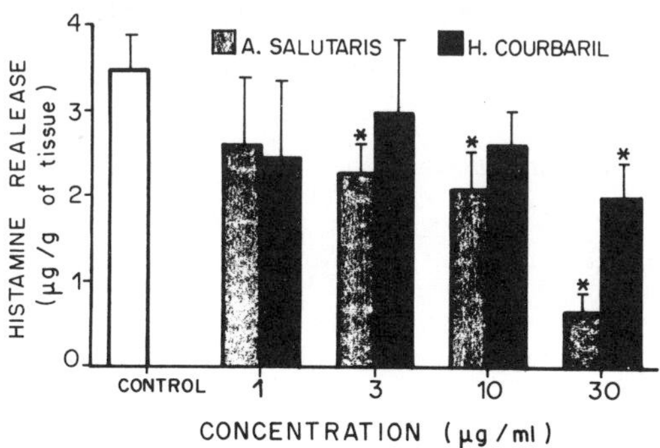

Fig. 2. Histamine release induced by cardiac anaphylaxis *in vitro* in guinea-pig hearts in the presence of *H. courbaril* or *A. salutaris*. Columns represent means of 4 to 11 experiments; vertical bars show S.E.M.. *Indicates values significantly different from control (*t* test for independent samples).

perfusion fluid of the former nearly abolished release. *H. courbaril* showed a weaker effect. Pre-treatment of guinea-pigs with *A. salutaris* extract (30 mg/kg i.p), inhibited histamine release induced by cardiac anaphylaxis *in vitro*. *H. courbaril* had no effect at 100 mg/kg. Following treatment, inhibition by *A. salutaris* increased during 12 hours. It had disappeared after 48 hours (Fig. 3). The high activity of extracts of *A. salutaris* in preventing histamine release in two animal species *in vivo* and *in vitro* points towards the interest of further studies on this subject. These are at present underway in this laboratory.

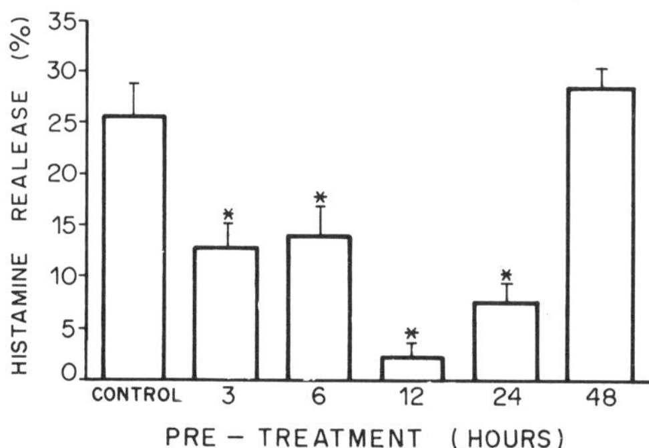

Fig. 3. Histamine release induced by cardiac anaphylaxis *in vitro* in hearts of guinea-pigs previously treated with *A. salutaris* (30 mg/kg i.p.). Columns represent the means of 5 to 13 experiments; vertical bars show S.E.M.. *Indicates values different from controls (*t* test for independent samples).

References

1. Riley, J.F. and G.B. West, The presence of histamine in tissue mast cells. J. Physiol. 120, 528-537 (1953).

2. Lagunoff, D., T.W. Martin and G. Read, Agents that release histamine from mast cells, Ann. Rev. Pharmacol. Toxicol. 23, 331-351 (1983).

3. Holgate, S.T. and A.B. Kay, Mast cell mediators and asthma, Clin. Allergy 15, 221-234 (1985).

4. Peters, S.P., R.P. Schleimer, R.M. Naclerio, D.N. MacGlashan, A.G. Togias, D. Proud, H.S. Freeland, C. Fox, N.F. Adkinson and L.M. Lichtenstein, The pathophysiology of human mast cells. *In vitro* and *in vivo* function, Am. Rev. Respir. Dis. 135, 1196-1200 (1987).

5. Holgate, S.T., Contribution of inflammatory mediators to the immediate asthmatic reaction. Am. Rev. Respir. Dis. 135, S57-S62 (1987).

6. Holgate, S.T. and J.P. Finnerty, Recent advances in understanding the pathogenesis of asthma and its clinical implication, Quartely J. Med. 66, 5-19 (1988).

7. Wasserman, S.I., Mast cell-mediated inflammation in asthma, Annals Allergy 63, 546-550 (1989).

8. Charlesworth, E.N., O. Iliopoulos, S.M. MacDonald, A. Kagey-Sobotka and L.M. Lichtenstein, Cells and secretagogues involved in the human late-phase response, Int. Arch. Allergy appl. Immunol. 88, 50-53 (1989).

9. Malone, D.G. and D.D. Metcalfe, Mast cells and arthritis, Ann. Allergy 61, 27-30 (1988).

10. Sweeney, G.D. and S.M. MacLeod, Anti-allergy and anti-asthma drugs. Disposition in infancy and childhood, Clin. Pharmacokinet. 17, 156-168 (1989).

11. Wasserman, S.I., Future pharmacologic agents and maneuvers in asthma therapy, J. Allergy Clin. Immunol. 76, 405-408 (1985).

12. Suschitzky, J.L., Antiasthmatic agents: the discovery of Intal, Chem. Britain 21, 554-555 (1985).

13. Foreman, J.C., J.L. Mongar, B.D. Gomperts and L.G. Garland, A possible role for cyclic AMP in the regulation of histamine secretion and the action of cromoglycate, Bioch. Pharmacol. 24, 538-540 (1975).

14. Marquardt, D.L., L.L. Walker and S.I. Wasserman, Cromolyn inhibition of mediator release in mast cells derived from mouse bone marrow, Am. Rev. Resp. Dis. 133, 1105-1109 (1986).

15. Barret, K.E. and D.D. Metcalfe, The histologic and functional characterization of enzymatically dispersed intestinal mast cells of non-human primates: effects of secretagogues and anti-allergic drugs on histamine secretion, J. Immunol. 135, 2020-2026 (1985).

16. Leung, K.B.P., K.C. Flint, J. Brostoff, B.N. Hudspith, N.M. Johnson and F.L. Pearce, Some properties of mast cells obtained by human bronchoalveolar lavage, Agents Actions 18, 110-112 (1986).

17. Pearce, F.L., A.D. Befus, J. Gauldie and J. Bienenstock, Mucosal mast cells II. Effects of anti-allergic compounds on histamine secretion by isolated intestinal mast cells, J. Immunol. 128, 2481-2486 (1982).

18. Kay, A.B., The mode of action of antiallergic drugs, Clin. Allergy 17, 153-164 (1987).

19. Church, M.K., Reassessment of mast cell stabilizers in the treatment of respiratory disease, Annals Allergy 62, 215-221 (1989).

20. Marone, G., The role of mast cell and basophil activation in human allergic reactions, Eur. Respir. J. 2, 446S-455S (1989).

21. Nishizuka, Y., The molecular heterogeneity of protein kinase C and its implication for cellular regulation, Nature 334, 661-665 (1988).

22. Gonzalez, J.P. and R.N. Brogden, Nedocromil sodium: A preliminary review of its pharmacodynamic and pharmacokinetic properties and therapeutic efficacy in the treatment of reversible obstructive airways disease, Drug Evaluation 34, 560-577 (1987).

23. Patalano, F. and F. Ruggieri, Sodium cromoglycate: a review, Eur. Respir. J. 2, 556S-560 S (1989).

24. Mota, I. and W. Dias da Silva, The anti-anaphylatic and histamine-releasing properties of the antihistaminics. Their effect on the mast cell, Br. J. Pharmac. 15, 396-404 (1960).

25. Lichtenstein, L.M. and E. Gillespie, The effects of H_1 and H_2 antihistaminics on allergic histamine release and its inhibition by histamine, J. Pharmacol. Exp. Ther. 192, 441-450 (1975).

26. Hahn, F., Antianaphylatic and antiallergic effects, In: Histamine and antihistaminics Part 2 - Handb. Exp. Pharm. XVIII/2, pp. 439-504 (Ed. M. Rocha e Silva). Springer-Verlag, Berlin, Heidelberg, N.Y. 1978.

27. Togias, A.G., D. Proud, A.K. Sobotka, L. Freidhoff, L.M. Lichtenstein and R.M. Naclerio, *In vivo* and *in vitro* effects of antihistamines on mast cell mediator release: a potentially important property in the treatment on allergic disease, Annals Allergy 63, 456-469 (1989).

28. Holgate, S.T. and J.P. Finnerty, Antihistamines in asthma, J. Clin. Immunol. 83, 537-547 (1989).

29. Lichtenstein, L.M. and S. Margolis, Histamine release *in vitro*: inhibition by catecholamines and methylxantines, Science 161, 902-903 (1968).

30. Skov, P.S., A. Geisler, R. Klysner and S. Norn, Allergic reactions, cyclic AMP and histamine release, Experientia 33, 965-966 (1977).

31. Fredholm, B.B., Are the action of methylxantines due to antagonism of adenosine?, TIPS 1, 129-132 (1980).

32. Marquardt, D.L., C.W. Parker and T.J. Sullivan, Potentiation of mast cell mediator release by adenosine, J. Immunol. 120, 871-878 (1978).

33. Fredholm, B.B. and A. Sydbom, Are the antiallergic actions of theophylline due to antagonism at the adenosine receptor?, Agents Actions 10, 145-147 (1980).

34. Nishibori, M., S. Shimamura, H. Yokoyama, K. Tsutsumi and K. Saeki, Differential effects of adenosine on histamine secretion induced by antigen and chemical stimuli, Arch. Int. Pharmacodyn. Ther. 265, 17-28 (1983).

35. Hughes, P.J. and M.K. Church, Inhibition of immunological and non-immunological histamine release from human basophils by adenosine analogues that act at P-sites. Biochem. Pharmacol. 35, 1809-1816 (1986).

36. Peachell, P.T., L.M. Lichtenstein and R.P. Schleimer, Inhibition by adenosine of histamine and leukotriene release from human basophils, Biochem. Pharmacol. 38, 1717-1725 (1989).

37. Londos, C. and J. Wolff, Two distinct adenosine-sensitive sites on adenylate cyclase, Proc. Natl. Acad. Sci. 74, 5482-5486 (1977).

38. Peachell, P.T., D.W. MacGlashan, L.M. Lichtenstein and R.P. Schleimer, Regulation of human basophil and lung mast cell function by cyclic adenosine monophosphate, J. Immunol. 140, 571-579 (1988).

39. Foreman, J.C., A.K. Sobotka and L.M. Lichtenstein, Modulation of the rate of histamine release from basophils by cyclic AMP, Eur. J. Pharmac. 63, 341-346 (1980).

40. Parker, W.L. and E. Martz, Calcium ionophore A23187 as a secretagogue for rat mast cells: Does it bypass inhibition by calcium flux blockers?, Agents Actions 12, 276-284 (1982).

41. Gomes, J.C., E.A. Gregorio and A. Antonio, Granular dissolution of mast cells and histamine release by compound 48/80 in isolated guinea-pig heart, J. Submicrosc. Cytol. 16, 659-664 (1984).

42. Assem, E.S.K. and H.O. Schild, Inhibition by sympathomimetic amines of histamine release induced by antigen in passively sensitized human lung, Nature, 224, 1028-1029 (1969).

43. Phillips, M.J., P.J. Barnes and W.M. Gold, Characterization of purified dog mastocytoma: autonomic membrane receptors and pharmacological modulation of histamine release, Am. Rev. Respir. Dis. 132, 1019-1026 (1985).

44. Undem, B.J., P.T. Peachell and L.M. Lichtenstein, Isoproterenol induced inhibition of immunoglobulin E-mediated release of histamine and arachidonic acid metabolites from the human lung mast cell, J. Pharmacol. Exp. Ther. 247, 209-217 (1988).

45. Soll, A.H. and M. Toomey, Beta adrenergic and prostanoid inhibition of canine fundic mucosal mast cells, Am. J. Physiol. 256, G727-G732 (1989).

46. Mongar, J.L. and H.O. Schild, The effect of calcium and pH on the anaphylatic reaction, J. Physiol. 140, 272-284 (1958).

47. Foreman, J.C., M.B. Hallett and J.L. Mongar, The relationship between histamine secretion and ^{45}calcium uptake by mast cells, J. Physiol. Lond. 271, 193-214 (1977).

48. Cerrina, J., A. Dejean; G. Alexander; A. Lockhart and P. Durox, Inhibition of exercise-induced asthma by a calcium antagonist nifedipine, Am. Rev. Respir. Dis. 123, 156-160 (1980).

49. Barnes, P.J., N.M. Wilson and M.J. Brown, A calcium antagonist, nifedipine, modifies exercise-induced asthma, Thorax 36, 726-730 (1981).

50. Ennis, M., P.W. Ind, F.L. Pearce and C.T. Dollery, Calcium antagonists and histamine secretion from rat peritoneal mast cells, Agents Actions 13, 144-148 (1983).

51. Tanizaki, Y., K. Akaji; K.N. Lee and R.G. Townley, Inhibitory effect of nifedipine and cromolyn sodium on skin reaction and ^{45}Ca uptake and histamine release in rat mast cells induced by various stimulating agents, Int. Archs. Allergy appl. Immunol. 72, 102-109 (1983).

52. Norn, S., C. Jensen and S.P. Stahl, *In vivo* and *in vitro* inhibition of histamine release by calcium antagonists, Eur. J. Respir. Dis. 64, 394-397 (1983).

53. Ford, D.A., J.A. Sharp and M.J. Rovetto, Erythrocyte adenosine transport effects of Ca^{2+} channel antagonists and ions, Am. J. Physiol. 248, H593-H598 (1985).

54. Katz, H.R., R.L. Stevens and K.L. Austen, Heterogeneity of mammalian mast cells differentiated *in vivo* and *in vitro*, J. Allergy Clin. Immunol. 76, 250-259 (1985).

55. Pearce, F.L., On the heterogeneity of mast cells, Pharmacology 32, 61-71 (1986).

56. Miller, J. and L.B. Schwartz, Heterogeneity of human mast cells, In: Biochemistry of the acute allergic reaction: Fifth International Symposium, p. 115-130, Alan R. Liss, 1989.

57. Galli, S.L., New insights into "The riddle of the mast cells": microenvironmental regulation of mast cell development and phenotypic heterogeneity, Lab. Invest. 62, 5-33 (1990).

AAS 36
Contributions to
Autacoid Pharmacology

HISTAMINE LEVELS IN TISSUES OF *TRYPANOSSOMA CRUZI*-INFECTED MICE

J.G.P. Pires, M.C. Milanez* and F.E.L. Pereira*

Department of Physiology and Pathology*, Biomedical Center, Federal University of Espírito Santo, 29001 Vitória, ES, Brazil

Abstract

Histamine levels of several organs from mice chronically infected with a myotropic strain of *Trypanossoma cruzi* were determined by bioassay. An increase in histamine content was observed in stomach, small intestine, colon, heart and skeletal muscle, when compared with noninfected weight and age-matched mice. These results suggest that mast cells, the main storage site of peripheral histamine, can play a role in the inflammatory and/or immunologic components of experimental trypanosomiasis.

Introduction

Mast cells have been implicated in inflammation[1,2,3] and could possibly play a role in Chaga's disease. Autopsy studies have shown an increased number of mast cells in the esophagus and heart of chagasic patients[4,5]. An increase in the number of mast cells was also described in skeletal muscle from mice chronically infected with a myotropic strain of *Trypanossoma Cruzi*[6]. Recently, a parallel increase in mast cell counts and histamine content in the stomach of acutely *T. cruzi*-infected rats has been reported[7]. In order to further investigate this subject, and accepting histamine content as a marker for mast cell content[2,3], we measured histamine levels in several tissues of chronically *T. cruzi*-infected mice.

Materials and Methods

Young adult albino mice of both sexes, weighing 25-35 g, were intraperitoneally innoculated with 10^4 trypomastigotes of a myotropic strain of *T. cruzi.* 140 days later, the animals were sacrificed by decapitation. Noninfected age and weight-matched mice served as controls. The following tissues were excised and studied: stomach (whole), small intestine (a 5 cm fragment of ileum, 10 cm distant from the ileocecal junction), colon (a 5 cm fragment located immediately after the cecum), skeletal muscle (quadriceps) and heart (atria plus ventricles). Tissues were cut into small pieces and heated in a boiling water for 30 min with 0.1NHCI to extract histamine. The solution was neutralized with 0.1NNaOH, filtered and assayed for histamine on the atropinized isolated guinea-pig ileum[9]. Results were expressed as micrograms of histamine (free base) per gram of tissue. Statistical analyses were made using Student's *t*-test. The level of significance was set at 5%.

Results

Table 1 shows a significant increase of the histamine content of the stomach, small and large intestines and skeletal muscle in *T. cruzi*-infected mice. In the heart, an observed tendency towards an increase in histamine levels was statistically non-significant.

Table 1. Histamine levels in tissues of *T. cruzi*-infected mice.

Tissue	Histamine, µg/g tissue	
	Controls (N = 4)	Infected (N = 5)
Stomach	1.3 ± 0.24	25.2 ± 9.0*
Small intestine	0.4 ± 0.06	4.9 ± 1.0*
Colon	0.9 ± 0.23	3.7 ± 0.7*
Skeletal muscle	< 0.02	7.2 ± 2.7*
Heart	0.2 ± 0.15	0.9 ± 0.5

Data reported are means ± SEM for N animals per group.

* = $P < 0.05$

These results demonstrate increases in the histamine content of skeletal muscle and of the gastrointestinal tract in mice chronically infected with *T. cruzi*. They suggest a parallelism with previously demonstrated increases in tissue mast cells in Chagas disease[4,5]. They also support the hypothesis[1,2,10] that histamine and other biologically active components of mast cells could play a role in inflammatory and/or immunologic components of clinical and experimental trypanosomiasis.

Acknowledgements

Research supported in party by SRPPG-UFES.

References

1. Liauw, L. and A.J. Lewis, Mast cells in inflammation and allergy, Agents Actions 17, 77-79 (1985).

2. Rocha e Silva, M. and J. Garcia Leme, Chemical Mediators of the Acute Inflammatory Reaction. Pergamon Press, Oxford 1972.

3. Wasserman, S.I., Mast cell-mediated inflammation in asthma, Ann. Allergy 63, 546-550 (1989).

4. Almeida, H.O. and F.E.L. Pereira, Estudo quantitativo dos mastócitos na cardiopatia chagástica crônica, Revista do Instituto de Medicina Tropical de São Paulo 17, 5-9 (1975).

5. Pereira, F.E.L., Estudo quantitativo dos mastócitos na musculatura do esôfago de chagásicos crônicos, Revista do Instituto de Medicina Tropical de São Paulo 14, 30-32 (1972).

6. Gomes, N.G.L. and F.E.L. Pereira, A quantitative study of the occurrence of mast cells in the skeletal muscle of mice infected with *Trypanossoma cruzi*, Proceedings of the Tenth Annual Meeting on Basic Research in Chaga's Disease, Caxambu, Brazil, abstr. nr. BI65 (1983).

7. Almeida, A.P., H. Gobbi, N.H. Toppa, E. Chiari, H.M.S. Gonzaga, M.V. Gomes, Freire Maia and J.R. Cunha-Melo, Gastric acetylcholine and histamine content of normal and *Trypanossoma cruzi*-infected mice, Braz. J. Med. Biol. Res. 22, 1229-1236 (1989).

8. Feldberg, W. and J. Talesnik, Reduction of tissue histamine by compound 48/80, J. Phys. 120, 550-555 (1953).

9. Vugman, I. and M. Rocha e Silva, Biological determination of histamine in living tissues and body fluids, In: Histamine and Anti-histamines. Handbook of Experimental Pharmacology, XVIII/1, pp. 81-115 (Ed. M. Rocha e Silva). Springer-Verlag, Berlin 1966.

10. West, G.B., Mast cells revisited, Agents Actions 18, 5-18 (1986).

AAS 36
Contributions to
Autacoid Pharmacology

INSULIN, GLUCOCORTICOIDS AND THE CONTROL OF INFLAMMATORY RESPONSES

J. Garcia-Leme, Z.B. Fortes, P. Sannomiya and S.P. Farsky

Department of Pharmacology, Institute of Biomedical Sciences, University of São Paulo, 05508 São Paulo, SP, Brazil

A. Mediation and Modulation of the Inflammatory Response

A significant aspect in the response of an organism to injury is its characteristic stereotypical pattern, dependent more on the species or the individual than on the nature of the damaging agent. It was from such stereotypical reaction that the idea of the response being mediated by endogenously mobilized materials arose. Ideally, a potential mediator should have the appropriate properties to bring about that part of the inflammatory reaction for which it is deemed to be responsible; it should be demonstrably present for a phase of the inflammatory response; and if it is possible to deplete the tissues of the mediator, this should also lead to a suppression of the inflammatory event for which it is responsible[1,2].

Mediators of the inflammatory response have a cellular origin or they originate from precursors in plasma. In the cells they may be preformed and stored, or may be synthesized *de novo* before release. In the plasma they are generally formed as a consequence of limited proteolysis involving multiple enzymatic steps. Inflammation, however, is also a modulated process in the sense that as an ongoing event, its amplitude varies in accordance with the intensity of the noxious stimulus. It is possible to identify local tissue factors, plasma factors, hepatic factors, neurogenic factors, and endocrine factors which act as modulators of the inflammatory response[3]. Hormone studies, from the early decades in this century, clearly indicated that many biological systems are subject to control by hormone actions. This is effected by binding of hormone molecules to specific receptors in target structures resulting in the generation of signals that influence cell functions. Inflammation evokes remarkable changes in the behavior of microvessels, hematogenous cells and other reacting components. Though these changes are mainly brought about by release or activation of endogenous mediators, hormones are an integral part of the control system of inflammation. Specific receptors are detected in the reacting structures and, in most instances, there is a striking similarity of the binding sites in these structures and those present in recognized target cells as far as the apparent affinity, specificity, and kinetics of interaction are concerned. Hormones, therefore, influence cell functions relevant for the development of inflammatory responses. Accordingly, inflammation is a hormone-controlled process.

Diversity of hormonal functions is likely to account for the recognized pro- and antiinflammatory effects exerted by these substances. The cooperative actions of different hormone systems provide the basis for a fine-tune adjustment of the response of the host in accordance with the intensity of the injury inflicted.

Most hormone systems are capable of influencing the development of inflammatory reactions(3). Insulin and glucocorticoids, however, appear to exert direct regulatory effects on the reacting structures in an inflamed area. The present discussion will be restricted, therefore, to the actions of these hormones on inflammation.

B. The Vascular Component of Inflammation

1. Insulin and the Endothelial Cell. Insulin receptors are demonstrable on the surface of endothelial cells which can internalize and release insulin with little degradation(4). Regional differences, however, are observed in insulin receptor concentration, as revealed by insulin-binding studies in primary cultures of endothelial cells. Both arterial and venous endothelial cells possess typical receptors for insulin on the basis of specificity of binding, curvilinear Scatchard plots, affinity profiles, pH dependence, and dissociation kinetics. Arterial cells, however, bind at least 2.5 times more insulin than do venous cells(5). The characterization of insulin uptake by microvascular tissues has been hampered by a lack of suitable preparations and by the complexity involved in analyzing binding studies in a tissue with more than one cell type. Notwithstanding, binding of insulin to microvessels isolated from adult bovine and neonatal porcine cerebral cortex is shown to be affected by pH, temperature, and other physiological conditions in much the same manner as the binding of this hormone to liver, adipose tissue, and muscle. Nevertheless, the binding capacity of isolated microvascular tissue is clearly lower than that of liver, fat, or muscle[6]. Chemical covalent cross-linking of insulin to its receptor in cerebral microvessels and the subsequent isolation of the hormone-receptor complex, indicate that the hormone is found associated with a peptide with a molecular weight which is indistinguishable from the *a*-subunit of the liver insulin receptor[6]. Though the mechanism of glucose entry into vascular endothelial cells is thought to be independent of the action of insulin[7], the hormone is likely to modulate functions of the endothelium[8,9].

2. *Vascular Responsiveness in Insulin-Deficient States.* The ability of insulin to restore altered vascular responsiveness in experimental *diabetes mellitus* is an indication that the alterations are a consequence of the diabetic state. This is observed not only in preparations of large vessels from diabetic animals receiving insulin[10,11], but also in microvascular beds of insulin-treated diabetic animals. Norepinephrine evokes a constrictor response of mesenteric microvessels *in situ*, the latency of which is analogous in normal and alloxan-diabetic rats. Histamine and bradykinin are capable of antagonizing this response in normal but not in diabetic animals, unless the minimum effective doses are increased about 20-fold. In contrast, acetylcholine and papaverine are equally effective in both groups of animals. The altered responses to histamine and bradykinin are not associated with hyperglycemia since fasting renders the diabetic animals normoglycemic and yet does not restore the reactivity of microvessels to these agents. Previous administration of insulin to diabetic animals corrects the impaired responses. The functional changes observed in the responses to histamine and bradykinin, under these conditions, are unlikely to be associated with a defective response of the smooth muscle. First, because in extravascular smooth muscles obtained from either normal or diabetic animals equivalent responses to histamine or bradykinin are observed. Second, because concentration-effect curves, constructed from the response of isolated aortae to norepinephrine, are similar in normal and diabetic animals, provided the endothelium is removed. Differences are only observed in preparations in which the endothelium is left intact. Since histamine and bradykinin are potent permeability-increasing agents in most species, whereas acetylcholine and papaverine are devoid of such an action, histamine and bradykinin might antagonize the constrictor response of microvessels to norepinephrine through an action on lining endothelial cells resulting in interendothelial gaps and increased vascular permeability with transitory changes in composition of extravascular fluid[12,13]. Induced changes in local steady-state conditions, if only from the osmotic point of view, can affect the reactivity of small vessels[14]. If the osmolarity of the extravascular fluid is increased, a significant increase in latency of the vasoconstrictor response to

norepinephrine is observed. Accordingly, endothelial cells may play a role when vasoactive substances, endowed with permeability-increasing properties, act on microvessels. That insulin is involved in such events is suggested by the restorative effect it exerts in diabetic animals, and by the finding that a similar condition of impaired responses to histamine and bradykinin is produced in normal animals by the injection of 2-deoxyglucose, the acute effects of which are the result of intracellular glucopenia secondary to inhibition of glucose utilization[(15)].

Data obtained with tyramine, an indirectly acting sympathomimetic amine, provide evidence that no abnormal release of norepinephrine from storage sites occurs at the early stages of *diabetes mellitus*. Furthermore, they indicate that uptake mechanisms into the adrenergic nerve terminal are unlikely to be altered since displacement of norepinephrine requires tyramine uptake. Interaction of norepinephrine with specific receptors to produce sympathomimetic effects is also unaffected as shown by equivalent arteriolar constrictor responses induced by the catecholamine in normal and diabetic animals. In addition, equal concentrations of phentolamine are capable of blocking such reponses in both groups of animals. Dilatation of arterioles and venules are observed in normal and diabetic animals with equivalent doses of acetylcholine, thereby suggesting that effector mechanisms for vasodilatation are preserved at the early stages of diabetes mellitus. Accordingly, release of endothelium-derived relaxing factor (EDRF) by acetylcholine does not appear to be altered, nor does the relaxing mechanisms in vascular smooth muscle, as shown by the responses to papaverine, an endothelium-independent vasodilatador[(16)].

The findings suggest that functional alterations of microvessels, characteristic of the early stages of the diabetic state, may occur in the absence of any noticeable dysfunction of the autonomic nervous system; that these alterations appear to involve the vascular endothelium; and that they may be linked to continuing insulin deficiency. Insulin, therefore, seems to play a relevant modulatory role on vascular function and reactivity.

3. *Insulin and the Response to Injury.* The observations described above point to the involvement of insulin in events that are of importance for the development of inflammatory responses. One should, therefore, expect that many aspects of inflammation will be altered by the diabetic state. Decreased inflammatory responses in alloxan-diabetic animals are related to the diabetic state, since they can be obtained for several days or months following the injection of alloxan and can be reversed by insulin treatment. Alloxan-diabetic rats fail to present the characteristic cutaneous edema (anaphylactoid response) which follows the intravenous injection of dextran or egg white. The histamine

content of the skin in these animals, however, is indistinguishable from that of controls. Pretreatment with insulin restores the ability of the animals to respond in a normal fashion to the injection of dextran or egg white. In addition, insulin considerably sensitizes rats to the dextran anaphylactoid reaction[17,18]. The edema which develops in an inflamed area following injection of chemical irritants or application of physical stimuli, is reduced when the animals are rendered diabetic by the administration of alloxan or subtotal pancreatectomy. This inhibition is reversed by previous injection of insulin and is not associated with increased blood glucose concentrations. *Diabetes mellitus*, however, does not interfere with the release or activation of inflammatory mediators. Diabetic animals also exhibit decreased responses to permeability factors such as histamine, bradykinin or serotonin injected into the skin, relative to controls. Accordingly, even when inflamatory mediators are formed in appropriate quantities in diabetic animals, their ultimate effect on the microvasculature is impaired, thereby suggesting that insulin exerts a facilitatory action at this level[19,20]. Activation of sensory neurons in unmyelinated fibers results in arteriolar dilatation and plasma exudation. The response is known as neurogenic inflammation and presumably involves the release of substance P and related substances. Neurogenic inflammation is reduced in alloxan-diabetic rats[20]. Furthermore, a marked reduction in plasma leakage evoked by substance P is observed in rats rendered diabetic by the administration of streptozocin. Determination of the content of substance P in sensory nerves and spinal ganglia, however, shows that it is not altered by the diabetic state. Similarly, nociception is unchanged in streptozocin-treated animals, relative to controls[21].

Light microscope investigation shows that microvessels of alloxan-diabetic animals, challenged with histamine or serotonin, exhibit less labeling by intravenously injected colloidal carbon particles than do vessels of normal animals. Insulin corrects this condition and also potentiates leakage of carbon induced by permeability factors in normal animals. The carbon particles label venules almost exclusively[22]. Electron microscopic studies reveal that labeling of microvessels with accumulation of carbon particles beyond the vascular endothelial barrier is observed in diabetic animals pretreated with insulin as much as in normal animals. The particles abandon the lumen of leaking vessels through interendothelial junctions[22]. Active contraction of endothelial cells has been favored as an acceptable explanation for the partial "disconnection" of the cells along the intercellular junctions. Metabolic effects of insulin may, therefore, be a relevant factor in the contractility of endothelial cells. The integrity of the microcirculatory responses to noxious stimuli may, consequently, depend on the availability of insulin.

4. Glucocorticoid Receptors in Vascular Endothelium. Glucocorticoid hormones have been reported to exert several effects on vascular endothelial cells. These include changes in morphology and protein synthesis[(23)]; induction of angiotensin-converting enzyme[(24)]; suppression of plasminogen activator production[(25,26)]; and inhibition of agonist-induced release of prostacyclin[(27)]. These actions are likely to be mediated by binding of glucocorticoid hormones to specific receptors in vascular endothelial cells. In the attempt to demonstrate the presence of glucocorticoid receptors in cultured bovine endothelial cells, the binding of dexamethasone to endothelial monolayers was studied. Scatchard analysis of the binding data gives results consistent with the presence of a population of high affinity binding sites in these cells[(27)].

5. *Glucocorticoids and Vascular Reactivity.* A given dose of corticosteroid may be physiological or pharmacological, depending on the activities of the organism. Therefore, widespread effects are expected unless investigations are conducted under rigidly comparable experimental conditions. Such conditions are not easily attained when endocrine influences are involved. Notwithstanding, glucocorticoids and adrenalectomy have long been known to interfere with vascular reactivity. Corticosteroids, particularly glucocorticoids, are suggested to play a role in the maintenance of the functional integrity of the microcirculation; to potentiate tension development of the vascular smooth muscle by vasoactive agents; or, to inhibit the constrictor action of a host of endogenous vasoactive factors. The magnitude of the permeability response to histamine and serotonin is subject to the influence of adrenal glucocorticoids. Corticosterone depresses the permeability effects of the above amines in normal rats, while the enhanced permeability response in adrenalectomized is decreased by corticosterone to levels somewhat lower than in control animals[(28)]. Eicosanoids and platelet-activating factor (PAF) are synthesized in response to stimulation. Precursors of eicosanoids are present in high concentrations in cells as esters, mainly in the form of membrane phospholipids. Before synthesis of eicosanoids can occur, the substrate must be released from cellular pools by acyl hydrolases. Deacylation of the precursor from cellular phospholipids is catalyzed by the activity of phospholipase A_2 acting on phosphatidylcholine and of phospholipase C plus diacylglycerol lipase acting on phosphatidylinositol[(29,30)]. PAF is synthesized from membrane lipids, and its formation involves the action of phospholipase A_2[(31)]. Most eicosanoids and PAF are vasoactive agents in most species. An interesting hypothesis has been that glucocorticoids inhibit phospholipase A_2 by a mechanism depending upon glucocorticoid receptor occupancy, followed by *de novo* RNA and protein synthesis thereby inducing the production and release of inhibitors of the enzyme (see below). It has been suggested that such inhibitors,

lipocortins, are not simply being produced under the influence of exogenous glucocorticoids. Blood contains circulating glucocorticoids in concentrations sufficient to induce the generation of lipocortins in normal tissues. These, in turn, would regulate the activity of membrane-bound phospholipases under resting conditions[32].

6. *Endogenous Glucocorticoids and the Vascular Component of Inflammation.* Increased blood concentrations of corticosteroids are observed after injection of endotoxins. This increase results from an enhanced release of steroids by the adrenal cortex rather than from decreased metabolism of the normally secreted adrenal steroids[33]. Hypophysectomy abolishes the adrenal cortical responses to endotoxins, thereby implying that endotoxins do not act directly upon the adrenal cortex. Since blockade of the hypothalamic release of corticotropin-releasing factor also abolishes the increase of plasma glucocorticoids resulting from the injection of endotoxins, the substances appear to cause an increase of plasma corticosteroids by action on the hypothalamic-pituitary adrenal axis at the level of the nervous system[34].

During the early stages of experimentally induced inflammatory responses, blood levels of glucocorticoids are consistently and markedly increased[35-37]. Evidence has been obtained that the development of acute inflammatory responses is regulated by a feedback mechanism which is induced comparatively early. In carrageenan or dextran lesions of the rat's paw, an antiinflammatory factor has been harvested in perfusions of lesions 2 to 3 h in age, though not less than 1 h old. The inhibitory effects of the factor are demonstrable by a decrease of exudation in other animals given the perfusate intravenously prior to injection of an irritant into the paw. Inhibition of edema formation is abolished by prior adrenalectomy or electrolytic lesions in the hypothalamic median eminence of the test animals. The perfusate also elevates the serum level of corticosterone, concomitantly depressing the content of ascorbic acid of the adrenal. On the other hand, the perfusate is effective in rats whose adrenal medula has been ablated, suggesting that adrenal catecholamines play no significant role in the inhibitory effect. Accordingly, the antiinflammatory factor harvested in perfusates from inflamed lesions seems to owe its effects to the release of glucocorticoids (corticosterone) via the hypothalamic-pituitary-adrenal axis. In addition, when both hind paws of the rat are injected simultaneously with an irritant, responses of the same magnitude and parallel time-course developments are observed. If the injections, however, are made at an interval of 2.5 h, the paw that is first injected exhibits a normal response, whereas the response in the other paw is reduced to about 50%. This attenuation is not observed in adrenalectomized animals. These data have been interpreted to indicate that glucocorticoids secreted in larger amounts during the early stages of an inflammatory reaction, apparently govern the development of such reaction. The increased secretion, induced via the hypothalamic-pituitary-adrenal axis under the influence of factors produced in the inflamed area would thus represent the last event of a feedback mechanism that regulates the progression of inflammatory responses(35). Recent investigations confirm the occurrence of a feedback mechanism governing the development of inflammation. First, a relationship between the temporal development of carrageenan-induced inflammatory lesions and pulsed release in plasma of increased amounts of corticosterone was reported(37). Second, it was shown that susceptibility of inbred Lewis female rats to develop an arthritis in response to streptococcal cell wall peptidoglycan polysaccharide (SCW) was related to a defective hypothalamic-pituitary-adrenal axis responsiveness to inflammatory mediators(38). Third, it was observed that resistance of histo-compatible Fischer rats to SCW arthritis is regulated by an intact hypothalamic-pituitary-adrenal axis – immune system feedback loop(38).

7. *Insulin, Glucocorticoids and Vascular Permeability Responses.* A possible interrelationship may exist between endogenous glucocorticoids and insulin in controlling the development of acute inflammation. The attenuation of an inflammatory response by a preexisting inflammatory lesion, as described above, can be abolished, in addition to adrenalectomy, by pretreatment of the animals with insulin(36). Insulin appears to facilitate the action of vasoactive substances on vascular endothelial cells, thus contributing to the formation of interendothelial gaps and to increased vascular permeability to plasma proteins. The activation of the hypothalamic-pituitary-adrenal axis by factors formed in the inflamed tissue results in increased levels of circulating glucocorticoids. These hormones, in increased concentrations, might antagonize the facilitatory effect of insulin, thereby limiting the development of the inflammatory responses. Estimates of vascular permeability changes to macromolecules occuring during the development of acute inflammation indicate that with mild stimuli vascular permeability increases are of short duration(39,40). The immediate opening of the endothelial intercellular junctions at the venular side of the microvasculature produced by inflammatory stimuli seems to close again after a short interval, even in the continuous presence of permeability-increasing agents(41). The progressive decay in vascular permeability observed in carrageenan or dextran-induced lesions in the rat's paw, closely coincides with the time interval over which glucocorticoids in blood start to increase. Accordingly, it is plausible that the roughly coincidental events reflect a stabilizing effect of increased concentrations of circulating glucocorticoids, evoked by a feedback mechanism, upon endothelial cells of the reacting vessels.

C. The Cellular Component of Inflammation

1. *Insulin Receptors in Inflammatory Cells.* Granulocytes, mononuclear leukocytes, granulocytic leukemic white cells, cultured human lymphocytes – and human erythrocytes and cultured fibroblasts as well – all have specific insulin-binding sites. These cells bind labeled insulin, and the bound hormone is displaced by nanogram quantities of unlabeled peptides. The ability of insulin and insulin derivatives to displace labeled insulin from these binding sites is proportional to their ability to stimulate glucose oxidation in isolated fat cells. In addition, there is a remarkable similarity of the binding sites in white cells and those that are present in the liver and fat cells, as far as the apparent affinity, specificity, kinetics, and temperature sensitivity are concerned. This strongly suggests that the molecular structures that recognize insulin in these different types of cells are very similar and possibly identical(42-46).

2. *Diabetes Mellitus and Leukocyte Functions in Inflammation.* Granulocyte dysfunction is a common finding in *diabetes mellitus*. Investigations in well-controlled diabetic subjects may fail to demonstrate any consistent defect that might predispose the patient to infection. However, in poorly controlled diabetic states, abnormalities in granulocyte chemotaxis, phagocytosis and microbicidal mechanisms are frequently described.

Studies on chemotaxis of polymorphonuclear leukocytes from diabetic subjects show that, while there are a few negative results, defective responses of the cells in the presence of a chemoattractant gradient can occur. The defect in chemotaxis is not correlated with plasma glucose levels, serum carbon dioxide, or blood urea nitrogen values(47-50). The early local exudative cellular reaction in an inflammatory lesion is impaired in alloxan-induced diabetic rats due to a reduced migration of neutrophils to the inflamed area. Neutrophils, however, are capable of moving from reserve compartments into blood in these animals, as much as in controls. Furthermore, an intrinsic cellular defect does not occur, because leukocytes obtained from diabetic animals are not devoid of chemotactic responsiveness when suspended in culture medium or normal serum. Suspended in the corresponding "diabetic" serum, blockade of chemotaxis to lipopolysaccharide (LPS)-activated serum is observed. Increasing concentrations of diabetic serum added to a suspension containing neutrophils from normal donors progressively inhibit the response of the cells to the activated serum. Hyperglycemia alone, or hyperosmolality secondary to hyperglycemia, the presence of ketone bodies, malnutrition, or a direct effect of alloxan do not explain the results. In addition, the capacity to generate chemotactic agents remains intact in serum of diabetic animals. The defect appears to be due to the presence of an inhibitory factor in plasma which is heat labile (56°C), is destroyed by incubation with trypsin, and is retained after dialysis with 10,000-Mr retention dialysis tubing. Pretreatment of the animals with insulin results in the recovery of the chemotactic response, either *in vitro* or *in vivo*(51). The inhibitory activity of chemotaxis is detected shortly after the onset of the diabetic state, being observed from the third day of alloxan administration (Fig. 1). The neutrophil migratory responses *in vitro* to the chemotactic peptide FMLP, and to LTB_4 are not affected by the presence of diabetic rat serum(52). Bacterial lipopolysaccharides have been demonstrated to activate both the classical and the alternative pathways of complement by a mechanism that does not require antibody to the LPS molecules. This results in the rapid appearance of chemotactic activity. Distinct subsets of chemotactic receptors mediate the response of neutrophils to FMLP, LTB_4 and complement-derived chemotaxins. Accordingly, the inhibitory activity of chemotaxis developing in alloxan-induced diabetic rat serum appears to be restricted to some stage of the interactive process between neutrophils and complement-derived chemoattractants. Overall, the findings agree with clinical evidence that disturbances of the inflammatory cycle evoked by *diabetes mellitus* – and characterized by a reduced leukocyte migration to the inflammed area – are not uncommon(53,54).

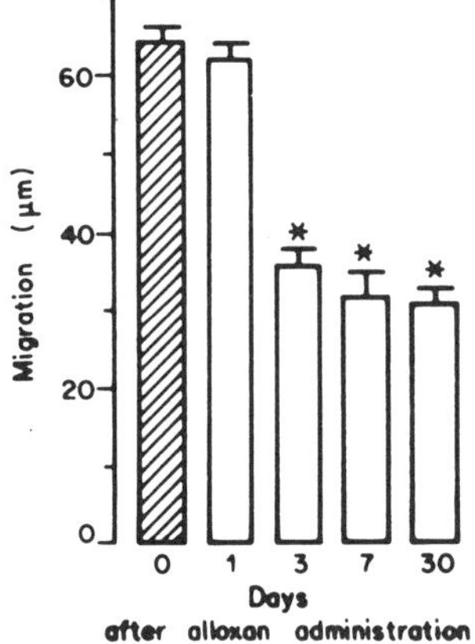

Fig. 1. Chemotactic responses of rat neutrophils assessed by the micropore filter system. Aliquots of cell suspensions containing 1.5×10^6 peritoneal neutrophils in serum of the corresponding donor were added to the upper compartment of a modified Boyden's chamber, separated from the chemotactic agent (10% of LPS-activated homologous serum in Hanks solution) in the lower compartment by a cellulose nitrate filter, 8 µm average pore size. The cells were incubated in humidified air at 37°C for 60 min, followed by removal of the filters for fixation and staining of the cells. Neutrophil migration within the filter was determined under light microscopy. Rats were rendered diabetic by the injection of 40 mg/kg alloxan. Values are means ± SE of 6-8 separate experiments. *$p < 0.01$ compared with value at time zero.

Much effort has gone into studies of the phagocytic and microbicidal function in *diabetes mellitus* and, with a few exceptions, results reveal impairment of these functions. The percentage of neutrophils actively engaged in phagocytosis is considerably less in diabetic rats and the average number of organisms phagocytized by these cells is reduced relative to cells of normal control animals. However, the differential cell counts of the peripheral blood of the alloxan-diabetic rats are equivalent to those of controls(55). In addition, alloxan-diabetic rats are more susceptible to experimental pneumococcal pneumonia than nondiabetic rats. The cumulative mortality in the diabetic group is significantly higher and more than ten times as many viable pneumococci are found in the pneumonic lesions of these animals as are present in the lesions of the nondiabetic controls. Serial histologic studies revealed that phagocytosis is strikingly depressed in the alveolar exudates of the diabetic animals[(56)]. To separate ingestion from killing in "diabetic" granulocytes, a technique was developed which distinguishes whether the altered efficiency of microbial killing is a consequence of an impairment in intracellular mechanisms or simply a consequence of a slower rate of microbial ingestion. From these studies it was concluded that diabetic subjects may have a neutrophil phagocytic defect, an impaired intracellular killing, or a combined phagocytic and intracellular killing defect[(57)]. Since a clearcut improvement in the microbicidal function of granulocytes is achieved following intensive diabetes management and reduction of fasting glucose concentrations, insulin may also participate in metabolic pathways regulating intracellular microbial killing. Glucose is freely permeable to the polymorphonuclear membrane. Most glucose, however, is metabolized via the glycolytic pathway and some enzyme reactions in this pathway are closely regulated by insulin availability. This suggests that the impairment in microbicidal functions, as well as other polymorphonuclear functions in *diabetes mellitus*, may have a metabolic basis[(58)].

Diabetes mellitus may also affect the mononuclear phagocytic system. Macrophages obtained from the peritoneal cavity of alloxan-diabetic rats exhibit a reduced capacity to engulf opsonized sheep erythrocytes when compared with the activity of cells obtained from matching controls. Recovery of the impaired response was attained by pretreatment of the animals with insulin. Details of the methods are described elsewhere[(59,60)]. Results are presented in Fig. 2.

Certain biochemical aspects of the lymphocyte may also be altered in diabetes. This raises the possibilty that normal antigenic recognition and satisfactory initiation of the immune response, as mediated by the lymphocyte, may be abnormal in diabetic subjects. Despite the fact that comparison of antibody responses in normal and diabetic animals has not always conclusively revealed a significant difference between both groups, more recent findings suggest that humoral responses may be affected in experimentally induced *diabetes mellitus*[(61)]. Cell-mediated immune responses are depressed in human insulin-dependent diabetes[(62)], as well as the production of interleukins[(63)]. Therefore, at least in part, a possibly impaired lymphocyte activity in diabetic subjects might be related to the insulin deficiency.

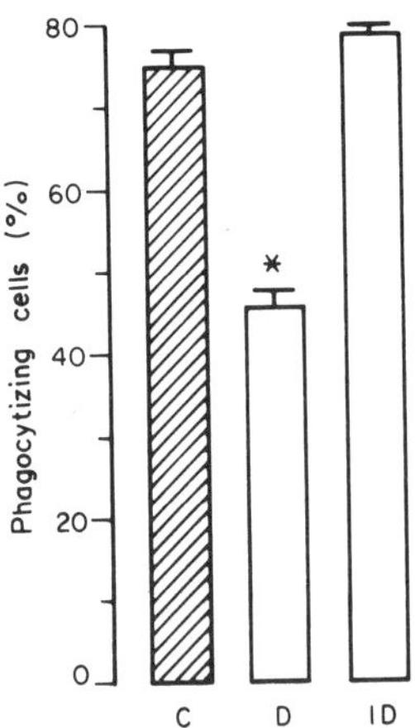

Fig. 2. Phagocytosis of IgG-coated sheep erythrocytes by peritoneal macrophages of normal (N), diabetic (D) and insulin-treated diabetic (ID) rats. Animals were rendered diabetic by the injection of 40 mg/kg alloxan 14 days before. Insulin-treated animals received 2 U NPH insulin, daily, for 4 days, by the subcutaneous route. Macrophages were made to adhere to glass cover slips, then incubated for 60 min at 37°C in the presence of a suspension of IgG-coated sheep erythrocytes. The cover slips were then washed and preparations fixed and stained for microscopic observation. Experiments were made in duplicate and 100 macrophages in each evaluated for determination of the percentage of phagocytizing cells. Values are means ± SE of 8 separate experiments in each group. $^*p<0.01$ compared with control value.

3. *Endogenous Glucocorticoids and the Control of Inflammatory Cell Functions.* Investigations on the participation of glucocorticoids in inflammatory responses have generally involved the parenteral administration of such substances to experimental animals and man. However, endogenous glucocorticoids play a role in the control of inflammation.

The immune response itself brings about changes in hormone levels. Increase in glucocorticoid concentration in blood has been reported during the course of an antigenic response. Moreover, adrenalectomy almost abolishes the so-called antigenic competition phenomenon in which injection of one antigen inhibits the immune response to a noncross-reactive antigen injected together. These changes may have significance in immunoregulation, and may imply that a flow of information occurs from the activated immune system to neuroendocrine structures, resulting in some type of regulation of the response(64).

The effect of the ablation of the adrenal glands on the acute inflammatory process has been recently reevaluated. The magnitude and duration of carrageenan-induced inflammation as estimated by fluid exudation and cell migration, is greatly increased in adrenalectomized rats compared with that in their sham-operated controls. In addition, the content of prostaglandin, thromboxane B_2, and leukotriene B_4 in inflammatory exudates from adrenalectomized animals is significantly greater than in controls. Moreover, resident macrophages obtained from adrenalectomized rats produce more eicosanoids per cell unit time when stimulated *in vitro* with zymosan than do cells from sham-operated controls. The findings are consistent with the notion that the increased secretion of glucocorticoids during the inflammatory response serves to check and control the development of inflammation[65]. Using television microscopy the number of leukocytes rolling along the venular endothelium of the vascular network of the internal spermatic fascia was determined in adrenalectomized, sham-operated and normal rats. A marked increase in the number of rolling cells was observed in adrenalectomized rats, relative to controls (Table 1). Blood leukocyte counts, however, were equivalent in the

Table 1. Rolling leukocytes in venules of adrenalectomized rats and matching controls.

Animals	Blood leukocyte counts (cells/mm^3)	Rolling leukocytes (number/10min/venule)
Adrenalectomized (14)	12,392 ± 1185	224.6 ± 17.3*
Sham-operated (5)	12,994 ± 620	115.6 ± 5.6
Normal (8)	12,988 ± 530	112.2 ± 11.5

Surgeries were performed 6 days before. Adrenalectomized animals were supplied with physiologic saline in addition to water. Blood leukocyte counts were carried out in samples obtained from the cut tip of the tail. The exteriorized spermatic fascia of the wall of the scrotal chamber was used for direct vital observation of microvessels in anesthetized animals. A 500-line television camera was incorporated to the microscope to facilitate observation of the enlarged image (× 3400) on the video screen. Vessels selected for study were postcapillary venules with resting diameters ranging from 12 to 16 μm. A given section of the vascular bed was tested only once and no more than two determinations were performed on a single animal. These were averaged for each animal. To measure vessel diameter an image splitting micrometer was adjusted to the prototube of the microscope. The image-splitter sheared the optical image into two separate images and displaced one with respect to the other. By rotating the image-splitter in the prototube the shearing was maintained in a direction at right angles to the axis of the vessel. The displacement of one image from the other allowed measurement of the vessel diameter. Leukocytes moving in the periphery of the axial stream, in contact with the endothelium, were considered to be "rollers" and their number determined in 10-min periods. These leukocytes moved sufficiently slowly to be individually visible and were counted as they rolled past a selected point on one side of the vessel. Values are mean ± SE. Figures within parentheses indicate number of animals used. *$p < 0.01$ compared with values in matching controls.

three groups of animals. No noticeable hemodynamic change occurred to explain the increase in number of rolling leukocytes in adrenalectomized rats. The rolling movement is presumably the result of two forces, one an adhesive force towards the wall and the other the shearing force of the flowing blood. In a given venule with approximately constant blood flow velocity the shear force also remains constant[66]. Adhesion changes affecting the primary leukocyte-endothelium interaction may, therefore, have occurred in adrenalectomized animals, resulting in an increased number of rolling leukocytes. The effect is likely to be under the control of glucocorticoids because metyrapone-treated rats also exhibited an enhanced number of cells rolling along the venular endothelium. Metyrapone through inhibition of the 11 β-hydroxylation reactions in the adrenal cortex markedly reduces the secretion of cortisol, corticosterone and aldosterone, while the secretion of 11-deoxycorticosteroids is relatively unimpaired. Accordingly, the administration of metyrapone results in a compensatory increase in ACTH secretion and in increased secretion of 11-deoxycortisol, a relatively inert steroid, and 11-deoxycorticosterone, a mineralocorticoid. Therefore, metyrapone blocks the production of glucocorticoids but does not typically cause a deficiency of mineralocorticoids. Under the influence of a local inflammatory stimulus, cells emerge into the perivascular tissue. The number of cells present in a standard area in the tissue was greater in adrenalectomized than in control animals (Table 2). At least in part, endogenous glucocorticoids might, therefore, control leukocyte migration to an inflamed area since the first visible change is a slowing of a proportion of these cells in the small veins.

Table 2. Leukocytes in perivascular tissue of adrenalectomized, metyrapone-treated and matching control rats 2h after the initiation of an inflammatory response.

Animals	Blood leukocyte counts (cells/mm^3)	Leukocytes in perivascular tissue (number/10000 μm^2)
Adrenalectomized	15,160 ± 576 / 19,530 ± 2362	33.5 ± 2.3*
Metyrapone-treated	11,783 ± 777 / 14,775 ± 1209	24.0 ± 1.8*
Sham-operated	14,000 ± 998 / 13,410 ± 1934	11.5 ± 1.5
Normal	12,490 ± 567 / 12,717 ± 1788	11.0 ± 1.4

The exteriorized spermatic fascia of the wall of the scrotal chamber was used. Details of the method are described in Table 1. Blood leukocyte counts were made before the initiation of the inflammatory response and 2 h thereafter. The number of leukocytes which accumulated in the perivascular tissue was estimated in a standard area of 1000 μm^2 at the connective tissue adjacent to a postcapillary venule. Images were recorded on a videorecorder and the area defined on the video screen, 10 μm in tissue corresponding to 3.4 cm on the screen (magnification × 3400). Five different fields were evaluated on a single animal to avoid variability based upon sampling. Data were averaged for each animal. The inflammatory reaction was evoked by the injection of 0.1 ml of a solution containing 100 μg carrageenan in physiologic saline into the scrotum of the animals. Values are mean ± SE of six animals in each group. *$p<0.01$ compared with values in matching controls.

4. *Lipocortins.* Lipocortin has been described as a glycoprotein whose synthesis or secretion is stimulated by glucocorticoids and which specifically inhibits phospholipase A_2 *in vitro* and *in vivo*[67]. It is now known that the substance belongs to a much larger class of

proteins which share the property of binding membrane phospholipids in a calcium-dependent manner. Due to inhibition of the phospholipase A_2 activity, a controlling enzyme in the production of eicosanoids, lipocortins have been suggested to act as mediators of the antiinflammatory effect of glucocorticoids. Recent findings, however, have raised some questions[68,69]. Lipocortins are thought to act extracellularly and must, therefore, be secreted but there is no direct evidence that they are, in fact, secreted proteins and it is not known whether they act as inhibitors of intracellular phospholipase. Purified lipocortins block the stimulated release of arachidonic acid from membrane phospholipids, but not basal release. It is not clear whether any of the recombinant or otherwise structurally characterized lipocortins are actually induced by glucocorticoids, particularly in a way that correlates with antiinflammatory activity. Clearly, effort must be expended to solve the question of whether lipocortins are primary agents of the antiinflammatory effect of glucocorticoids.

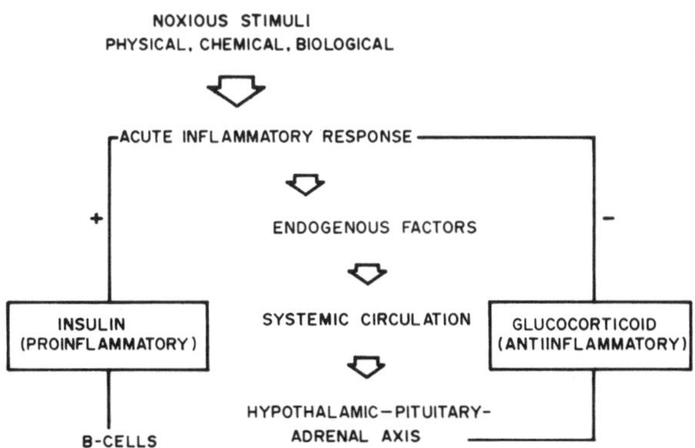

Fig. 3. Proposed hormonal mechanisms controlling the development of inflammatory responses. Insulin acts as a proinflammatory hormone. Glucocorticoids are secreted in increased amounts and act as antiinflammatory hormones. Secretion of glucocorticoids results from stimulation of the hypothalamic-pituitary-adrenal axis by compounds formed in the inflamed area (feedback mechanism).

D. Conclusions

There is evidence to show that insulin and glucocorticoids play an integrative role in inflammation. Specific binding sites for these hormones are recognized in vascular structures and cells involved with the development of inflammatory responses. Furthermore, endocrine disorders, characterized by altered levels of circulating insulin or glucocorticoids, may affect fundamental features of inflammation. The action of these hormones should be distinguished from the effects of chemical mediators of the inflammatory process. Apparently, insulin and glucocorticoids are involved with the control system of inflammation (Fig. 3). Much of the defensive character of the inflammatory process appears to reside in the integrative function of these hormones. Overall, the findings seem to indicate that inflammation is not merely a local event, but is rather a complex response of the organism, requiring a high level of integration.

Acknowledgement. This work was supported in part by FAPESP grants, São Paulo, Brazil.

References

1. Willoughby, D.A., Mediation of increased vascular permeability in inflammation, In: The Inflammatory Process, vol.2, 2nd ed., pp. 303-331 (Eds. B.W. Zweifach, L. Grant and R.T. McCluskey). Academic Press, New York 1973.

2. Wilhelm, D.L., Chemical mediators, In: The Inflammatory Process, vol.2, 2nd ed., pp. 251-301 (Eds. B.W. Zweifach, L. Grant and R.T. McCluskey). Academic Press, New York 1973.

3. Garcia-Leme, J., Hormones and inflammation, pp. 1-238, CRC Press, Boca Raton 1989.

4. Bar, R.S., J.C. Hoack and M.L. Peacock, Insulin receptors in human endothelial cells: identification and characterization, J. Clin. Endocrinol. Metab. 46, 699-702 (1978).

5. Bar, R.S., M.L. Peacock, R.G. Spanheimer, R. Veenstra and J.C. Hoack, Differential binding of insulin to human arterial and venous endothelial cells in primary culture, Diabetes 29, 991-995 (1980).

6. Haskell, J.F., G. Meezan and D.J. Pillion, Identification of the insulin receptor of cerebral microvessels, Am. J. Physiol. 248, E115-125 (1985).

7. Corkey, R.F., B.E. Corkey and M.A. Gimbrone Jr., Hexose transport in normal and SV40-transformed human endothelial cells in culture, J. Cell Physiol. 106, 425-434 (1981).

8. Meezan, E. and D.J. Pillion, Direct demonstration that cerebral and retinal micro-vessels respond to insulin, Fed. Proc. Fed. Am. Soc. Exp. Biol. 40, 366 (1981).

9. Pillion, D.J., J.F. Haskell and E. Meezan, Cerebral cortical microvessels: an insulin-sensitive tissue, Biochem. Biophys. Res. Commun. 104, 686-692 (1982).

10. Pfaffman, M.A., C.R. Ball, A. Darby and R. Hilman, Insulin reversal of diabetes-induced inhibition of vascular contractility in the rat, Am. J. Physiol. 242, H490-495 (1982).

11. McLeod, K.M., The effect of insulin treatment on changes in vascular reactivity in chronic experimental diabetes, Diabetes 34, 1160-1167 (1985).

12. Fortes, Z.B., J. Garcia-Leme and R. Scivoletto, Influence of diabetes on the reactivty of mesenteric microvessels to histamine, bradykinin and acetylcholine, Br. J. Pharmacol. 78, 39-48 (1983).

13. Fortes, Z.B., J. Garcia-Leme and R. Scivoletto, Vascular reactivity in *diabetes mellitus:* role of the endothelial cell, Br. J. Pharmacol. 79, 771-781 (1983).

14. Vanhoutte, P.M., Heterogeneity in vascular smooth muscle, In: Microcirculation, vol. 2, pp. 181-309 (Eds. G. Kaley and B.M. Altura). University Park Press, Baltimore 1978.

15. Fortes, Z.B., J. Garcia-Leme and R. Scivoletto, Vascular reactivity in *diabetes mellitus:* possible role of insulin on the endothelial cell, Br. J. Pharmacol. 83, 635-643 (1984).

16. Fortes, Z.B., R. Scivoletto and J. Garcia-Leme, Functional changes in the micro-circulation of alloxan-induced diabetic rats, Gen. Pharmacol. 20, 615-620 (1989).

17. Goth, A., W.L. Nash, M. Nagler and J. Holman, Inhibition of histamine release in experimental diabetes, Am. J. Physiol. 191, 25-28 (1957).

18. Adamkiewicz, V.W. and Y. Langlois, Sensitization by insulin to the dextran anaphylactoid reaction, Can. J. Biochem. Physiol. 35, 251-256 (1957).

19. Garcia-Leme, J., L. Hamamura, R.H. Migliorini and M.P. Leite, Influence of *diabetes mellitus* upon the inflammatory response of the rat. A pharmacological analysis, Eur. J. Pharmacol. 23, 74-81 (1973).

20. Garcia-Leme, J., G.M. Böhm, R.H. Migliorini and M.Z.A. Souza, Possible participation of insulin in the control of vascular permeability, Eur. J. Pharmacol. 29, 298-306 (1974).

21. Gamse, R. and G. Jancsó, Reduced neurogenic inflammation in streptozotocin-diabetic rats due to microvascular changes but not to substance P depletion, Eur. J. Pharmacol. 118, 175-180 (1985).

22. Llorach, M.A.S., G.M. Böhm and J. Garcia-Leme, Decreased vascular reaction to permeability factors in experimental diabetes, Br. J. Exp. Pathol. 57, 747-754 (1976).

23. Maca, R.D., G.L. Fry and J.C. Hoack, The effects of glucocorticoids on cultured human endothelial cells, Br. J. Haematol. 38, 501-509 (1978).

24. Mendelsohn, F.A.O., C.J. Lloyd, C. Kachel and J.W. Funder, Induction by glucocorticoids of angiotensin converting enzyme production from bovine endothelial cells in culture and rat lung in vivo, J. Clin. Invest. 70, 684-692 (1982).

25. Levin, E.G. and D.J. Loskutoff, Regulation of plasminogen activator production by cultured endothelial cells, Ann. N.Y. Acad. Sci. 401, 184-194 (1982).

26. Lang, W.E., Glucocorticoids inhibit plasminogen activator production by endothelial cells, Thromb. Haemost. 50, 888-892 (1983).

27. Crutchley, D.J., U.S. Ryan and J.W. Ryan, Glucocorticoid modulation of prostacyclin production in cultured bovine pulmonary endothelial cells, J. Pharmacol. Exp. Ther. 233, 650-655 (1985).

28. Garcia-Leme, J. and D.L. Wilhelm, The effects of adrenalectomy and corticosterone on vascular permeability responses in the skin of the rat, Br. J. Exp. Pathol. 56, 402-407 (1975).

29. P. Davies, P.J. Bailey, M.M. Goldenberg and A.W. Ford-Hutchinson, The role of arachidonic acid oxygenation products in pain and inflammation, Ann. Rev. Immunol. 2, 335-357 (1984).

30. Smith, W.L., Prostaglandin biosynthesis and its compartmentation in vascular smooth muscle and endothelial cells, Ann. Rev. Physiol. 48, 251-262 (1986).

31. Snyder, F., Biochemistry of platelet-activating factor: a unique class of biologically active phospholipids, Proc. Soc. Exp. Biol. Med. 190, 125-135 (1989).

32. Flower, R.J., The mediators of steroid action, Nature (London) 320, 20 (1986).

33. Melby, J., R. Egdahl and W. Spink, Secretion and metabolism of cortisol after injection of endotoxin, J. Lab. Clin. Med. 56, 50-62 (1960).

34. Moberg, G.P., Site of action of endotoxins on hypothalamic-pituitary-adrenal axis, Am. J. Physiol. 220, 397-400 (1971).

35. Garcia-Leme, J. and E.E.S. Schapoval, Stimulation of the hypothalamic-pituitary-adrenal axis by compounds formed in inflamed tissue, Br. J. Pharmacol. 53, 75-83 (1975).

36. Moraes, F.R. and J. Garcia-Leme, Endogenous corticosteroids and insulin in acute inflammation, Microvasc. Res. 23, 281-293 (1982).

37. Stenberg, V.I., M.G. Bouley, B.M. Katz, K.J. Lee and S.S. Parmar, Negative endocrine control system for inflammation in rats, Agents Actions 29, 189-195 (1990).

38. Sternberg, E.M., J.M. Hill, G.P. Chrousos, T. Kamilaris, S.J. Listwak, P.W. Gold and R.L. Wilder, Inflammatory mediator-induced hypothalamic-pituitary-adrenal axis activation is defective in streptococcal cell wall arthritis- susceptible Lewis rats, Proc. Natl. Acad. Sci. USA 86, 2374-2378 (1989).

39. Garcia-Leme, J., L. Hamamura, M.P. Leite and M. Rocha e Silva, Pharmacological analysis of the acute inflammatory process induced in the rat's paw by local injection of carrageenin and by heating, Br. J. Pharmacol. 48, 88-96 (1973).

40. Zanin, M.T. and S.H. Ferreira, Relationship between oedema and plasma exudation in rat paw carrageenin inflammation, Agents Actions 8, 606-609 (1978).

41. Casley-Smith, J.R. and J. Window, Quantitative morphological correlations in capillary permeability following histamine and moderate burning, in the mouse diaphragm and the effects of benzopyrones, Microvasc. Res. 11, 279-305 (1976).

42. Gavin, J.R., J. Roth, P. Jen and P. Freychet, Insulin receptors in human circulating cells and fibroblasts, Proc. Natl. Acad. Sci. USA 69, 747-751 (1972).

43. Fussganger, R.D., C.R. Kahn, J. Roth and P. De Meyts, Binding and degradation of insulin by human peripheral granulocytes. Demonstration of specific receptors with high affinity, J. Biol. Chem. 251, 2761-2769 (1976).

44. Krug, U., F. Krug and P. Cuatrecasas, Emergence of insulin receptors on human lymphocytes during in vitro transformation, Proc. Natl. Acad. Sci. USA 69, 2604-2608 (1972).

45. Olefsky, J. and G.M. Reaven, The human lymphocyte: a model for the study of insulin-receptor interaction, J. Clin. Endocrinol. Metab. 38, 554-560 (1974).

46. Gavin, J.R., D.N. Buell and J. Roth, Water-soluble insulin receptors from human lymphocytes, Science 178, 168-169 (1972).

47. Mowat, A.G. and J. Baum, Chemotaxis of polymorphonuclear leukocytes from patients with *diabetes mellitus*, N. Engl. J. Med. 284, 621-624 (1971).

48. Miller, M.E. and L. Baker, Leukocyte functions in juvenile *diabetes mellitus:* humoral and cellular aspects, J. Pediatr. 81, 979-982 (1972).

49. Hill, H.R., H.S. Sauls, J.L. Dettloff and P.G. Quie, Impaired leukocyte responsiveness in patients with juvenile *diabetes mellitus*, Clin. Immunol. Immunopathol. 2, 395-403 (1974).

50. Mohandes, A.E., J.L. Touraine, M. Osman and B. Salle, Neutrophil chemotaxis in infants of diabetic mothers and in preterms at birth, J. Clin. Lab. Immunol. 8, 117-120 (1982).

51. Pereira, M.A.A., P. Sannomiya and J. Garcia-Leme, Inhibition of leukocyte chemotaxis by factor in alloxan-induced diabetic rat plasma, Diabetes 36, 1307-1314 (1987).

52. Sannomiya, P., M.A.A. Pereira and J. Garcia-Leme, Inhibition of leukocyte chemotaxis by serum factor in *diabetes mellitus:* selective depression of cell responses mediated by complement-derived chemoattractants, Agents Actions 30, 369-376 (1990).

53. Kontras, S.B. and M.T. Bodenbender, Studies of the inflammatory cycle in juvenile diabetes, Am. J. Dis. Child. 116, 130-134 (1968).

54. Perillie, P.E., J.P. Nolan and S.C. Finch, Studies of the resistance to infection in *diabetes mellitus:* local exudative cellular response, J. Lab. Clin. Med. 59, 1008-1015 (1962).

55. Wertman, K.F. and M.R. Henney, The effects of alloxan diabetes on phagocytosis and susceptibility to infection, J. Immunol. 89, 314-317 (1962).

56. Drachman, R.H., R.K. Root and W.B. Wood Jr., Studies on the effect of experimental nonketotic *diabetes mellitus* on antibacterial defence. I. Demonstration of a defect in phagocytosis, J. Exp. Med. 124, 227-240 (1966).

57. Tan, J.S., J.L. Anderson, C. Watanakunakorn and J.P. Phair, Neutrophil dysfunction in *diabetes mellitus*, J. Lab. Clin. Med. 85, 26-33 (1975).

58. Bagdade, J.D., Phagocytic and microbicidal function in *diabetes mellitus*, Acta Endocrinol. 83 (Suppl. 205), 27-34 (1976).

59. Edelson, P.J. and Z.A. Cohn, Effects of conconavalin-A on mouse peritoneal macrophages. I. Stimulation of endocytic activity and inhibition of phagolysosome formation, J. Exp. Med. 140, 1364-1386 (1974).

60. Bagasra, O., A. Howeedy and A.K. Balla, Macrophage function in chronic experimental alcoholism. I. Modulation of surface receptors and phagocytosis, Immunology 65, 405-409 (1988).

61. Ptak, W., M. Hanczakowska, R. Rozycka and D. Rozycka, Impaired antibody responses in alloxan diabetic mice, Clin. Exp. Immunol. 29, 140-146 (1977).

62. MacCuish, A.C., S.J. Urbaniak, C.J. Campbell, J.J.P. Duncan and W. J. Irvine, Phytohaemagglutinin transformation and circulating lymphocyte subpopulations in insulin-dependent diabetic patients, Diabetes 23, 708-712 (1974).

63. Zier, K.S., M.R. Leo, R.S. Spielman and L. Baker, Decreased synthesis of interleukin-2 (IL-2) in insulin-dependent *diabetes mellitus*, Diabetes 33, 552-555 (1984).

64. Besedovsky, H.O., E. Sorkin, M. Keller and J. Muller, Changes in blood hormone levels during the immune response, Proc. Soc. Exp. Biol. Med. 150, 466-470 (1975).

65. Flower, R.J., L. Parente, P. Persico and J.A. Salmon, A comparison of the acute inflammatory response in adrenalectomized and sham-operated rats, Br. J. Pharmacol. 87, 57-62 (1986).

66. Atherton, A. and G.V.R. Born, Quantitative investigations of the adhesiveness of circulating polymorphonuclear leukocytes to blood vessel walls, J. Physiol. 222, 447-474 (1972).

67. Flower, R.J., Background and discovery of lipocortins, Agents Actions 17, 255-262 (1985).

68. Davidson, F.F. and E.A. Dennis, Biological relevance of lipocortins and related proteins as inhibitors of phospholipase A_2, Biochem. Pharmacol. 38, 3645-3651 (1989).

69. Whitehouse, B.J., Lipocortins, mediators of the anti-inflammatory action of corticosteroids?, J. Endocrinol. 123, 363-366 (1989).

AAS 36
Contributions to
Autacoid Pharmacology

FROM HISTAMINE TO IR-GENES TO THE IDIOTYPIC NETWORK

N.M. Vaz

Departament of Biochemistry and Immunology, Institute of Biological Sciences, Federal University of Minas Gerais, 31270 Belo Horizonte, MG, Brazil

Scope

In this tribute to Mauricio Rocha e Silva, I would like to sketch the pathway I have followed in science, starting in the laboratory of one of his dearest friends, Haity Moussatché, to whom I owe my initial and most valuable insights into the nature of science and scientific activity. In those early years of acquaintance with physiology in his laboratory, the ideas of Rocha e Silva were often present. So, I am very honored to submit my personal contribution to this event.

It turned out that this pathway lead me into immunology, and away from physiology and pharmacology. Thus, my work had little to do with Rocha e Silva's ideas – except for the essential first steps.

From Histamine to Ir Genes

When I first arrived at Dr. Moutssaché's laboratory, in 1959, he was interested in the relationships between cellular metabolism and the release of histamine from guinea pig lung slices during *in vitro* anaphylaxis. Experiments were conducted in a huge Warburg apparatus, to determine oxygen consumption during the anaphylactic reaction. The histamine released from the slices was assayed in the guinea pig ileum preparation. Before the experiment was actually performed, Schultz-Dale reactions were triggered in ileum fragments to assess the magnitude of anaphylactic sensitization of the particular guinea pig used that day. Guinea pigs were actively sensitized by previous injections of horse serum.

I became immediately puzzled by the phenomenon of anapylaxis itself, and especially, by its immunological aspects. There was very little work in immunology going on in Brazil at that time, and my first incursions in its terrain were done with Moussatché himself, studying the Schultz-Dale reaction in the guinea pig ileum preparations. We found that after the reaction was triggered, the ileum underwent a transient period of depression in its responsiveness to various agonists, including histamine. My first published observations described these experiments[(1)].

Anaphylactic reactions, as damaging as they may be to the organism in which they are triggered, are ratifications of individuality. And that was what interested me the most: *what is individuality?* Immunology seemed to be a door for that question.

I spent a short time in Antonio Oliveira Lima's laboratory, which was about the only place where experiments in basic immunology were performed in Rio at that time. I also made a short trip to Otto Bier's laboratory in São Paulo, but I was not interested in the problems they were tackling at the moment. I preferred working in anaphylaxis, and I soon returned to Rio.

In Oliveira Lima's laboratory, I met the laboratory mouse for the first time. Immunologists in the fifties and the sixties used to work with rabbits and guinea pigs, not mice. Lima's laboratory, at the Santa Casa de Misericórdia, was small and crowded. He raised a few mice in round, cute, glass cages. They looked like pets, rather than experimental animals, but I started to work with mice then.

In 1963, mice were not supposed to undergo anaphylaxis, because they were considered insensitive to histamine. With Junia Peixoto, I developed standard methods of anaphylactic sensitization of Swiss mice, using crystallized ovalbumin as an antigen, and calcium phosphate as an adjuvant[(2)]. That was great progress over the erratic sensitization of guinea pigs to horse serum. With Ezio Iff and Junia Peixoto, we showed that massive amounts of histamine were released to the blood of mice undergoing anaphylaxis[(3)], and that mixtures of histamine and serotonin were highly toxic and mimicked symptoms of anaphylaxis in mice[(4)]. In Moussatché's laboratory, Annie Danon had started to work with rat mast cells, which Ivan Mota had shown to be the source of the histamine released during anaphylactic phenomena. We did a few experiments together, using mouse mast cells instead of rat mast cells, and demonstrated that mice had two kinds of anaphylactic antibodies: one that stuck very firmly to mast cells, another that could be very easily washed off. Today we know that they correspond to the IgE and IgG1 isotypes[(5)].

I worked for 6 years in Moussatché's laboratory. In Europe, and in the United States, immunology was becoming an independent branch of experimental biology. In Rio, I lived across Guanabara Bay, in Niteroi, and I used to take the Journal of Immunology with me to read in the ferry boat. Everything was happening in those years. Immunoglobulins were characterized by different isotypes, their biological properties were being defined. Plasma cells were identified as the source of antibodies, and lymphocytes were clearly involved in immune responsiveness. I read all this in silence; nobody I knew could share my enthusiasm, except when I went, every morning, to Moussatché's office, under a stairway, and he would ask: "So...?" And we would talk for hours.

These were the early sixties. Brazil was in a political turmoil. The University of Brasilia was being built, and many young scientist were attracted by the new educational projects. I was supposed to organize a laboratory of immunology in Brasilia for Victor and Ruth Nussenzweig, who would soon return from New York. But this was 1964, the year of the military coup d'etat.

In 1965, I moved to Brasilia, but soon was compelled to resign together with dozens of other professors and scientists. Instead of receiving the Nussenzweigs in Brasilia, I was invited by Victor Nussenzweig to join the Department of Pathology of NYU, in New York.

At NYU, Baruj Benecerraf, and his coworkers were building what was to become the foundations of cellular immunology. In that Department, I met many investigators which in the next few years were to become quite famous in immunology. I joined Zoltan Ovary's laboratory. Zoltan, who is still alive and well, working at NYU, is a very peculiar character, extremely clever in using his method of passive cutaneous anaphylaxis (PCA) in guinea pigs in a variety of basic immunological problems. My skills in working with mice and mast cells and the evidence I had for the existence of two kinds of sensitizing antibodies were very welcome in his lab, and we did quite a few things together(5).

I was very unhappy in New York as I missed Brazil very much, and after two years I returned to Rio. Our laboratory in Manguinhos had been virtually destroyed by political repression. Moussatché was not even allowed to enter the library of the Institute. Thus, Rio was worse than New York, and soon I returned to New York.

But before I returned, I met Thales Torres at the Cancer Institute in Rio, and he introduced me to inbred mice and the problems of immunogenetics of transplantation. He taught me about the H-2 system, and congenic-resistant mice for the first time. I decided I would use only inbred mice in my experiments from then on.

Ir Genes

I returned to NYU, invited by Bernard Levine to work on the production of IgE in mice. The main problem with the induction of IgE formation in experimental animals at that time was its weakness and transience. On the other hand, human allergic symptoms often are based on the persistent formation of high titers of specific IgE antibodies. Where was the trick to reproduce this vigorous, persistent synthesis of IgE in animals? How could laboratory animals be made truly allergic? An efficient animal model of allergy would be extremely useful.

Levine and I started a huge experiment with inbred mice. We reasoned that humans become allergic by breathing or contacting very small amounts of allergenic materials. We also knew that there is a familial tendency in allergy, suggesting the operation of genetic factors. Thus, we started this huge experiment with several inbread strains of mice and several different antigens, which we injected in very low doses at monthly intervals. At that time, animals were immunized with milligram amounts of antigen. We were using thousand-fold lower doses.

I tested the production of IgE with the methods I had developed to work on mouse anaphylaxis. Levine used a sensitive hemagglutination method he had developed for penicillin-derived haptens. Nothing happened for a while, and we entertained the thought that the huge experiment had been simply a huge failure. But, then, some strains of mice started to make IgE antibodies for some antigens. Others remained totally unresponsive. The IgE responses, to our delight, were not the transient peaks obtained after the injection of higher doses of antigen, but the persistent pattern of IgE formation found in allergic human patients. The experiments were showing us exactly what we expected: the persistent synthesis of IgE antibodies resulted from repeated contact with small doses of antigen; only individuals with certain genetic characteristics would respond under these conditions. This explained the familial tendency of allergy(6). But, obviously, there was more to it. The total amounts of antibodies formed, not only the IgE antibodies, followed the same patterns. Mice either formed progressive amounts of antibodies at each repeated contact with a low dose, or did not respond at all.

A few years before, Levine and Benacerraf had characterized the Poly-L-lysine (PLL) gene in the guinea pig(7). There are two inbred strains of guinea pig; one of them can be immunized to linear polymers of L-lysine, and the other cannot. Crossings and backcrossing between these animals revealed that the ability to respond to PLL is under control of a single, autosomal, dominant gene. The gene was called an immune-responsiveness gene, or ir-gene. Victor Nussenzweig called my attention to experiments that Hugh MacDevitt and co-workers were doing in Stanford. They had characterized an ir-gene in mice, which controlled the response to branched synthetic polymers of aminoacids. By chance, they included in the experiments a pair of mouse strains that comprise a congenic-pair, strains that differ only by the H-2 complex. One of these strains responded well to one of his polymers, the other strain did not. Crosses and backcrosses between the strains, characterized an ir-gene[8]. In summary, ir-genes had been recently discovered in the control of immune responses of guinea pigs and mice to synthetic polypeptides, but their significance remained unknown.

When I looked at our huge experiment, and tried to match characteristics of the strains with their responsiveness to some of the antigens, I found a hint that the H-2 complex might be involved. I ordered several mouse strains selected by their H-2 type from the Jackson Laboratory, and included in this panel several congenic-resistant pairs of strains. The results were sharp and clear: the H-2 type controlled the pattern of immune responsiveness of the strains to repeated low doses of protein antigens. Crosses and backcrosses revealed that also here, there was a single autosomal dominant gene controlling immune responsiveness, and that this gene was linked to the H-2 complex. Something fundamental at H-2 had to do with the control of all types of immune responses[9,10].

My feelings about the importance of individuality were being substantiated in unexpected ways. Genes coding for transplantation antigens were important for immune responsiveness. Ir-genes were soon involved in the key problems of cellular immunology. "MHC-restriction" was discovered[11,12]. Vertebrate organisms interact with materials from their environment using not only immunoglobulins and T-cell receptors, but also products of the genes at the MHC. And the MHC was somehow involved in the ratification of their individuality.

Meanwhile, I was again becoming very unhappy about being in New York. So I returned to Rio in 1970, and applied for a professorship in immunology in my home town, Niteroi. I brought to Brazil several inbred strains of mice. Thales Torres joined us in Niteroi to organize the animal houses, and we managed to do some experiments. But it was very hard to work, and soon I was again longing to return to the States.

This time I went to Denver, invited by Kimishige Ishizaka to head the immunology unit at the Childrens's Asthma Research Institute and Hospital (CARIH). At CARIH, I met Donald Hanson, then a young experimental psychologist, who wanted to work with me. And that was going to change my whole career.

Oral Tolerance

As an experimental psychologist, Don Hanson was familiar with the drinking habits of experimental animals. We planned to investigate whether mice which were made allergic to ovalbumin (Ova) would still drink from a bottle containing a dilute Ova solution, although they had access to Ova-free water.

Don used the trick of adding saccharin, as a marker taste, to the Ova solution. Laboratory mice eagerly drink saccharin solutions and, thus, these mice ingested a lot of Ova. On the other hand, mice which had been made allergic (low dose immunized) to Ova, avoided drinking Ova, despite the presence of saccharin. There was a stark contrast between the behaviour of the two groups of animals. We were very happy with these results.

But then, in a control group of mice, Don made an observation which made me forget this and everything else. He found that mice which drank Ova and subsequently were intraperitoneally immunized with Ova in adjuvant, totally failed to make circulating anti-Ova antibodies. They had become immunologically tolerant. The ingestion of a protein, as in normal feeding, was blocking the development of specific immune responses to it[(13,14)]. This simply failed to fit everything else I knew about immunology. I was perplexed.

However, the phenomenon of "oral tolerance" was not new in immunology. Actually, it is the oldest recorded information of an immunologic intervention performed with the specific intention of preventing allergic dermatitis. In 1826, Dakin published his observations on the life of North American Indians. Indian children were given an extract of poison ivy to drink when very young, to avoid the development of contact dermatitis by subsequent contacts with this sensitizing plant. Louis Pasteur was six years old when this was published. And there were many other findings in the early and the recent literature describing oral tolerance[(15)]. I, myself, "knew" it. I was simply not aware of it.

When I became aware of it, my interpretation of virtually all the basic problems of immunology changed. But nobody I knew saw it the way I did. Even today, when "mucosal immunology" has become very fashionable, oral tolerance is as yet seen as a way to control the magnitude of specific immune responses initiated through the gut and other mucosal surfaces[(15)]. And that is not the way I see it.

To tell you the way I see it, I will have to tell you about some parallel developments. This was 1977. In Denver, I had met a bright young Chilean neurobiologist, Francisco Varela, who kept talking about "self-referential systems". I became progressively more interested in what he said.

From Ir Genes to the Idiotypic Network

In 1974, three years before my encounter with oral tolerance and Francisco Varela, Niels Jerne had published a theoretical paper describing the immune system as a complex network of molecular and cellular interactions[(16)]. That paper came to be very important in immunology.

Lymphocytes differ from all other cell types, because they "invent" the genes they use for coding their most important molecular products: their clonal receptors. By special processes of gene rearrangement, B lymphocytes "invent" the genes that code for the variable regions of the immunoglobulin molecules; T lymphocytes to the same with the variable regions of Ti receptors. Each lymphocyte generates their most important receptors *somatically*, each lymphocyte is unique, each is a clone.

The survival of emergent lymphocytes depends on whether their clonal receptors allow them to engage in cellular interactions in which essential growth factors are produced (interleukins). Therefore, the invention of clonal receptors is equivalent to the invention of new lines of lymphocytes.

Niels Jerne was the first to realize that, sooner or later, immunologists would have to tackle the problem of organizing the activities of all those "invented" cell types into a coherent whole, to constitute the immune system. He then proposed that the connections among lymphocytes were made exactly through determinants on the molecules which made each one of them unique. He called these determinants *idiotopes* and his theory became known as the idiotypic network theory[(16)].

To tell you how I blended the ideas of Niels Jerne on idiotypic networks with those of Francisco Varela on self-referential systems, would take longer than we can afford here. I would rather refer you to a paper I published with Varela, in 1978[(17)]. But I want to tell you how this solved the enigma of oral tolerance, and explain what is an organism-centered approach to immunology, as opposed to the traditional antigen-centered approach.

My contention is that antigen-centered views confound *domains of description* of immunological events. I will illustrate this with a very simple example which, nevertheless, may have profound consequences in our notions about what is the immune system and what are immunological events. What I will say now derives directly from Humberto Maturana's ideas on the organization of living systems. Maturana had been Varela's teacher, in Chile, a few years before[(18-22)].

When human blood is "typed" – i.e., classified preceding blood transfusions, an anti-A serum is used to detect the presence of the "A-antigen" on red cells by agglutination.

When exposed to the anti-A serum, A^+ cells (A, AB) agglutinate and A^- cells (B,O) fail to agglutinate. The procedure is rather specific, as it must be, if transfusion accidents are to be avoided.

The test is specific. However, the anti-A serum is *not* specific for A^+ red cells; tested with a variety of other materials, ranging from bacteria, to plant extracts, to pollen grains, it may show positive reactions. The same serum which reacts with A^+ cells, also reacts with many unrelated materials.

These "cross-reactions" occur because: a) there are similar epitopes in these "unrelated" materials; and b) there is a multitude of different "specific" antibodies in the serum. The same antibody reacts with multiple polysacharide epitopes, and many different antibodies react with the same epitope with varying degrees of binding affinity.

The anti-A test is specific, but anti-A antibodies are not. They are used *as if* they were specific. The operations performed by immunologists during blood typing, and many other procedures, restrict which antibodies may react and thus are, or may be, highly specific. We are then seduced to believe that antibodies play specific roles *as components of the immune system*. Whenever we do this, we confound the operation of immunologists with the operations of immune systems. We confound *domains of description* of immunological phenomena.

We have the option to describe immunoglobulins as specific antibodies. We have also the option to describe immunoglobulins as components of the immune system. The specificity of immunoglobulins as antibodies (e.g., as reagents in immunological tests) is created by the conditions (restrictions) in which the tests are made; tested outside these conditions, immunoglobulins are no longer specific, and may react with many other materials. Under natural circumstances, immunoglobulins occur under conditions (restrictions) determined by the organization of living vertebrate organisms. These conditions are very different from those prevailing during the performance of serological tests. However, because we see immunoglobulins playing the role of specific antibodies (reagents) in these tests, we are led to believe that immunoglobulins play specific roles in the organism that produced them.

This is a difficult point to grasp because basic immunologists claim to be describing the inner workings of the immune system. However, if these descriptions are based on the belief that immunological phenomena are specific, they are confounding domains of description.

The Operational Closure of the Immune System

The immune system may be defined as a closed network of production of cellular and molecular components in which relative states of lymphocyte activation can only lead to other relative states of lymphocyte activation. This definition of the immune system is a literal transcription of the definition of the nervous system as a closed network of neuronal relations, as proposed by Maturana[18].

As a closed network of lymphocyte relations, the immune system is totally unable to discriminate between "self" and "nonself" materials, unable to discriminate between the "inside" and the "outside" of the organism. We, as observers of immune systems, positioned externally to the immune system, can easily make these distinctions. But the immune system cannot make them. To the system, there are only materials which can, or cannot interact with its components and trigger changes in the relative states of lymphocyte activation. Both "self" and "nonself" materials include elements of both categories. Plastics and synthetic polymers of d-aminoacids are examples of immunologically inert "foreign" materials; immunoglobulins, themselves, are examples of "self" components which are efficient in triggering changes in lymphocyte activation.

Self/nonself discrimination is indispensable in traditional immunology because healthy organisms seen to be unable to undertake immune responses against their own components, whereas they seem to respond vigorously to foreign elements. Specific immune responses, however, belong to our domain of operations as observers of immune systems, not to the domain of operations of immune systems. The specificity of immune responses, as assayed in immunological tests, is created by the conditions (restrictions) in which these tests are made. All these tests utilize the specific antigen (or idiotype) to assess the magnitude of the immune response. Assessed outside these conditions – i.e., *without* the specific antigen – "immune responses", as a consequence of events conducting to an increase in the concentration of immunoglobulins, or activated lymphocytes, are no longer specific. For example, injections of an antigen usually trigger the activation of many more lymphocytes than those specifically reactive with the antigen[23] – and probably trigger the inhibition of many others[24].

In an organism-centered perspective, the perturbation caused by penetration of antigen molecules is compensated by changes in the whole structure of the immune system in order to preserve its organization as a self-regenerating network of cellular and molecular relations[17,25]. The perturbations triggered by antigens are not qualitatively different from those continuously generated by the internal dynamics of the immune system itself. Thus, from the point of view of the system itself, what happens after the penetration of an antigen is not qualitatively different from what was happening before its penetration. There are no specific events in the life of immune system. Specificity lies in the operations of immunologists as observers of immune systems.

Oral Tolerance in the Idiotypic Network

After the induction of oral tolerance, for example, to ovalbumin (Ova)[26,27], mice:
a) fail to form specific anti-Ova antibodies upon injection of Ova plus adjuvants by parenteral routes;
b) show only background levels of lymphocyte blast transformation upon in vitro exposure to Ova;
c) clear Ova from plasma at normal or slower than normal rates.

These, and other related observations, show that oral tolerant mice behave *as if* they were unreactive to Ova. Therefore, these animals should have very few Ova-reactive lymphocytes. That this is not the case is demonstrated by several observations:
a) exposed to B-lymphocyte mitogens, oral tolerant mice form higher than normal levels of anti-Ova antibodies[28];
b) in limiting dilution assays, the spleens of oral tolerant mice show higher frequencies of Ova-specific precursors of antibody forming cells than normal mice[29];
c) the concomitant injection of Ova may inhibit the initiation of immune responses to an unrelated antigen in Ova-tolerant mice, but not in normal mice[30];
d) the induction of oral tolerance to Ova may trigger a significant increase in the total number of immunoglobulin-secreting cells in the spleen[31,32].

These and other observations demonstrate that oral tolerant mice have normal, or higher than normal, numbers of precursors of Ova-reactive cells, but these cells fail to undergo clonal expansion upon immunization with Ova. A similar situation exists concerning lymphocytes reactive with self-components[33-36]. Oral tolerance and self-tolerance are maintained by similar mechanisms and are dependent on global properties of the idiotypic network.

Natural Immunity by Self-Copying

When Niels Bohr proposed his modification for Rutherford's model of the atom, he stated that electrons spinning around the nucleus did not dissipate energy. This statement was contrary to the laws of electromagnetism. In a way, Bohr was saying "This should be so, but it is not so"[37]. When Niels Jerne proposed the idiotypic network theory[16], he also contradicted the fundamental tenets of traditional immunology[*]. The contradiction stems from the fact that lymphocytes cannot discriminate between idiotopes on other lymphocytes and epitopes on foreign molecules and, thus, the immune system cannot discriminate between self and nonself. Actually, Jerne proposed that the immune system reacts with foreign epitopes *because* it was previously reacting with immunoglobulin idiotopes which mimic these epitopes; in Jerne's nomenclature, these idiotopes are *internal images* of the epitopes[16].

Because it reacts with its own components – and components of the organism, and is able to "copy" these components in immunoglobulin idiotopes – i.e., make internal images of them – the immune system may protect the organism from the invasion of foreign materials, including virus and microorganisms. This protection is not based on the prediction of what each of these invading materials will look like. It is based of the premise that the invading materials will initially bind to plasma membrane of body cells. This is known to occur in infections by viruses and bacteria. For example, certain viruses use molecules of MHC products as their cellular "receptors"[38]; the HIV bind to CD4 molecules on T cells[39]; many bacteria adhere to cell membranes by specialized pilli[40]. Furthermore, in the mouse, there is direct evidence that "major" idiotopes in immunoglobulins may be internal images of MHC products[41]. If immunoglobulin idiotopes mimick epitopes present on the cell membrane and these membrane epitopes are "receptors" for invading materials, then these immunoglobulins play a natural protective role, because the invading materials will bind to them before they bind to the cell membranes.

This same internal copying mechanism may be important in the prevention of auto-immune diseases. There is now ample evidence that normal organisms produce immunoglobulins that react with other components of the organism[42]. Disease results from an imbalance in the network of interactions among antibodies[43], not from the simple presence of "forbidden" types of auto-antibodies[44].

An important recent development in clinical immunology has been the use of intravenous injections of large doses of normal immunoglobulins in the treatment of many auto-immune diseases. There is evidence that the restoration of health achieved with this

(*) I am not sure whether Jerne really intended to do this or not because, in subsequent papers, he made statements that neutralized this radical interpretation of his original statements. For example, he asked whether all immunoglobulins belonged to the idiotypic network[26]. If you see the immune system as an idiotypic network you do not raise issues like this one.

therapy depends on idiotypes which permit the articulation of healthy patterns of lymphocyte connections[45,46].

In schistosomiasis[47] and in Chagas' disease[48] severe clinical forms are associated with the presence of certain idiotypes and certain patterns of T-lymphocyte stimulation. "Healthy" carriers of these infections, therefore, are characterized by certain patterns of network organization. Disease is not "caused" by invading virus and parasites; in many instances, these invaders may be accommodated in the organism without major ill effects. Disease occurs when there are failures in the harmonic flux of body processes, when there are troubles with the reassertment of individuality.

References

1. Vaz, N.M. and H. Moussatché, Observações preliminares sobre fenômenos depressivos de natureza reversível desencadeados na fibra muscular lisa pela reação de Schultz-Dale, An. Acad. Bras. Cj.33, 83 (abstr.) (1961).

2. Vaz, N.M. and J.M. Peixoto, Gellified suspensions of tricalcium phosphate as adjuvants in the sensitization of the mouse, An. Acad. Bras. Cj.35, 139-144 (1963).

3. Vaz, N.M., E.T. Iff and J.M. Peixoto, Histamine release in vivo during anaphylaxis in the mouse, Int. Arch. Allergy 30, 268-280 (1966).

4. Vaz, N.M. and E.T. Iff, Mechanisms of anaphylaxis in the mouse. Similarity of shock induced by anaphylaxis and by mixtures of histamine and serotonin, Int. Arch. Allergy 30, 313-322 (1966).

5. Vaz, N.M., Anaphylactic sensitization of mouse tissues with IgG1 and reaginic antibodies, In: Biochemistry of the Acute Allergic Reactions, pp. 91-109 (Eds. K.F. Austen and E.L. Becker), Blackwell, Oxford 1971.

6. Levine, B.B. and N.M. Vaz, Effect of combinations of inbred strain, antigen and antigen doses on immune responsiveness and reagin production in the mouse, Int. Arch. Allergy 39, 156-171 (1970).

7. Benacerraf, B. and H.O. McDevitt, Histocompatibility-linked-immune-response genes, Science 175, 273-279 (1972) PLL.

8. McDevitt, H.O. and B. Benacerraf, Genetic control of immuneresponsiveness, Adv. Immunol. 11, 31-74 (1969).

9. Vaz, N.M. and B.B. Levine, Immune responsiveness of mice to low doses of antigen. Relationship to histocompatibility (H-2) type, Science 168, 852-854 (1970).

10. Vaz, N.M., J.M. Phillips-Quagliatta, B.B. Levine and E.M. Vaz, H-2 linked genetic control of immune responsiveness to ovalbumin and ovomucoid, J. Exp. Med. 134, 1335-1348 (1971).

11. Kindred, B. and D.C. Shreffler, H-2 dependence of cooperation between B and T cells in vivo, J. Immunol. 109, 940-943 (1972).

12. Lorenz, R.G. and P.M. Allen, Processing and presentation of self-proteins, Immunol. Rev. 106, 115-127 (1988).

13. Mowat, A. Mcl., The regulation of immune responses to dietary protein antigens, Immunology Today 8, 93-98 (1987).

14. Vaz, N.M., L.C.S. Maia, D.H. Hanson and J.M. Lynch, Inhibition of homocytotropic antibody responses in adult inbred mice by previous feeding of the specific antigen, J. Allergy Clin. Immunol. 60, 110-115 (1977).

15. Vaz, N.M., Immunological tolerance and dogma, Medical Hypotheses 5, 1037-1043 (1979).

16. Jerne, N.K., Towards a network theory of the immune system, Ann. Immunol. (Paris) 125C, 373-389 (1978).

17. Vaz, N.M. and F.J. Varela, Self and nonsense: an organism-centered approach to immunology, Medical Hypotheses 4, 231-258 (1978).

18. Maturana, H.R., Biology of Cognition, reprinted in Autopoiesis and Cognition, Reidel, Dordrecht, 1980, pp.2-58 (1970).

19. Maturana, H.R., The organization of the living. A theory of living organization, J. Man-Machine Studies. 17, 313-332 (1975).

20. Maturana, H.R. and F.J. Varela, Autopoiesis and Cognition. The Realization of the Living, Reidel, Dordrecht 1980.

21. Maturana, H.R. and F.J. Varela, The Tree of Knowledge. Biological Basis of Human Understanding, New Science, Boston 1983.

22. Maturana, H.R., Reality: the search for objectivity or the quest for the cogent argument, Irish. J. Psychology 9, 25-82 (1988).

23. Rosenberg, Y. and J.M. Chiller, Ability of antigen-specific helper cells to effect a class-restricted increase in total Ig-secreting cells in spleen after immunization with the antigen, J. Exp. Med. 150, 517-530 (1979).

24. Lundkvist, I., D. Portnoï and A. Coutinho, Idiotype-specific regulation might contribute to specific unresponsiveness in dextran-primed mice, Res. Immunol. 140, 7-18 (1989).

25. Vaz, N.M. and A.M.C. Faria, Ordem e desordem: uma abordagem imunológica, Ciência e Cultura 40, 452-457 (1988).

26. Richman, L.K., J.M. Chiller, W.M. Brown, D.G. Hanson and N.M. Vaz, Enterically-induced immunological tolerance. I. Induction of suppressor T cells by intragastric administration of soluble proteins, J. Immunol. 122, 2429-2435 (1978).

27. Hanson, D.G., N.M. Vaz, L.C.S. Maia and J.M. Lych, Inhibition of immune responses by feeding proteins antigen. III. Evidence against maintenance of tolerance to ovalbumin by orally-induced antibodies, J. Immunol. 123, 2337-2344 (1979).

28. Titus, R.G. and J.M. Chiller, Orally-induced tolerance. Definition at the cellular level, Int. Arch. Allergy 65, 323-338 (1981).

29. Portnoï, D. and N.M. Vaz, Unpublished observations (1987).

30. Vaz, N.M., L.C.S. Maia and D.G. Hanson, Cross-suppression of specific immune responses after oral tolerance, Mem. Inst. Oswaldo Cruz. 76, 83-91 (1981).

31. Carvalho, C.R. and N.M. Vaz, Immune responses to two unrelated antigens in mice orally-tolerant to one of them, Braz. J. Med. Biol. Res. (1990).

32. Faria, A.M.C., L.M. Lopes, M.A.C. Pereira and N.M. Vaz, A tolerância imunológica adquirida por via oral em camundongos envolve ativação linfocitária inespecífica, IV Reunião Fesbe, Caxambú (Abstr.) (1989).

33. Winchester, G., G.H. Sunshine, N. Nardi and N.A. Mitchinson, Antigen-presenting cells do not discriminate between self and nonself, Immunogenetics 19, 487-495 (1984).

34. Coutinho, A., Tolerance to self as a global behaviour of the immune system based upon the connectivity of auto-reactive lymphocytes, In: The Tolerance Workshop, Vol. 3, pp. 54-74 (Eds. P. Matzinger, M. Flajnik, H.-G. Rammensee, G. Stockinger, T. Polnik, L. Nicklin). Editiones Roche, Basel 1988.

35. Avrameas, S., B. Guilbert, W. Mahana, P. Matsiota, T. Ternynck. Recognition of self and non-self constituents by polyspecific autoreceptors, Inter. Rev. Immunol. 3, 7-18 (1988).

36. Vaz, N.M. e A.M.C. Faria, Imunologia: o externo e o estranho, IDEA 1, 61-70 (Rio de Janeiro) (1989).

37. Moore, R., Niels Bohr: The Man, his Science & the World they Changed. The MIT Press, Cambridge 1985.

38. Inada, T. and C.A. Mims, Mouse Ia antigens are receptors for lactate dehydrogenase virus, Nature P 309, 59-61 (1984).

39. Koff, W.C. and D.F. Hoth, Development and testing of AIDS vaccines, Science 241, 426-432 (1988).

40. Lindley, M., Adhesion of pathogenic microorganisms, Nature 286, 556-557 (1980).

41. Holmberg,D., S. Forsgren, L. Forni, F. Ivars and A. Coutinho, Idiotypic determinants of natural IgM antibodies resemble self Ia antigens, Proc. Natl. Acad. Sci. USA 81, 3175-3179 (1984).

42. Avrameas, S., Natural auto-reactive B cells and auto-antibodies. The know-thyself of the immune system, Ann. Immunol (Paris) 137D, 150-156 (1986).

43. Holmberg, D. and A. Coutinho, High connectivity of natural antibodies and auto-immunity, Immunol. Today 6, 356-357 (1985).

44. Burnet, M.F., Immune Surveillance. Pergamon Press, Oxford 1970.

45. Nydegger, V.E., Y. Sultan, and M.D. Kazatchkine, The concept of anti-idiotypic regulation of selected autoimmune diseases by intravenous immunoglobulins, Clin. Immunol. Immunopathol. 53, S72-S73 (1989).

46. F. Rossi, G. Dietrich and M.D. Kazatchkine, Antiidiotypic suppression of autoantibodies with normal polyspecific immunoglobulins, Res. Immunol. 140, 19-31 (1989).

47. Parra, J.C., M.S. Lima, G. Gazzinelli and D.G. Colley, Immune responses during human schistosomiasis mansoni. XV. Anti-idiotypic T cells can recognize and respond to anti-SEA idiotypes directly, J. Immunol. 140, 2401-2406 (1988).

48. Gazzinelli, R.T., J.C. Parra, R. Correa-Oliveira, J.R. Cançado, R.S. Rocha, G. Gazzinelli and D.G. Colley, Idiotypic anti-idiotypic interactions in schistosomiasis and/or Chagas' disease, Am. J. Trop. Med. Hyg. 39, 288-291 (1988).

I thank José Reinaldo Magalhães for the critical reading of this manuscript.

(Supported by grant CNPq 50.0265/88-7)

AAS 36
Contributions to
Autacoid Pharmacology

MAURICIO ROCHA E SILVA AND THE DISCOVERY OF BRADYKININ

W.T. Beraldo

Department of Physiology and Biophysics, Institute of Biological Sciences, Federal University of Minas Gerais, 30000 Belo Horizonte, MG, Brazil

Mauricio Rocha e Silva was born in Rio de Janeiro on September 19, 1910. In 1933 he obtained his M.D. from the Faculty of Medicine of Rio de Janeiro; in 1934 he moved to São Paulo, where he started his scientific career at the Biological Institute, working with Otto Bier on hemolysis, the photodynamic action of grazing plants, and the role of histamine in inflammation. As a result of these studies, Rocha e Silva clarified the etiology of a photosensitizing disease of cattle caused by a leguminosa (*Holocalyx glaziovii*) that grows in the northwestern region of the state of São Paulo, Brazil.

From 1938 to 1940, he worked on the pharmacology of trypsin in histamine and anaphylactic shock. As a Fellow of the Guggenheim Foundation, he went to Northwestern University Medical School, Chicago, in 1941, where he worked with Dragstedt on pancreatic necrosis, measuring histamine in the blood of dogs. He also studied the effects of histamine and proteolytic enzymes on capillary permeability. In 1941 he spent some time at the Mayo Clinic in Rochester, where he worked with C.F. Code studying changes in histamine content in rabbit blood, under the action of different venoms.

When his Guggenheim Fellowship was extended, he went to New York to work with M. Bergmann at the Rockefeller Institute. At the time, Rocha e Silva strongly believed that trypsin could displace histamine from its binding sites in liver and lung cells. He hoped to set up an experimental model where histamine would be artificially combined with proteins; and which would respond to the action of trypsin, freeing histamine.

Upon his return in 1942, the Biological Institute in São Paulo under the direction of H. Rocha Lima was undergoing its "golden" period. As head of the Section of Biochemistry and Pharmacodynamics, Rocha e Silva had the opportunity to train several promising young scientists. Among them was a very intelligent young chemist, Silvia Andrade, which trained by him in the techniques of protein chemistry acquired at the Rockefeller Institute, was the first person to use paper chromatography in Brazil. Another young scientist working in his laboratory, Alfonso Grana from Uruguay, was interested in studying vascular shock produced by the fluid of tapeworm larvae. An extensive study of this type of allergic shock was developed.

In 1946, as a British Council Fellow, Rocha e Silva spent the summer in Toronto working with L.B. Jaques, who had become interested in Mauricio's studies on the activation of the fibrinolytic system during peptone and anaphylactic shock. Using siliconized glassware to prevent blood clotting, they showed that large amounts of histamine were released either when the liver of sensitized dogs was perfused with antigen, or when the liver of normal dogs was perfused with peptone. This showed that whole blood participates in histamine release in dog liver during peptone or anaphylactic shock.

In 1947, Rocha e Silva worked with C. Rimington at University College of London on the preparation of the fibrinolytic enzyme of plasma; with H.O. Schild in the Department of Pharmacology of the College he studied quantitative aspects of agonist and antagonist action using the pA2 scale to classify antagonists according to their potency. Through Schild, Rocha e Silva met many reputed pharmacologists of Dale's school, like G.L. Brown, J.H. Gaddum, W. Feldberg, J.H. Burn, Edith Bulbring. Such contacts strengthened his belief on the value of biossay to tackle problems that could not be solved by purely biochemical means. This concept was of great help in studies on active polypeptides derived from blood; its importance was soon to be demonstrated by the discovery of bradykinin. When Rocha e Silva returned to Brazil, I had the privilege of collaborating with him at the Biological Institute of São Paulo, in a study of antihistamine actions on smooth muscle preparations.

The discovery of bradykinin was made on a day in 1948, when Dr. G. Rosenfeld of the Butantan Institute of São Paulo brought a sample of venom from *Bothrops jararaca*, an extremely poisonous pit viper found only in South America, to Rocha e Silva's laboratory, asking for a study of the mechanism of the vascular shock produced by this venom in dogs. We tested the blood of the shocked animals on the isolated guinea pig gut expecting a contraction due to histamine, because Feldberg and Kellaway[1] had shown that venoms of many Australian and Indian snakes release this amine. The blood from dog injected with *Bothrops jararaca* venom, however, showed no increased histamine content: it had no effect on the guinea pig gut. I was at the time working on histamine bioassay and decided to reapply the blood that had shown no effect on the guinea pig gut after it had been left on the bench for a few minutes. Surprised to see that now the guinea pig gut did respond with a contraction, I called Prof. Rocha e Silva to show this result. He repeated the addition of the blood sample to the organ bath; contractions were again observed, the first evoked by bradykinin on the isolated guinea pig ileum. We knew right away that they were not caused by histamine or acetylcholine, because the test gut had been pretreated with an antihistaminic and with atropine. However, we were still conditioned to think in terms of histamine and decided to give the venom another chance by performing a liver perfusion using defibrinated blood as vehicle. To our great surprise, enormous activity was observed when such perfusates were tested on the guinea pig gut. Again it was clear that this activity could not be due to histamine or acetylcholine and it took but a few days to realize that the liver had nothing to do with its formation: the addition of venom directly to defibrinated blood "in vitro", was sufficient to evoke the appearance of activity, which however, was noted to disappear within a few minutes. Pseudoglobulin, precipitated by the addition of 35 to 50% ammonium sulfate to plasma produced active material when incubated with the venom.

The appearance of a slow gut-contraction agent when precursor plasma pseudoglobulin was incubated with *B. jararaca* venom was a completely new result. Rocha e Silva decided to coin a Greek name for this substance using the word *kinin* (indicating movement) with the prefix *brady* (indicating slow), thus describing its effect on the guinea pig gut. The term *Bradykinin* had been created. Dr. J. Reis, also of the Biological Institute and an expert in linguistics gave his approval to this choice.

The action of *B. jararaca* venom on the plasma precursor recalled the action of the enzyme renin releasing angiotensin from a globulin fraction of plasma. Angiotensin raises blood pressure; bradykinin causes it to fall. Very soon we found that we could use pure trypsin rather than venom to release bradykinin from the pseudoglobulin fraction and that the agent acting on smooth muscle (guinea pig gut and uterus, rabbit intestine), caused a fall in blood pressure of the cat, the rabbit and the dog. The fundamental report on bradykinin was published by M. Rocha e Silva, myself and G. Rosenfeld[(2)]. Bradykinin was thus launched on its long and continuing career. Its road was paved with many obstacles and much discouragement. Prof. H. Rocha Lima, Director of the Biological Institute, used to say: "every discovery must go through three phases; in the first, people do not believe in it, or if they do, they think it is not important; in the second, it has become important but somebody has seen it before; in the third, if you are lucky, people recognize the real value of your contribution. Bradykinin was no exception in this respect: we had to fight for one and a half years to prove its existence. First presented at the International Congress of Physiology in Copenhagen in 1950, it was subsequently discussed at the Istituto Superiore di Sanitá in Rome, at the Pasteur Institute in Paris and at the National Institute of Pharmacology, Madrid.

Until then nobody had claimed that bradykinin resembled any previously identified naturally occurring chemical substance. Yet, German scientific literature contained many reports about incompletely identified active factors which, judging from their properties, might have been bradykinin. The claim by Werle and his co-workers, that kallikrein, an enzyme extracted from urine by Frey and Kraut in 1930, could be an endogenous releaser of bradykinin only appeared in a convincing way in 1950[(3)]. Much later it was rumored that bradykinin had been discovered in Germany in 1936 and named factor DK ("Darmkontrahierender Faktor"). No evidence was presented showing that it originated from the globulin fraction of plasma. During one discussion, professor J.H. Gaddum, at the London Symposium on Vaso-active peptides in 1959, stated: "Bradykinin was described by Rocha e Silva in 1948 and it proved a very potent stimulus to research. People who had not really been attracted to this field, took up work on this substance because Rocha's results were so clear-cut and simple. He performed a very great service to us by drawing our attention to substances of this group". From that stage on, the story of bradykinin can be read in many Proceedings of Symposia on Kinins held in: Canada, 1953; London, 1960; New York, 1962; Florence, 1965; Ribeirão Preto, 1966; Fiesole, 1970; San Francisco, 1972; Bethesda, 1974; Tokyo, 1978; Munich, 1981; Savannah, 1984 and Tokyo, 1987. A coming Symposium will be held in Munich in 1991.

Another important contribution to this area was made by Sergio Ferreira, a disciple of Rocha e Silva who isolated from the venom of *Bothrops jararaca*, a factor that strongly potentiated the action of bradykinin; he named it BPF (bradykinin potentiating factor)[(4)]. In 1970, Ferreira, Bartelt and Greene isolated and identified this factor as one of a family of related peptides. Later on, in 1977, Cushman and Ondetti, of the Squibb Institute for Medical Research, used BPF to develop Captopril, a drug used in the treatment of high blood pressure. Thus, this story starts with bradykinin discovered when *Bothrops jararaca* venom was used to study histamine release, is followed by the discovery of BPF also isolated from the venom of *Bothrops jararaca*, and culminates in the development of synthetic angiotensin converting enzyme inhibitors currently in use for the treatment of high blood pressure. What had started out as mere curiosity resulted in an important therapeutic application.

During the time I worked at the Biological Institute in São Paulo, I never heard Rocha e Silva complain that materials or equipment were insufficient or that his salary was too low. However, we could get an idea of his economic situation by the quality of his cigars; it tended to oscillate, especially when, at one time, a governor decided to freeze the salary of scientists and employees at a certain level, in order to solve the difficult situation of the Treasury of the State of São Paulo.

In 1948, together with J. Reis, P. Sawaya, G. Rosenfeld and H. Moussatché, Rocha e Silva founded the Brazilian Society for the Advancement of Science (SBPC) modeled after the British and American Societies founded in 1832 and 1848, respectively. The SBPC is now 42 years old and is the third largest Society for the Advancement of Science in the world. The founding of the Society coincided with a change in orientation by the administration of the Butantan Institute in São Paulo. The new director decided to ban so-called basic scientific research from the Institute to emphasize, instead, the production of vaccines and sera. He said that basic research is a privilege of rich countries. To this Rocha e Silva replied that if those countries are rich it is because they developed basic research and were thus able to create their own industrial technology.

In 1957, Rocha e Silva was appointed full professor of Pharmacology at the Faculty of Medicine of Ribeirão Preto, a newly created Campus of the University of São Paulo. There he formed a very active group involved in the study of kinins. This group has made very important contributions. They include the characterization of bradykinin potentiating factors, studies on new central nervous system peptides, of cyto-and chemical mediators of the antiinflammatory reaction, and on the action of bradykinin on the central nervous system and on cardiac circulation. Today, the Department of Pharmacology of the Faculty of Medicine of Ribeirão Preto is one of the largest in Latin America. Rocha e Silva always had an exceptional ability to attract students towards a scientific career. In Ribeirão Preto he had the efficient collaboration of Hanna Rothschild whose name appears in several books as coauthor.

One of the most outstanding aspects of Rocha e Silva's personality was the diversity of his intellectual interests and curiosity. He once said: "to begin a career in science as in any other creative branch of life, is always an adventure. I might have become a better physicist or a better writer than a pharmacologist". His interest in theoretical physics was a constant one: in 1978–1979 he published articles on the hydrogen line spectrum, electrostatic fields, and the Rydberg constant in "Speculations in Science and Technology". As a medical student he wrote short stories and novels during the free intervals of his clinical work. He published a book "Bonecos de Porcelana" and was working on a play when he decided to move to São Paulo in 1934. He was a philosopher of science and published articles and several books on the subject. He also painted and often gave his pictures to friends as presents.

Rocha e Silva was a very intelligent and extraordinarily gifted man, interested in the most diverse fields. Today we appreciate his contributions, not only as a famous pharmacologist but, as a highly creative human being involved in other fields of human activity.

References

1. Feldberg, W. and C.H. Kellaway, Liberation of histamine and formation of lysolecithin-like substances by snake venom, J. Physiol. 94, 187-226 (1938).

2. Rocha e Silva, M., W.T. Beraldo and G. Rosenfeld, Bradykinin, a hypotensive and smooth muscle stimulating principle released from plasma globulin by snake venoms and by trypsin, Amer. J. Physiol. 156, 261-273 (1949).

3. Werle, E., R. Kehl and K. Koebke, Ueber Bradykinin, Kallikin und Hypertensin, Bioch. Z. 320, 372-383 (1950).

4. Ferreira, S.H., A bradykinin-potentiating factor (BPI) present in the venom of *Bothrops jararaca*, Br. J. Pharmacol. 24, 163-169 (1965).

AAS 36
Contributions to
Autacoid Pharmacology

CHARACTERIZATION OF TWO ENZYMES OF BROAD SUBSTRATE SPECIFICITY, THAT CLEAVE BRADYKININ

E.G. Erdös

Departments of Pharmacology and Anesthesiology, University of Illinois, College of Medicine, Chicago, Illinois 60612

The name bradykinin (BK), given to an active material released from a plasma protein that contracted the isolated guinea pig ileum(1), implies movement, as it comes from the Greek *kinisis*, meaning motion. Considering the ever increasing number of reports on the various actions attributed to BK, the naming was prescient. BK, a nona-peptide, is inactivated by enzymes collectively called kininases(2). With the increase in the reported activities of BK – especially in triggering intracellular events – there has been a parallel growth in the number of additional kininases characterized.

In blood, kallidin (Lys-Bk) is probably converted to Bk either prior or simultaneously with inactivation(3,4). Because the $Arg^1Pro^2Pro^3$ sequence lends stability and resistance to many peptidases, inactivation at the C-terminus of Bk has been encountered most. Indeed, major kininases have been divided into two groups: kininase I and II(5). Kininase I-type enzymes cleave Arg^9 and kininase II enzymes liberate the dipeptide Phe^8-Arg^9 (Fig. 1). With the finding of two different Bk receptors(6), it is recognized that both types of enzymes eliminate the action of the peptide on the more common B_2 receptor, but des-Arg^9-Bk is active on the B_1 receptor. Thus, the carboxypeptidase-type kininases in addition to abolishing most of the actions of Bk, also convert its receptor specifically from B_2 to B_1(7).

Obviously these enzymes do not act on Bk exclusively, but have many other functions. For example, the neutral endopeptidase 24.11 (a kininase II type enzyme), inactivates enkephalins(8) or the atrial natriuretic peptide(9). However, in some organs or

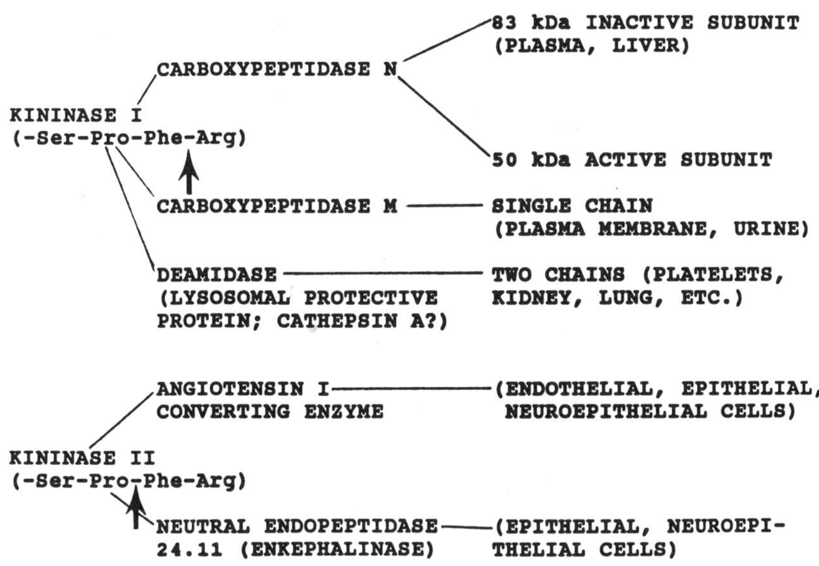

cells, for example in rat kidney[10] or human neutrophils[11], it appears to be a major kininase.

Recently, our laboratory characterized two human enzymes that cleave bradykinin, although their importance does not rest with the kinin system alone. Carboxypeptidase N of human plasma was originally called kininase I[2]. This blood-borne enzyme is a complex molecule, consisting of a tetramer formed from two heterodimers. The dimer consists of a 50 kDa active subunit and an 83 kDa regulatory subunit, which keeps the active subunit in circulation and protects it at 37°C [12,13]. The enzyme is also a major inactivador of anaphylatoxins which are released after the activation of the complement system[7]. However, whether carboxypeptidase N has any role outside the circulation is questionable. The finding of a carboxypeptidase in urine[14], on plasma membranes of cultured cells[7] and in tissues[15,16] was initially thought to be due to the presence of the 50 kDa active subunit. Subsequent purification of the enzyme first from human urine[14] and then from placental microvilli[17] revealed that there is a carboxypeptidase which cleaves basic amino acids, but is different from other known carboxypeptidases. For example the kinetics of Bk hydrolysis are more favorable than with carboxypeptidase N. Because of its presence on membranes it was named carboxypeptidase M. Indeed carboxypeptidase M differs from the similar enzymes not just in kinetics of substrate hydrolysis, but also in its size and immunological reactivity[7,17].

Finally, cloning of the enzyme from placental library and the sequencing of the cDNA indicated that the amino acid sequence of the 62 kDa protein has only a partial homology with other basic carboxypeptidases[18]. For example, it has 41–49% sequence identity with plasma carboxypeptidase N (active subunit) or with secretory granular carboxypeptidase H that is active at acid pH, but only 15% with the pancreatic carboxypeptidases. Concerning its importance and its presence in many organs or in urine, carboxypeptidase M very likely inactivates Bk and anaphylatoxins both on the vascular endothelial cells, and when these compounds appear outside the circulation. This idea was strengthened by some recent experiments where carboxypeptidase M was detected in cultured Madin-Darby Canine Kidney or MDCK Cells[19]. Here, the enzyme is anchored to the luminal membrane of the cells via a phosphatidylinositol-glycan group at its C-terminus. It follows that a phospholipase cleaving this bond can release it. MDCK cells are considered to originate from the distal part of the nephron. Presumably kallikrein, also located in the distal nephron[20], could release kinins into the lumen; thus, carboxypeptidase M is a major kininase in the distal tubules. This is in addition to the inactivation of kinins (filtered by the glomerulus) on the proximal tubular brush border[10] by kininase II-type enzymes, angiotensin I converting enzyme[2] and neutral endopeptidase 24.11[21].

The peptide bond of Arg^9 in Bk is also the target of another enzyme, but its properties differ from those of the basic carboxypeptidases. Recent advances in the techniques of protein purification and sequencing revealed that frequently a single protein may have two or more totally unrelated functions. This certainly is the case with the deamidase enzyme that we named after one of its very important functions[22]. This enzyme deamidates tachykinins by cleaving the C-terminal $CONH_2$ bond at neutral pH. For example, deamidase hydrolyzes the Met^{11}-NH_2 in substance P, converting it from the amide into substance P free acid (Met^{11}-OH), which is inactive in most tests. In addition, it cleaves many other substrates, by liberating free and protected C-terminal amino acids. The deamidase action is prevalent at neutral pH, but below neutrality the deamidase acts more as a carboxypeptidase, e.g., at pH 5.5. This acidic pH optimum of carboxypeptidase is quite sharp with short peptide substrates. With longer peptides, however, the enzyme acts as a carboxypeptidase at both neutral and acidic pH. Thus, it releases Arg^9 of bradykinin or $GlyNH_2$ of oxytocin at either pH value. Nevertheless, it is not a basic carboxypeptidase as it cleaves both basic and hydrophobic C-terminal amino acids. Specificity depends also on the penultimate amino acid; it does not hydrolyze peptides if the C-terminal amino acids is linked to arginine or, in case of des-Arg^9-Bk, to proline. Hence, it does not cleave vasopressin with -Arg-Gly-NH_2, in contrast to oxytocin (Leu-Gly-NH_2). Although it is an active carboxypeptidase, it does not absolutely require a free COOH group, as pancreatic, blood, or tissue carboxypeptidases do.

We purified the enzyme after releasing it from human platelet lysosomal granules with thrombin and epinephrine(22). It is a 52 kDa protein consisting of two chains of about 33 and 21 kDa. The high mol. wt. chain contains the active site serine. We sequenced the first 25 amino acids in each chain. Although searching for sequence identity by computer did not reveal homology with other enzymes or proteins, we found in a recent publication(23) that this sequence is identical with that of the so called lysosomal protective protein. This proteins binds *B*-galactosidase and neuraminidase in a high mol. wt. complex. A deficiency of this protein causes the lack of lysosomal *B*-galactosidase and neuraminidase activity, resulting in galactosialidosis, a genetically determined metabolic storage disease that can be fatal in infants. Thus protection and complexing functions of the enzyme do not depend on the enzymatic activity of this protease according to d'Azzo and colleagues (personal communication).

Deamidase also occurs in many other tissues including the kidney, brain, lung, etc. Many of its properties resemble those of the so called cathepsin A which has never been completely characterized. Judging from sequence similarities and the mode of hydrolysis of some substrates it is also probably related through evolution, to yeast carboxypeptidase Y and to the KEX I gene product(22,23). The enzyme is released from a very rich source, platelets, by endogenous agents; platelets have a variety of functions in non-thrombotic processes. Possibly, the release of this enzyme may lead to the inactivation of bradykinin or substance P, for example in inflammation.

This brief review attempted to point out that as we learn more and more about the various functions of bradykinin, we find that it can be inactivated by different but well characterized enzymes. The enzymes discussed in this review are the latest additions to a group collectively called kininases.

References

1. Rocha e Silva, M., W.T. Beraldo and G. Rosenfeld, Bradykinin, a hypotensive and smooth muscle stimulating factor released from plasma globulin by snake venoms and by trypsin, Am. J. Physiol. 156, 261-272 (1949).

2. Erdös, E.G., Kininases, In: Bradykinin, Kallidin and Kallikrein. Handb. Exp. Pharmac., Supplement to vol. XXV, pp. 427-487 (Ed. E.G. Erdös). Springer-Verlag, Heidelberg (1979).

3. Erdös, E.G., A.G. Renfrew, E.M. Sloane and J.R. Wohler, Enzymatic studies on bradykinin and similar peptides, Ann. N.Y. Acad. Sci. 104, 222-234 (1963).

4. Webster, M.E. and V. Pierce, The nature of kallidin released from human plasma by kallikreins and other enzymes, Ann. N.Y. Acad. Sci. 104, 91-107 (1963).

5. Erdös, E.G., Some old and some new ideas on kinin metabolism, J. Cardiovasc. Pharmacol. 15 (Suppl. 6), S20-S24 (1990).

6. Regoli, D. and J. Barabe, Pharmacology of bradykinin and related kinins, Pharmacol. Rev. 32, 1-46 (1980).

7. Skidgel, R.A., Basic carboxypeptidases: Regulators of peptide hormone activity, Trends Pharmacol. Sci. 9, 299-304 (1988).

8. Schwartz, J.-C., B. Malfroy and S. De La Baume, Biological inactivation of enkephalins and the role of enkephalin-dipeptidyl-carboxypeptidase ("enkephalinase") as neuropeptidase, Life Sci. 29, 1715-1740 (1981).

9. Olins, G.M., K.L. Spear, N.R. Siegel and H.A. Zurcher-Neely, Inactivation of atrial natriuretic factor by the renal brush border, Biochim. Biophys. Acta 901, 97-100 (1987).

10. Ura, N., O.A. Carretero and E.G. Erdös, The role of renal endopeptidase 24.11 in kinin metabolism, Kidney Internat. 32, 507-513 (1987).

11. Skidgel, R.A., Jackman, H.L. and Erdös, E.G., Metabolism of substance P and bradykinin by human neutrophils, Biochem. Pharmacol. (in press).

12. Tan, F., D.K. Weerasinghe, R.A. Skidgel, H. Tamei, R.K. Kaul, I. Robinson, J.W. Schilling and E.G. Erdös, The deduced protein sequence of the human carboxypeptidase N high molecular weight subunit reveals the presence of leucine-rich tandem repeats, J. Biol. Chem. 265, 13-19 (1990).

13. Levin, Y., R.A. Skidgel and E.G. Erdös, Isolation and characterization of the subunits of human plasma carboxypeptidase N (kininase I), Proc. Nat. Acad. Sci. USA 79, 4618-4622 (1982).

14. Skidgel, R.A., R.M. Davis and E.G. Erdös, Purification of a human urinary carboxypeptidase (kininase) distinct from carboxypeptidases A, B or N, Anal. Biochem. 140, 520-531 (1984).

15. Johnson, A.R., R.A. Skidgel, J.T. Gafford and E.G. Erdös, Enzymes in placental microvilli: Angiotensin I converting enzyme, angiotensinase A, carboxypeptidase, and neutral endopeptidase ("enkephalinase"), Peptides 5, 769-776 (1984).

16. Skidgel, R.A., A.R. Johnson, E.G. Erdös, Hydrolysis of opioid hexapeptides by carboxypeptidase N. Presence of carboxypeptidase in cell membranes, Biochem. Pharmacol. 33, 3471-3478 (1984).

17. Skidgel, R.A., R.M. Davis and F. Tan, Human carboxypeptidase M. Purification and characterization of a membrane-bound carboxypeptidase that cleaves peptide hormones, J. Biol. Chem. 264, 2236-2241 (1989).

18. Tan, F., S.J. Chan, D.F. Steiner, J.W. Schilling and R.A. Skidgel, Molecular cloning and sequencing of the cDNA for human membrane-bound carboxypeptidase M. Comparison with carboxypeptidases A, B, H and N, J. Biol. Chem. 264, 13165-13170 (1989).

19. Deddish, P.A., R.A. Skidgel, V.B. Krilho, R.P. Becker and E.G. Erdös, Carboxypeptidase M in cultured Madin-Darby canine kidney cells. Evidence that carboxypeptidase M has a phosphatidylinositol glycan anchor, J. Biol. Chem. 265, 15083-15089 (1990).

20. Scicli, A.G., O.A. Carretero, A. Hampton, P. Cortes and N.B. Oza, Site of kininogenase secretion in the dog nephron, Am. J. Physiol. 230, 533-536 (1976).

21. Gafford, J.T., R.A. Skidgel, E.G. Erdös and L.B. Hersh, Human kidney "enkephalinase", a neutral metalloendopeptidase that cleaves active peptides, Biochemistry 22, 3265-3271 (1983).

22. Jackman, H.L., Tan, F., Tamei, H., Erdös, E.G., Beurling-Harbury, C., Li, X.Y. and Skidgel, R.A., A peptidase in human platelets that deamidates tachykinins: probable identity with the lysosomal "protective protein", J. Biol. Chem. 265, 11265-11272 (1990).

23. Galjart, N.J., N Gillemans, A. Harris, G.T.J. van der Horst, F.W. Verheijen, H. Galjaard and A. d'Azzo, Expression of cDNA encoding the human "protective protein" associated with lysosomal *B*-galactosidase and neuraminidase: homology to yeast proteases, Cell. 54, 755-764 (1988).

AAS 36
Contributions to
Autacoid Pharmacology

THE TONIN-KININ SYSTEM

J.L. Pesquero, G.W. Araujo, M.P. Lima and W.T. Beraldo

Department of Physiology and Biophysics, Institute of Biological Sciences, Federal University of Minas Gerais, 31270 Belo Horizonte, MG, Brazil

Abstract

Observed oxytocic effects of a rat mandibular gland tonin preparation are shown to be due to a contaminating tonin-like serine protease, which chromatographic and pharmacological evidence indicates to predominantly release bradykinin from rat uterine horn preparations.

Introduction

Tonin (EC 3.4.99. –) is a serine protease which directly cleaves the vasoconstrictor peptide angiotensin II from angiotensinogen (AG), the natural renin substrate[1,2]. In rat submandibular gland (SMG) two mRNAs, designated S2 and S3 which encode two proteins of the serine proteinase family, have been described[3]. S2 encodes the enzyme tonin, while S3 encodes a protein closely related to tonin. This protein has 84% homology with tonin and retains identical amino acids at key positions; these are believed to be the determinants of substrates cleavage preferences.

In order to verify the S3 mRNA expression and the activity of the expressed protein, the purification of the angiotensin-forming enzyme of rat SMG was performed[4]. In the last step of the procedure, using DEAE-cellulose chromatography, two enzymes with atypical angiotensin-forming activity were isolated. These enzymes, designated rSMT3 and rSMT4, had different physical and chemical properties. Both apparently hydrolysed AG, liberating angiotensin II, had negligible activity on the synthetic kallikrein substrate Ac-

Phe-Arg-Nitroanilide and were strongly inhibited by serine proteinase inhibitors, but not by EDTA nor enaprilate. Their molecular weights determined by polyacrylamide gel electrophoresis, were 31,700 for rSMT3 and 29,800 for rSMT4. The physico-chemical properties of rSMT4 suggested that this enzyme is tonin, whereas rSMT3 appeared to be a tonin-like enzyme which accounts for 8% and 20% of the total oxytocic activity of the submandibular glands of the weaned and aged rat, respectively.

A partially purified tonin preparation from rat submandibular gland, was capable of eliciting a contraction of the rat uterus; dose-dependent desensitization of the uterine horn was observed(5). Desensitization of the uterine horn to kallikrein, had little or no effect on the contraction elicited by tonin. After desensitization of the uterine horn to tonin, the contraction due to kallikrein was reduced by about 80%. These results suggested that the rat uterus may have two different substrates, one relatively specific for the action of kallikrein and the other for tonin. In view of experiments showing kininogenase activity of rat SMG tonin(5,6), we present results of a comparative study of rSMT3 and rSMT4 oxytocic activity.

Results and Discussion

When rSMT4 was applied to an organ bath containing a rat uterine horn, no response was observed even after the addition of concentrations as high as 10 μg/ml (Fig. 1). In contrast, 2 μg/ml of rSMT3 caused the preparation to contract after a period of latency of 1 to 2 minutes. After 4–5 further additions at 2 min intervals, the same dose of rMST3 elicited little or no response. However, when a double dose of rMST3 was applied, the muscle again presented a contraction. A dose-dependent desensitization had occurred. Figure 1 illustrates one of these experiments.

In order to determine the nature of the response, i.e., whether due to a direct action of the enzyme or by way of the liberation of a bradykinin or an angiotensin-like product, we carried out experiments utilizing the parallel uterus preparation. In these experiments, one uterine horn was desensitized by several additions of rMST3 to the organ bath. Another horn not desensitized, was then mounted in the same bath at a short distance from the desensitized horn, which remained in connection with the recording lever. When the same dose of rMST3 used for desensitization was now added to the organ bath, the desensitized horn presented a contraction (Fig. 2). These experiments strongly suggest an indirect action of the enzyme. The product released from the non-depleted horn acts on the depleted one. The characterization of the product liberated by rSMT3 was

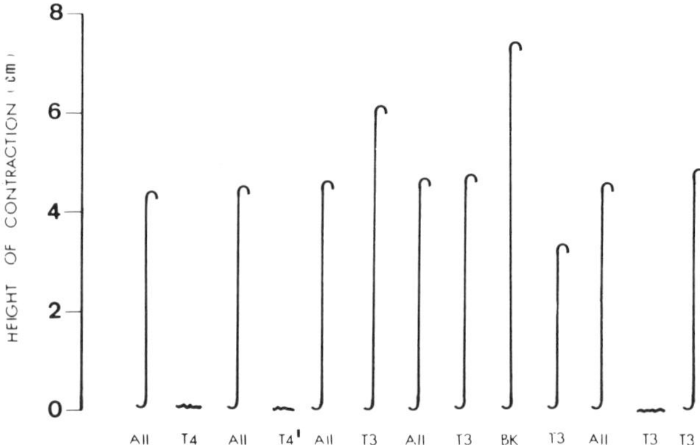

Fig. 1. Effect of repeated additions of 10 μg of rSMT3 (T3) to the isolated rat uterus; the last addition was of a doubled dose (20 μg). The uterine horn was suspended in a 5 ml bath of Tyrode solution, pH 7.4 at 37°C. Air was bubbled through the bath fluid. AII, angiotensin II (1 ng); BK, bradykinin (1 ng); T4 and T4', 25 and 50 μg of rSMT4, respectively.

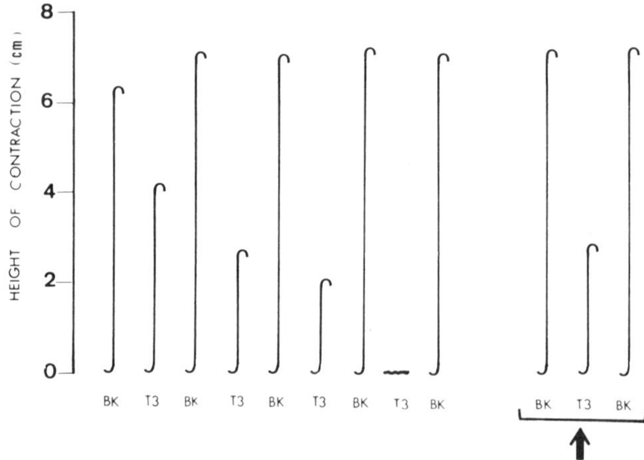

Fig. 2. Effect of repeated additions of 10 μg of rSMT3 (T3) to the organ bath containing the parallel uterus preparation. BK, 5 ng bradykinin; ↑ contractions of a desensitized horn in the presence of the not desensitized horn.

made by incubating the enzyme with a rat uterus homogenate, and submitting the incubate to high performance liquid chromatography (HPLG), utilizing a Mino-RPC column (Fig. 3). Fractions obtained were characterized by radioimmunoassay (RIA) and by

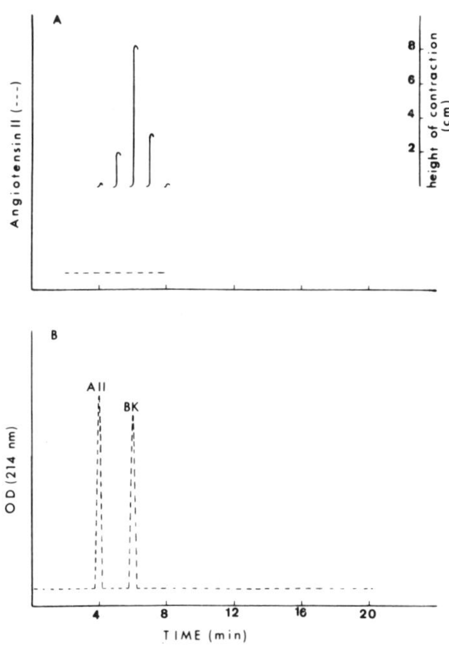

Fig. 3. HPLC elution profile of, A) products of the uterus homogenate incubated with rSMT3 and B) standard angiotensin II (AII) and bradykinin (BK). AII was determined by RIA; contractions recorded are of the isolated rat uterus.

bioassay on the isolated rat uterus. The HPLC profile was compared with that of a mixture of synthetic standards of angiotensin II and bradykinin. The retention times of the standard peptides under the HPLC conditions were determined by bioassay and optical density in the case of bradykinin, and by bioassay, RIA and optical density in the case of angiotensin II. Figure 3 shows that angiotensin II was not detected in any of the fractions of HPLC. On the other hand, the possibility that the released active product is bradykinin, was provided by the retention times of the active HPLC fractions: they coincided with those of the bradykinin standard; furthermore, their oxytocic activity was not inhibited by saralasin, a specific inhibitor of angiotensin II (Fig. 4).

The present results lead us to conclude that the kininogenase activity and the oxytocic effect observed, previously related to tonin[5,6], may be due to rSMT3 which probably was contaminating the preparations used. Furthermore, our results show that rSMT3 is a rat SMG enzyme having possible angiotensin II and definite bradykinin-generating activity. Although not part of the present experiment, we restate that the rat uterus must have two different kininogens: one is relatively specific for the action of kallikrein: both however, are attacked by rSMT3, a tonin-like enzyme.

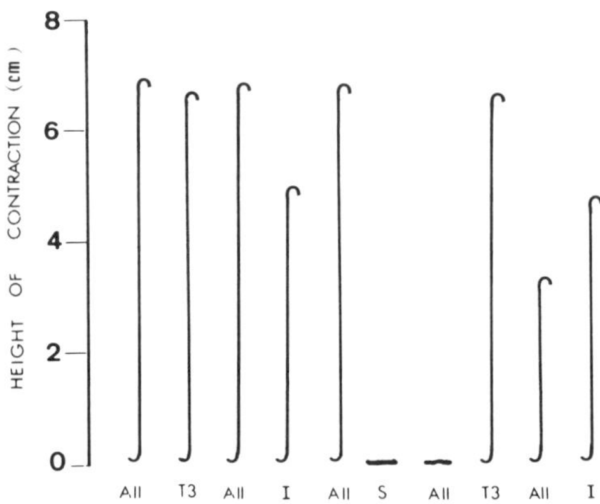

Fig. 4. Effect of 0.2 μg/ml of saralasin (S) on the contraction of the isolated rat uterus evolved by AII (4 ng/ml); T3, rSMT3 (2 μg/ml) and the active fraction obtained from HPLC (I).

References

1. Boucher, R., J. Asselin and J. Genest, A new enzyme leading to the direct formation of angiotensin II, Circ. Res. (Supl. 1) 34/35, 1203-1212 (1974).

2. Grise, C., R. Boucher, G. Thibault and J. Genest, Formation of angiotensin II by tonin from partially purified human angiotensin, Can. J. Biochem. 59, 250-255 (1981).

3. Ashley, P.L. and R.J. MacDonald, Kallikrein-related mRNAs of the rat submaxillary gland: nucleotide sequences of four distinct types including tonin, Biochemistry, 24, 4512-4520 (1985).

4. Araujo, G.W., J.B. Pesquero, C.J. Lindsey, A.C.M. Paiva and J.L. Pesquero, Identification of serine proteses with tonin-like activity in the rat submandibular and prostate glands, Biochim. Biophys. Acta (Accepted for publication, 1991).

5. Feitosa, M.H., J.L. Pesquero, M.A.D. Ferreira, G.M.L. Oliveira, E. Rogana and W.T. Beraldo, Tonin and kallikrein-kinin system, In: Kinins V, part A, pp. 573-580 (Eds. K. Abe, H. Moriya and S. Fujii). Plenum, New York 1989.

6. Ikeda, M. and K. Arakawa, Kininogenase activity of tonin, Hypertension 6, 222-228 (1984).

AAS 36
Contributions to
Autacoid Pharmacology

MECHANICAL AND NEURO-HUMORAL FACTORS IN ACUTE AORTIC COARCTATION HYPERTENSION

H.C. Salgado, R. Fazan Jr., B.H. Machado and M.C.O. Salgado*

Departments of Physiology and *Pharmacology, School of Medicine of Ribeirão Preto, USP, 14049 Ribeirão Preto, SP, Brazil

Abstract

The hemodynamic responses and the role of renal nerves in the physiopathogenesis of acute (45 min) aortic coarctation hypertension were studied in conscious rats. The hemodynamic responses elicited by aortic constriction in intact and bilaterally nephrectomized rats were analyzed by means of miniaturized pulsed-Doppler flow probes. Anephric rats presented a smaller increase in mean carotid pressure (MCP) and calculated aortic resistance during aortic coarctation than did intact animals. Reflex bradycardia throughout the experiment did not differ significantly between the two groups. The pressor response following aortic coarctation in untreated renal-denervated rats was similar to that found in intact subjects. Renal-denervated rats previously treated with V_1-vascular arginine vasopressin antagonist [$d(CH_2)_5$Tyr(Me)AVP] showed the same hypertensive response as control renal-denervated rats. Previous treatment of renal-denervated rats with saralasin (an angiotensin II antagonist) produced a significant reduction in the hypertensive response throughout the experiment when compared to untreated renal-denervated rats. Similarly, rats treated with the vasopressin antagonist plus saralasin showed a blunted hypertensive response following aortic coarctation. The results for rats previously treated with vasopressin antagonist plus saralasin did not differ from those obtained with saralasin alone. Overall, the results of aortic coarctation hypertension obtained in the present study indicate that: 1) Anephric rats showed a blunted hypertensive response due to the lack of neuro-humoral release of vasopressor substances (e.g. angiotensin II and vasopressin) triggered by the kidneys, when only the mechanical factor of constriction was present; 2) The lack of afferent feedback from the kidneys in renal-denervated rats for vasopressin release from the central nervous system allowed angiotensin II to play the major physiopathological role associated with the mechanical factor in the hypertensive response.

Introduction

The hypothesis that a mechanical factor may explain the pathogenesis of hypertension in aortic coarctation was originally proposed by Blumgart(1). Later, Goldblatt *et al.*(2) suggested that increased peripheral resistance in dogs with suprarenal abdominal aortic constriction was of renal origin. However, in suprarenal aortic constriction, augmented aortic resistance might share a physiopathological role with humoral factors in the increase of arterial pressure.

A technique developed in our laboratory for chronic implantation of a pneumatic cuff around arterial vessels (aortic or carotid), permits the study of cardiovascular responses to aortic constriction in conscious instrumented rats(3). Using this technique, we(4) have demonstrated that the renin-angiotensin system (RAS) plays a significant role in the maintenance of acute partial aortic coarctation hypertension in conscious rats and that bilateral nephrectomy abolishes the increase in plasma renin activity (PRA) and blunts the increase in arterial pressure caused by partial aortic constriction. However, removal of the kidneys eliminates not only hypertensive mechanisms other than the RAS, such as renal chemoreceptors(5-7), but might also cause important hemodynamic changes by the elimination of a vascular territory responsible for approximately 20% of the cardiac output.

To further study the role of humoral factors in the physiopathogenesis of acute aortic coarctation hypertension, without the undesired effect of a bilateral nephrectomy, we investigated, by using pharmacological blockade of the pressor effect of endogenous arginine vasopressin (AVP) and of angiotensin II (AII), the time course of action of these pressor peptides in acute (45 min) partial aortic coarctation hypertension. The results obtained demonstrated that, in addition to the mechanical effect of aortic constriction, AII acts on the prompt (5 min) rise in pressure, whereas AVP is responsible for the maintenance (30–45 min) of arterial pressure elevation(8).

Since the AVP antagonist [d(CH_2)$_5$Tyr(Me)AVP] abolishes the late rise in arterial pressure elicited by electrical stimulation of the afferent renal nerve in anesthetized cats(9), in the present study we investigated the role of the renal nerves in the acute (45 min) hypertension caused by partial aortic coarctation in conscious renal-denervated rats. Hemodynamic responses elicited by partial aortic constriction in intact and bilaterally nephrectomized conscious rats were also investigated using a pulsed-Doppler flowmeter(10).

Methods

Male Wistar rats (250–300 g) were used. Surgical procedures were performed under pentobarbital sodium (40 mg/kg, i.p.), or thiopental sodium (40 mg/kg, i.p.) anesthesia. All experiments were conducted with conscious unrestrained animals kept in individual cages.

Arterial and venous cannulation. The day before the experiment, the rats were anesthetized with pentobarbital sodium (hemodynamic studies) or thiopental sodium (renal denervation studies) and polyethylene catheters (Clay-Adams, Parsippany, NJ) were inserted into the femoral artery (PE 10 connected to PE 50) and into the ascending aorta via the left carotid artery (PE 50) for arterial pressure measurements, and into the femoral vein for drug administration. Both carotid and femoral arterial pressures were recorded continuously with a Statham pressure transducer (Model P23-Db; Hato Rey, PR) attached to a Hewlett-Packard recorder (Model 7848; Palo Alto, CA). Heart rate (HR) was measured by counting arterial pulses at high recorder speed.

Pneumatic cuff implantation. A pneumatic cuff was placed around the aorta immediately below the diaphragm following ample laparotomy and was exteriorized through the animal's back together with the catheters. Cuff preparation has been described(3). After control measurements of arterial pressures and HR, the balloon inside the cuff was filled with liquid to constrict the aorta. By controlling the amount of liquid, arterial pressure distal to the cuff (mean femoral arterial pressure) was maintained at precisely 50 mm Hg. This level of renal perfusion pressure was chosen because it is well below the lower limit of renal blood flow autoregulation(11) and can provide a potent stimulus for renin release.

Renal-denervation. The denervation procedure, performed three days prior to the experiment, consisted of stripping all visible renal nerves and painting the renal vessels with phenol (10%). After the experiment, the animals were anesthetized with thiopental sodium and their renal artery electrically stimulated to check the efficacy of denervation.

Implantation of Pulsed-Doppler Flow Probes. The day before the experiment a flow probe was implanted in intact or bilaterally nephrectomized rats for assessment of the flow in the abdominal aorta above the pneumatic cuff and immediately below the diaphragm(10). Briefly, a midline abdominal incision was made, and a 4–6 mm length of the abdominal aorta was carefully isolated immediately below the diaphragm. A miniaturized pulsed-Doppler flow probe was placed around the aorta and the cuff closed with 6-0 cotton sutures. The wire leads from the probe were exteriorized through the animal's back together with the catheters, and connected to an ultrasonic, pulsed-Doppler flowmeter (University of Iowa Bioengineering Department), which allows measurement of changes in blood velocity recorded as the Doppler shift, in kHz. Aortic resistance was calculated as the quotient of mean carotid pressure (MCP) and aortic blood flow Doppler shift.

Protocol. The experimental protocol consisted of producing an acute (45 min) hypertensive response by partial aortic coarctation in conscious freely moving rats after a control period of 10 to 15 min during which arterial pressure and HR were recorded.

Partial aortic coarctation in intact and bilaterally nephrectomized rats. Groups of 7 intact and of 7 bilaterally nephrectomized rats, respectively, were submitted to partial occlusion of the aorta during 45 min. The day before the experiment, bilateral nephrectomy had been performed after the pneumatic cuff and the pulsed-Doppler flow probes had been placed around the aorta.

Partial aortic coarctation in renal-denervated rats. Four groups of renal-denervated rats and one group of seven intact rats were submitted to partial occlusion of the aorta during 45 min.

Animals of group 1 had no previous treatment. Group 2 animals received an intravenous infusion of the AII receptor antagonist, saralasin, at 3 mg kg^{-1} min^{-1} using a peristaltic pump supplying 100 μl/min. Rats of group 3 were pre-treated with an AVP V_1-receptor antagonist, $d(CH_2)_5Tyr(Me)AVP$(10 μg/kg, i.v.). Group 4 consisted of rats pre-treated with the AVP/antagonist (10 μg/kg, i.v.) and subsequently infused with saralasin (3 mg kg^{-1} min^{-1}). Antagonists were administered 15 min prior to aortic coarctation; the effectiveness of blockade was tested immediately before aortic constriction and at the end of the experiment by verifying inhibition of the pressor response to 10 ng of AII (group 2), to 10 mU of AVP (group 3), or to both drugs (group 4), injected as a bolus into the venous catheter.

Drugs were dissolved in 0.9% NaCl. AII and saralasin were synthesized by Dr. A.C.M. Paiva, Escola Paulista de Medicina, SP, Brazil; AVP was purchased from Parke-Davis (Detroit, MI) and AVP antagonist from Bachem (Torrance, CA).

Statistics. Data were examined by analysis of variance using a split-plot model for each experimental protocol[12,13]. When differences were observed, responses during periods after coarctation of the aorta of treated groups were compared with their controls using Dunnett's T test[14]. Differences from controls were considered significant when $p < 0.05$.

Results

Hemodynamics of Aortic Coarctation. The effects of aortic constriction on the MCP and calculated aortic resistance (% change) of intact and nephrectomized rats are shown in Fig. 1. Nephrectomized rats showed a basal MCP (104 ± 3 mm Hg) similar to the MCP (109 ± 4 mm Hg) of intact rats. In both groups MCP presented a prompt rise and reached a plateau 15 min after the constriction. Nevertheless, after coarctation bilaterally nephrectomized rats showed a substantially smaller hypertensive response (10–16%) than intact animals (25–36%). Calculated aortic resistance presented a gradual rise in both groups of rats. However, the relative increase in the intact rats (167–292%) was about two-fold that observed in the nephrectomized rats (92–156%) throughout the experiment. Reflex bradycardia did not differ significantly throughout the experiment in either intact or nephrectomized animals.

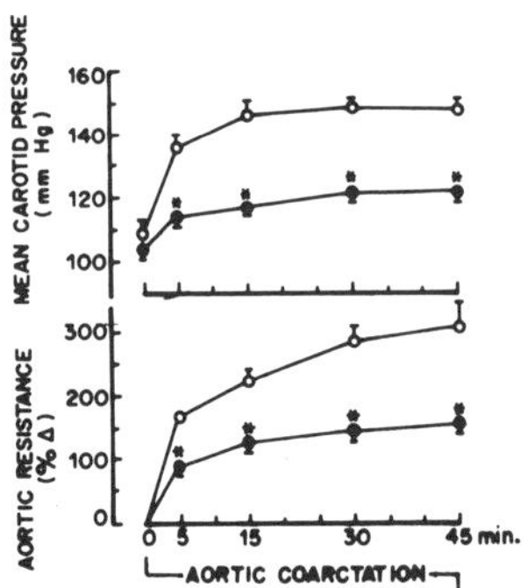

Fig. 1. Effect of acute aortic coarctation on mean carotid pressure (upper panel) and aortic vascular resistance (lower panel) in conscious unrestrained intact (○ — ○) and bilaterally nephrectomized (●—●) rats. Data are means ± SEM. *Significant difference ($p < 0.05$) compared with corresponding point in the intact group. Basal values (0 min) were recorded before coarctation.

Aortic Coarctation Hypertension After Renal Denervation. Hypertensive responses after partial aortic coarctation maintained for 45 min in untreated, AVP antagonist-, AVP antagonist plus saralasin- and saralasin-treated renal-denervated rats are shown in Fig. 2.

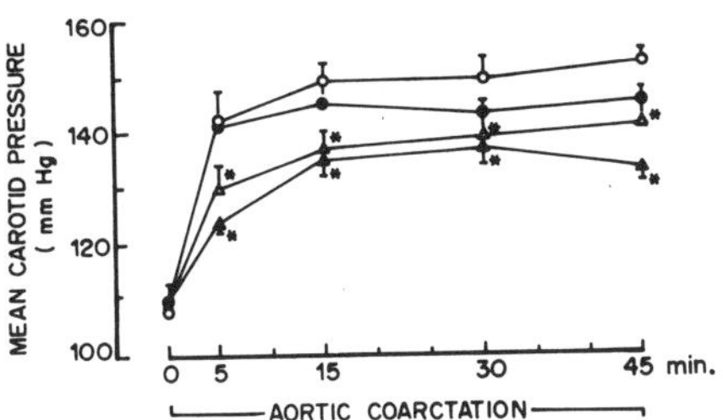

Fig. 2. Effect of acute aortic coarctation on mean carotid pressure of conscious unrestrained renal-denervated rats. Data are means ± SEM. *Significant difference ($p<0.05$) compared with corresponding point in the untreated renal-denervated group. Basal values (0 min) were recorded before coarctation. ○ — ○, untreated group; •—•, group pretreated intravenously with d(CH_2)$_5$Tyr(Me)AVP (10 μg/kg); Δ–Δ, group given a continuous intravenous infusion of saralasin (3 mg kg^{-1} min^{-1}); ▲–▲, group intravenously treated with d(CH_2)$_5$Tyr(Me)AVP (10 μg/kg), concomitantly with an intravenous infusion of saralasin (3 mg kg^{-1} min^{-1}).

Untreated renal-denervated rats presented basal MCP of 108±2 mm Hg and HR of 387±26 bpm, which did not differ significantly from those obtained in intact animals (113±2 mm Hg and 388±19 bpm, respectively). The hypertensive response observed in the intact rats (147±5, 151±3, 150±3 and 153±3 m Hg, at 5, 15, 30 and 45 min after coarctation, respectively) (not shown) was similar to that observed in the untreated renal-denervated group. The renal-denervated rats treated with AVP antagonist presented a MCP of 110±3 mm Hg and HR of 434±16 bpm before coarctation; these values are similar to those observed in untreated denervated rats. Constriction of the aorta in AVP antagonist-treated animals elicited a hypertensive response similar to that observed in untreated renal-denervated animals (Fig. 2). The effectiveness of the AVP antagonist was confirmed by the blockade of the hypertensive response to i.v. administration of AVP. Under basal conditions, the injection of AVP caused a transient increase in MCP of 27±3 mm Hg, whereas immediately before coarctation and after administration of the AVP antagonist, the pressor response to AVP was reduced to zero mm Hg (not shown). Renal-denervated rats treated with saralasin showed a MCP of 110±2 mm Hg and a HR of 427±9 bpm before coarctation. Both values were similar to those observed in the untreated renal-denervated group. Renal denervation plus saralasin significantly blunted the hypertensive response elicited by aortic constriction when compared to that of untreated renal-denervated rats throughout the experiment (Fig. 2). Saralasin effectively inhibited the pressor response to exogenous iv AII (from 27±2 mm Hg before saralasin to 1±1 mm Hg before coarctation, not shown). Renal-denervated rats treated with saralasin plus AVP antagonist, showed a MCP of 110±2 mm Hg and HR of 421±21 bpm before coarctation, values not different from those observed in untreated renal-denervated controls. Treatment with saralasin plus AVP antagonist again significantly blunted the hypertensive response observed after aortic constriction. The increase in MCP obtained was similar to that found after saralasin-treatment alone. Prior to the double blockade with saralasin and AVP antagonist, the transient hypertensive response to bolus iv administration of AII and AVP was 33±4 mm Hg and 32±4 mm Hg, respectively. The antagonist doses used fully blocked the pressor response to AII and reduced the pressor response to AVP to 2±1 mm Hg. Reflex bradycardia observed in the rats treated with saralasin and/or AVP antagonist was similar to that observed in untreated renal-denervated rats.

Discussion

The experimental model of aortic coarctation hypertension has been extensively studied, under both acute and chronic conditions. Chronic experiments have been carried out in rats[15,16] and, especially, dogs[17,18]. Acute experiments lasting minutes or a few hours have been performed mainly in anesthetized dogs[19]. In our laboratory, the model of partial aortic constriction in conscious, freely moving rats has been used to study the relative role of mechanical and neuro-humoral (AII and AVP) factors in the physiopathogenesis of aortic coarctation hypertension[4,8]. The prompt and sustained hypertensive response in the nephrectomized rat indicates that the mechanical factor plays a significant role in the physiopathogenesis of this model of hypertension. These data confirm previous observations[4] and support the notion that humoral factors (e.g. AII, AVP, etc.) are released in response to the lowered perfusion pressure present below the coarctation site in the intact rat[8]. For instance, measurement of the activity of the RAS, 45 min after coarctation, revealed a four-fold increase in PRA levels of intact rats versus no change in bilaterally nephrectomized animals, thus evidencing the role played by AII in the proximal hypertensive response. Pharmacological blockade of AII with saralasin and of AVP with $d(CH_2)_5Tyr(Me)AVP$ in conscious rats[8] not only confirmed the role played by the mechanical factor in the proximal hypertensive response, but also revealed that AII acts on the prompt (5 min) rise in pressure, whereas AVP is responsible for the (30–45 min) maintenance of the arterial pressure elevation. The objective in studying the hemodynamic changes elicited by acute (45 min) aortic constriction in conscious intact or bilaterally nephrectomized rats was to compare the degree of resistance imposed by the constriction of the aorta in both groups (intact or nephrectomized) when the pneumatic cuff reduced the distal pressure to 50 mm Hg. Actually, this is how the degree of aortic constriction was monitored in both groups. The hemodynamic studies demonstrated a greater resistance imposed by the constricted aorta in intact subjects, compared to nephrectomized ones (Fig. 1), indicating an important neuro-humoral role played by the kidney. It is worth pointing out that acute resetting of the sinoaortic baroreceptors[20] may play a role in the profile of gradual increase in resistance when the baroreceptors progressively cease to counteract the rise in pressure.

Because bilateral nephrectomy excludes an important vascular territory responsible for approximately 20% of the cardiac output, a methodological error would be masked by assuming that the same degree of aortic constriction was imposed on intact and nephrectomized rats. In order to circumvent this problem, preliminary experiments carried out in anephric animals showed that when aortic constriction is controlled by reducing the aortic blood flow Doppler shift to the same percentual extent as in the intact animals, the rise in pressure in the anephric rats does not attain the hypertensive levels observed in the former. These data also support the conclusion that the arterial pressure of the anephric animals does not rise to the same levels as in the intact animals, because anephric animals lack important hypertensive neuro-humoral factors such as AII and AVP[4,8] to increase resistance, being left with only the mechanical component of aortic constriction. Also favoring our methodological approach are findings[21] showing that 85% to 95% constriction of the aortic lumen is necessary to reduce the distal pressure of anesthetized dogs to 50 mm Hg. Moreover, unpublished results from our laboratory, comparing the proximal hypertensive response caused by total aortic occlusion with that evoked by partial occlusion, indicate that the degree of constriction necessary to reduce distal pressure to 50 mm Hg, as in the current protocol, is near maximal, as was also observed in anesthetized dogs[21].

In recent years, it has become increasingly evident that the renal nerves contribute to the control of renal function and to homeostasis under normal conditions and are important in the pathogenesis of hypertension[22]. It seems that renal nerves are involved in the early stages of hypertension in the spontaneously hypertensive rat; their importance in other forms of experimental hypertension is controversial[23]. There is evidence that afferent renal fibers carry mechanical and chemical information from the kidneys to specific brain nuclei which may influence neuro-humoral control of the kidney itself, or the circulation in general[23,24]. More recently, it has been demonstrated that sensory information from the kidney alters the release of AVP from the neurohypophysis, suggesting that afferent renal nerves (ARN) are an important component of the neural circuitry controlling arterial pressure[9]. In previous studies[8,4], it has been shown that in addition to AII, AVP participates in the onset of acute aortic coarctation hypertension. In the present study, experiments performed in conscious renal-denervated rats permitted us to investigate the contribution of sensory information originating in the kidneys to the release of AVP during an acute hypertensive response to partial aortic occlusion. The hypertensive response observed in renal-denervated rats did not differ significantly from that observed in intact animals. Moreover, the previous intravenous administration of the AVP V_1-vascular receptor antagonist $d(CH_2)_5Tyr(Me)AVP$ to renal-denervated rats did not change the hypertensive response of these animals when compared to that of untreated renal-denervated subjects. The lack of an effect of the V_1-vascular receptor antagonist on the hypertensive response of renal-denervated subjects indicates that AVP is not playing a role in this response, presumably due to the absence of sensory information from the kidneys to the central nervous system (CNS) needed to release AVP. In contrast, when renal-denervated rats were treated with saralasin, the hypertensive response following partial aortic coarctation was significantly blunted throughout the (45 min) experiment. These data are consistent with those previously observed in anephric rats[(4)] and also in intact animals treated with $d(CH_2)_5Tyr(Me)AVP$ plus saralasin[(8)]. Taken together, the data from 3 different models, i.e., anephric, intact animals treated with $d(CH_2)_5Tyr(Me)AVP$ plus saralasin and renal-denervated rats treated with saralasin only or saralasin plus $d(CH_2)_5Tyr(Me)AVP$, reveal a partial role for the mechanical component in the pathogenesis of acute aortic coarctation acting in concert with neuro-humoral (AVP and AII) factors. In addition, the results obtained with renal-denervated rats treated with saralasin permit one to hypothesize that when one of the pathophysiological mechanisms responsible for the hypertensive response is hampered, in the present case AVP due to lack of signalling from the kidneys, other mechanism, e.g. RAS, can assume a major role in increasing the arterial pressure associated with the mechanical component of constriction.

Total renal denervation is not selective in eliminating renal sensory input to the CNS, affecting also efferent axons to the kidney. Moreover, if compared to dorsal rhizotomy, total renal denervation is less permanent, damaged axons beginning to grow again within a few days[(25)]. Accordingly, care must be taken in the interpretation of results obtained with total renal-denervated rats. Nevertheless, Whitlow and Katholi[(26)] demonstrated that the attenuation of chronic coarctation in dogs, produced by renal denervation, did not involve changes of sodium excretion or PRA, thus providing indirect evidence that renal afferent feedback plays a role in the pathogenesis of this form of hypertension. In the present study, we associated an acute protocol (45 min duration) of aortic coarctation with total renal denervation performed 3 days earlier. The hypertensive response observed presumably did not involve water or salt reabsorption, but does not rule out a certain loss of renal function leading to the accumulation of AVP[(27)], or other vasoactive peptides, under low renal perfusion pressure. Although total renal denervation was ineffective in determining the final level of hypertension following chronic infusion of AII[28], it did significantly attenuate the pressor response during the first 6 days. The results of the current study indicate that renal denervation, performed 3 days before the acute aortic constriction, was able to prevent the sensory information from the kidneys to the CNS required for AVP release. The lack of sensory information was inferred from the failure of the AVP antagonist to attenuate the late (30–45 min) hypertensive response promoted by aortic constriction in renal-denervated rats, contrary to what had previously been observed in intact animals[8].

Because aortic constriction above the renal arteries exposes a large territory to low perfusion pressure, a role for afferent innervation from other visceral organs signalling the CNS to release AVP cannot be ruled out. Splanchnic receptors are physiologically involved in the regulation of AVP release in conscious rats, following salt and water intake[29]. These data indicate a role for renal afferents controlling AVP release and presumably regulating arterial pressure in conscious rats.

Acknowledgements

We thank Dr. M.A.P. Franco (Department of Genetics and Mathematics Applied to Biology, FMRP–USP) and Mrs. Denise B.P. Jorge for assistance with the statistical analysis, and Mr. M. Oliveira and Mr. J.A. Castania for technical support.

This work was supported by FAPESP (Fundação de Amparo à Pesquisa do Estado de São Paulo, grant nº 88/2522-0), FINEP (Financiadora de Estudos e Projetos, grant nº 43.87.0656.00) and CNPq (Conselho Nacional de Desenvolvimento Científico e Tecnológico, grant nº 30168£4/87-1/BF/BV).

References

1. Blumgart, H.L., J.S. Lawrence and A.C. Ernstene, The dynamics of the circulation in coarctation (stenosis of the isthmus) of the aorta of the adult type. Arch. Intern. Med. 47, 806-823 (1931).

2. Goldblatt, H., J.R. Kahn and R.F. Hanzal, The effect on blood pressure of constriction of the abdominal aorta above and below the site of origin of both main renal arteries, J. Exp. Med. 69, 649-674 (1937).

3. Maio, A.A., E.D. Moreira, H.C. Salgado and E.M. Krieger, Cardiovascular responses of conscious rats due to arterial occlusion (Abstr.), Braz. J. Med. Biol. Res. 14, 115 (1981).

4. Salgado, H.C. and E.M. Krieger, Mechanical and renin-angiotensin system components in acute aortic coarctation hypertension, Hypertension 8, I133-I136 (1986).

5. DiBona, G.F., The functions of the renal nerves, Rev. Physiol. Biochem. Pharmacol. 94, 75-181 (1982).

6. Recordati, G.M., N.G. Moss and L. Waselkov. Renal chemoreceptors in the rat, Circ. Res. 43, 534-543 (1978).

7. Recordati, G.M., N.G. Moss, S. Genovesi and P.R. Rogenes, Renal receptors in the rat sensitive to chemical alterations of their environment, Cir. Res. 46, 395-405 (1980).

8. Salgado, H.C. and M.C.O. Salgado, Acute aortic coarctation hypertension: role of vasopressin and angiotensin II, Am. J. Physiol. 257 (Heart Cir. Physiol. 26), H1480-H1484 (1989).

9. Caverson, M.M. and J. Ciriello, Effect of stimulation of afferent renal nerves on plasma levels of vasopressin, Am. J. Physiol. 252 (Regulatory Integrative Comp. Physiol. 21), R801-R807 (1987).

10. Haywood, J.R., R.A. Shaffer, C. Fastenow, G.D. Fink and M.J. Brody, Regional blood flow measurement with pulsed-Doppler flowmeter in conscious rat, Am. J. Physiol. 241 (Heart Circ. Physiol. 10), H273-H278 (1981).

11. Arendshorst, W.J., W.F. Finn and C.W Gottschalk, Autoregulation of blood flow in the rat kidney, Am. J. Physiol. 228, 127-133 (1975).

12. Gill, J.L., Repeated measurement: sensitive tests for experiments with few animals, J. Anim. Sci. 63, 943-954 (1986).

13. Gill, J.L., Repeated measurement: split-plot trend analysis versus analysis of first differences, Biometrics 44, 289-297 (1988).

14. Dunnett, C.W., A multiple comparison procedure for comparing several treatments with a control, J. Am. Stat. Association 50, 1096-1121 (1965).

15. Eklof, A.-C. and A. Aperia, Renal function in different forms of renovascular hypertension in rats, Acta. Physiol. Scand. 136, 487-492 (1989).

16. Eklof, A.-C. and A. Aperia, Renal hypertension following aortic constriction is abolished by angiotensin II converting enzyme inhibitor, but not by low-salt diet, Acta. Physiol. Scand. 139, 435-440 (1990).

17. Whitlow, P.L. and R.E. Katholi, Neurohumoral mechanisms in acute aortic coarctation in conscious and anesthetized dogs, Am. J. Physiol. (Heart Circ. Physiol. 13), H614-H621 (1983).

18. Bagby, S.P. and E.F. Fuchs, Chronic MK421 fails to modify evolution of hypertension in neonatally coarcted pups, Hypertension 13, 91-101 (1989).

19. Stene, J.K., B. Burns, S. Permutt, P. Caldini and M. Shannoff, Increased cardiac output following occlusion of the descending thoracic aorta in dogs, Am. J. Physiol. (Regulatory Integrative Comp. Physiol. 12), R152-R158 (1982).

20. Moreira, E.D., F. Ida and E.M. Krieger, Extent of rapid baroreceptor resetting during the first hours of hypertension, Am. J. Physiol. 257 (Heart and Cir. Physiol.26), H711-H716 (1989).

21. Katholi, R.E., Renal nerves in the pathogenesis of hypertension in experimental animals and humans, Am. J. Physiol. 245 (Renal Fluid Electrolyte Physiol. 14), F1-F14 (1983).

22. Gupta, T.C. and C.J. Wiggers, Basic hemodynamic changes produced by aortic coarctation of different degrees, Circulation III, 17-31 (1951).

23. Kline, R.L., Renal nerves and experimental hypertension: evidence and controversy, Can. J. Physiol. Pharmacol. 65, 1540-1547 (1987).

24. Moss, N.G., Renal function and renal afferent and efferent nerve activity, Am. J. Physiol. 243 (Renal Fluid Electrolyte Physiol.12), F425-F433, (1982).

25. Wyss, J.M., N. Aboukarsh and S. Oparil, Sensory denervation of the kidneys attenuates renovascular hypertension in the rat, Am. J. Physiol. 250 (Heart Circ. Physiol. 19), H82-H86 (1986).

26. Whitlow, P.L. and R.E. Katholi, Neuro-humoral activity and the role of the renal nerves in canine coarctation of the aorta (Abstr.), Am. J. Cardiol. 49, 888 (1982).

27. Rabkin, R., P.A. Payne, J. Young and J. Crofton, The handling of immunoreactive vasopressin by the isolated perfusate rat kidney, J. Clin. Invest. 63, 6-13 (1979).

28. Vari, R.C., S. Zinn, K.W. Verburg and R.H. Freeman, Renal nerves and the pathogenesis of angiotensin-induced hypertension, Hypertension 9, 345-349 (1987).

29. Kwon, S.C., R. McCarty and A.J. Baertschi, Splanchnic osmoreceptors control plasma vasopressin (AVP) in conscious rats (Abstr.), The FASEB Journal 3, A245 (1989).

AAS 36
Contributions to
Autacoid Pharmacology

FROM BRADYKININ AND SNAKE VENOM PEPTIDES TO NEUROPEPTIDE CONVERSION AND INACTIVATION

A.C.M. Camargo

Department of Pharmacology, Biomedical Sciences Institute, University of São Paulo, 05508 São Paulo, SP, Brazil

In many aspects, the work developed by Professor Maurício Rocha e Silva is connected to the history of the biologically active polypeptides. Besides his direct involvement with the discovery of bradykinin(1), Rocha e Silva's name is associated with two additional aspects of the biochemistry and pharmacology of neuropeptides: first of all the concept of partial proteolysis in the generation of bioactive peptides and secondly, the discovery of inhibitors of kinin inactivation and angiotensin conversion(2,3). His views on these two subjects underlied my initial scientific engagement in 1964. I was very lucky to be among the researchers who had the privilege to start their scientific carriers in the Department of Pharmacology directed by Rocha e Silva and I believe that there has not been a similar opportunity in the past 30 years. Indeed, twenty years ago when the neuropeptide revolution was just getting under way, research on metabolism of biologically active peptides was still quiet and relatively inactive in the area of biomedical sciences.

I graduated in Medicine from the Faculty of Medicine of Ribeirão Preto, University of São Paulo, in 1964. In 1962 as a student, I had been engaged in a research project in the Department of Pharmacology under the supervision of Dr. Sergio Steiner Cardoso. My initial research project was related to the control of cell multiplication in the liver of partially hepatectomized rats. In 1965, after having been appointed Assistant of Pharmacology by professor Rocha e Silva, I was still working on the same subject. I was the

Abbreviations used: **BK**, Bradykinin, **DFP**, Diisopropylfluor phosphate, **EDTA**, Ethylenediaminete, **LHRH**, Luteinizing Hormone-Releasing Hormone, **BAM-12P**, Bovine Adrenal Medulla Duodecapep.

only member of the Department of Pharmacology not working on any subject related to bradykinin or histamine. Professor Rocha e Silva was not happy with the development of my research project specially after reading the outline of my plans for the doctorate. He not only disapproved of those plans but also gave me an ultimatum to move to one of the research projects being pursued in the Department in 1966. The project which I found to suit my motivations was being carried out by Frederico Graeff who had discovered that the neurovegetative and behavioural effects of bradykinin injected into the fourth ventricle of rabbit brain were substantially potentiated by peptides extracted from *Bothrops jararaca* venom. The most logical interpretation of this result was that snake venom peptides could somehow protect bradykinin from degradation in the brain. Using the isolated guinea pig ileum as a biossay to monitor bradykinin inactivation, I was surprised to find a high kinin-destroying (kininase) activity in rabbit brain homogenates. At the time, less than a dozen reports on proteolytic activity in nervous tissue at neutral pH were known. I felt that brain bradykinin inactivating enzymes were involved in the mechanism of neuronal communication rather than being part of the overall protein turnover mechanism. I asked Professor Rocha e Silva whether he would agree with a new research project, ultimately aimed at studying the role of brain peptidases in the process of neurotransmission. This hypothesis was rather naive but it generated the strength which I am still using in my research activity. Professor Rocha e Silva agreed with this project provided that I accepted him as adviser. I cannot state that he was a good adviser; he certainly did not act as the classical prototype. Nevertheless, his approval of my thesis project represented a guarantee that I had initiated a promising line of research, in which I knew that I would have to do everything by myself. Within a few weeks, I found that the enzymes which were responsible for bradykinin degradation were active at neutral or slightly alkaline pH; they were probably cysteine-proteinases, because they were activated by thiols, inactivated by heavy metals and p-hydroxy-mercuribenzoate but not affected by **EDTA** or **DFP**. I also found 70% of the kininase activity of the brain homogenates to be concentrated in the cytosol. The remaining activity was present in the mitochondrial fraction. These preliminary observations were published[(4)]. More detailed data[(5)] included results of my doctorate thesis. The main tool for the determination of enzyme activity was biossay on the isolated guinea pig ileum; it allowed us to show that besides kininases, the cytosol contained aminopeptidases which convert [Lys^1]-BK and [Met^1, Lys^2]Bk into BK and were partially separated from kininase-endopeptidases, by gel filtration on Sephadex G-100.

In January 1970, I was compelled to rapidly leave Brazil to escape political persecution. I had been invited by Dr. Lewis J. Greene to spend 6 months in his laboratory at Brookhaven National Laboratory, USA, purifying brain enzymes responsible for kinin conversion and degradation. With the help of Dr. Warwick Kerr, then Scientific Director of Research Foundation of the State of São Paulo (FAPESP), I obtained a post-doctoral fellowship within less than one week, and went to Brookhaven, my wife 7-8 months pregnant and my two boys 5 and 6 years old. It was my first trip abroad. We left São Paulo at a temperature of 32°C, to arrive in New York at −5°C. To illustrate how dramatic the change was, I remember my older son seriously asking me as soon as we got to Brookhaven, whether we had moved to another planet. The biology unit at Brookhaven National Laboratory was rather small, but an excellent place to learn protein chemistry and to develop a research project involving isolation and characterization of peptidases. Dr. Lewis Greene had a well equipped laboratory and the help of two very good technicians, Nicholas Alonzo and Roslyn Shapanka. Two other laboratories of Drs. Elliott Shaw and Darrel Liu, offered an exceptional environment to discuss and delineate research projects related to proteolytic enzymes. With the help of all of these persons, specially Dr. Greene, Nicholas Alonzo and Roslyn Shapanka it became possible to isolate and partially characterize a first enzyme, now classified as endooligopeptidase A (E.C.3.4.22.19). This cysteine protease is responsible for 70% of the degradation of bradykinin in the cytosol fraction of rabbit brain(6,7).

Returning to Brazil in January 1972, I hoped to set up a protein chemistry research laboratory and simultaneously train students and technicians. I was sure that this kind of laboratory would also help in the development of many other areas of research in the biomedical sciences. With the help of Dr. Lewis Greene, Nicholas Alonzo, Roslyn Shapanka and Eduardo B. Oliveira, the support of Professors Mauricio Rocha e Silva and Carlos Diniz and funds from FAPESP, the Protein Chemistry Laboratory of the School of Medicine of Ribeirão Preto was set up. After one year of intensive activity to organize minimum facilities, we were able to continue studies on brain peptidases. Eduardo Oliveira, Antonio R. Martins and myself were able to isolate a second endopeptidase, responsible for part of the remaining 30% of bradykinin degradation activity taking place in cytosol of rabbit brain(8), endooligopeptidase B(9). In February of 1973, Nicholas Alonso, Eduardo B. Oliveira and myself had good reasons to enjoy a Brazilian carnival: the first automatic aminoacid analyzer so far instaled in this half of the globe, gave its initial reliable amino acid analysis results.

Bradykinin-degrading enzymes from nervous tissue, seem to differ from other endopeptidases, in special from pancreatic proteinases, by being selectively active towards oligopeptides. This selectivity is in agreement with the hypothesis that these enzymes modulate the action of biologically active polypeptides, rather than merely partaking in overall protein metabolism in brain. Up to now, all experimental results have demonstrated that only peptides ranging in size between 7 and 13 aminoacid residues, are susceptible to hydrolysis by these brain endopeptidases[7,9,10]. Therefore, the name endooligopeptidases is justified to distinguish this class of enzymes from endopeptidases which hydrolyse proteins and larger peptides.

The seventies were marked by the discovery of a number of neuropeptides, whose size made most of them potential substrates for brain endooligopeptidases. However, substance P and [Leu^5] enkephalin were resistant to hydrolysis by endooligopeptidase A (data not published); LHRH was hydrolysed at the Tyr-Gly bond but only after endooligopeptidase B had previously removed the C-terminal Gly-NH_2 [11]. Angiotensin I and II were resistant to endooligopeptidase A (data not published), but susceptible to hydrolysis by endooligopeptidase B[12]. In 1980 we succeeded in purifying both endooligopeptidase A and B to apparent homogeneity; policlonal antibodies against either enzymes were raised[7].

In 1981, I visited several laboratories in Europe looking for a place where the immunocytochemical distribution of these enzymes in the central nervous system could be studied. In November of 1981, I gave a seminar to Dr. Leslie Iversen's group at the Neurochemical Pharmacology Unit (NPU) - MRC - Cambridge. After the seminar, Dr. Iversen invited me to spend 6 months at his laboratory to exploit the possible involvement of endooligopeptidase A and B in the metabolism of neurotensin and substance P. I started working with Dr. Pears Emson at NPU-Cambridge, in May of 1982. At the very first day of work at NPU, we found that both endooligopeptidase A and B were able to hydrolyse neurotensin. As expected, endooligopeptidase B was able to split off both proline residues of this neuropeptide; to our surprise however, endooligopeptidase A caused only one single cleavage at the Arg^8-Arg^9 bond[13]. This unexpected finding led us to question whether endooligopeptidase A could be involved in the processing of neuropeptides since, according to Steiner *et al.*[14], enzymes with this specificity could act as neuropeptide-processing endopeptidases. To test this hypothesis, we decided to try BAM-12P, a proenkephalin-derived peptide as a putative substrate. BAM-12P contains a pair of arginine residues following the [Met^5] enkephalin sequence; we expected to obtain [Met^5] enkephalin-Arg as one of the products of its hydrolysis. Again we were surprised to find that instead of cleaving the Arg^6-Arg^7 bond of the peptide, the enzyme directly released [Met^5] enkephalin by single cleavage[15]. This enkephalin-forming activity of endopeptidase 22.19 was further exploited in collaboration with Dr. Jean Rossier at the "Laboratorie de Physiologie Nerveuse", CNRS, Gif-sur-Yvette, France. In June of 1985, we were able to demonstrate that most enkephalin-containing peptides ranging in size between 7 and 13 aminoacid residues derived from pro-enkephalin and from prodynorphin, are converted to enkephalin by single cleavage[10,16,17]. The physiological role of endooligopeptidase A may be to participate in the metabolism of a number of oligopeptides; it is noteworthy however, that the immunohistochemical regional distribution of this enzyme in the rat CNS coincides with regions presenting high density of enkephalin containing neurons[18]. Recently it could be demonstrated, that the enzyme co-exists with enkephalin in neurones and is not present in neurones where enkephalin could not be found[19]. In collaboration with Dr. Luiz Juliano, Escola Paulista de Medicina) a quenched fluorescent enkephalin-derived peptide useful as an operational substrate, has been synthesized[20]. This is important because bradykinin had until now been the only reliable substrate available for endooligopeptidase activity determinations rendering them expensive and time consuming. The sequence of the endooligopeptidase A gene is being determined by Dr. O. Toffoletto, in collaboration with Dr. Jean Rossier, Gif-sur-Yvette, France.

We would like to conclude, by emphasizing the importance of Professor Mauricio Rocha e Silva as the most significant scientific referential for the beginning of my professional career. This work which had its origin in the Department of Pharmacology in Ribeirão Preto, was relatively fruitful if we consider all the difficulties of developing research in Brazil, specially in areas which demand technical and scientific support of good quality. Over 40 full papers and 15 doctorate projects on different aspects of neuropeptide metabolism, have been carried out. This line of research is increasingly motivating students and researchers among the Brazilian and international scientific community.

Acknowledgment

I thank Dr. Beatriz L. Fernandes for reviewing the manuscript and Mrs. Selma R.M. Regionati for typing it. Almost 100% of the financial support of the research developed in my laboratory was provided by FAPESP (Fundação de Amparo à Pesquisa do Estado de São Paulo).

References

1. Rocha e Silva, M., W.T. Beraldo and G. Rosenfeld, Bradykinin a new hypotensive and smooth muscle stimulating factor released from plasma globulin by snake venoms and by trypsin, Amer. J. Physiol. 156, 261, 1949.

2. Ferreira, S.H. and M. Rocha e Silva, Potentiation of bradykinin by dimercaptopropanol ('BAL) and other inhibitors of its destroying enzyme in plasma, Biochem. Pharmacol. 11, 1123-1128, 1962.

3. Ferreira, S.H. and M. Rocha e Silva, Potentiation of bradykinin and eledoisin by BPF (bradykinin potentiating factor) from *Bothrops jararaca* venom, Experientia 21, 347-349, 1965.

4. Camargo, A.C.M. and F.G. Graeff, Subcellular distribution and properties of the bradykinin inactivation system in rabbit brain homogenates, Biochem. Pharmacol. 18, 548-549, 1969.

5. Camargo, A.C.M., F.J. Ramalho and L.J. Greene. Brain peptidase: conversion and inactivation of kinin hormones. J. Neurochem. 119, 37-49, 1972.

6. Camargo, A.C.M., R. Shapanka and L.J. Greene, Preparation, assay and partial characterization of a neutral endopeptidase from rabbit brain, Biochemistry 12, 1838-1844, 1973.

7. Carvalho, K.M. and A.C.M. Camargo, Purification of rabbit brain endooligopeptidase and preparation of anti-enzyme antibodies, Biochemistry 20, 7082-7088, 1981.

8. Oliveira, E.B., A.R. Martins and A.C.M. Camargo, Isolation of brain endopeptidases. Influence of size and sequence of substrates structurally related to bradykinin, Biochemistry 16, 1967-1974, 1976.

9. Camargo, A.C.M., M.L. Reis and H. Caldo, Susceptibility of a peptide derived from bradykinin to hydrolysis by brain endo-oligopeptidases and pancreatic proteinases, J. Biol. Chem. 254, 5304-5307, 1979.

10. Camargo, A.C.M., E.B. Oliveira, O. Toffoletto, K.M. Metters and J. Rossier. Brain endo-olipeptidase A, a putative enkephalin converting enzyme, J. Neurochem. 48, 1258-1263, 1987.

11. Camargo, A.C.M., M.J.V. da Fonseca, H. Caldo and K.M. Camargo, Influence of the carboxyl terminus of luteinizing hormone-releasing hormone and bradykinin on hydrolysis by brain endo-oligopeptidases, J. Biol. Chem. 257, 9265-9267, 1982.

12. Greene, L.J., A.C. Spadaro, A.R. Martins, W.D. Perussi de Jesus and A.C.M. Camargo, Brain endo-oligopeptidase B. A post proline cleaving enzyme that inactivates angiotensin I and II, Hypertension 4(2), 178-184, 1982.

13. Camargo, A.C.M., H. Caldo and P.C. Emson, Degradation of neurotensin by rabbit brain endo-oligopeptidase A and endo-oligopeptidase B (Proline-endopeptidase), Biochem. Bioph. Res. Comm. 166(3), 1151-1159, 1983.

14. Steiner, D.F., D.S. Quinn, S.J. Chan, J. Marsh and H.S. Tager, Processing mechanisms in the biosynthesis of protein, Ann. N.Y. Acad. Sci. 343, 1-16, 1980.

15. Camargo, A.C.M., M.J.V.F. Ribeiro and W. Schwartz, Conversion and inactivation of opioid peptides by rabbit brain endo-oligopeptidase A, Biochem. Biophys. Res. Comm. 130, 932-938, 1985.

16. Toffoletto, O., K.M. Metters, E.B. Oliveira, J. Rossier and A.C.M. Camargo, Enkephalin is liberated from [Met^5] enkephalin-R-R-V-NH2 and Dynorphin A_{1-8} by endo-oligopeptidase A but not by metalloendopeptidase EC 3.4.24.15, Biochem. J. 252, 35-38, 1988.

17. Cicilini, M.A., M.J.V.F. Ribeiro, E.B. Oliveira, R.A. Mortara and A.C.M. Camargo, Endo-oligopeptidase A activity in rabbit heart, generation of enkephalin from enkephalin-containing peptides, Peptides 9, 945-946, 1988.

18. Oliveira, E.S., P.E.P. Leite, M.G. Spillarini, A.C.M. Camargo and S.P. Hunt, Localization of endo-oligopeptidase (E.C.3.4.22.19) in the rat nervous tissue, J. Neurochem. 55, 1114-1121, 1990.

19. Ferro, E.S., D.E. Hamassaki, A.C.M. Camargo and L.R.G. Britto, Endooligopeptidase A, a putative enkephalin-generating enzyme in the vertebrate retina, J. Neurochem. (in press).

20. Juliano, L., J.R. Chagas, I.Y. Hirata, E. Carmona, M. Sucupira, E.S. Oliveira, E.B. Oliveira and A.C.M. Camargo. A selective assay for endo-oligopeptidase A based on the cleavage of fluorogenic substrate structurally related to enkephalin, Biochem. Biophys. Res. Comm. 173, 647-652, 1990.

AAS 36
Contributions to
Autacoid Pharmacology

THE LIVER AND THE KALLIKREIN-KININ SYSTEM: A BRIEF REVIEW

D.R. Borges

Gastroenterology Division, Escola Paulista de Medicina, São Paulo, SP, Brazil

A. Introduction

A review on liver modulation of the kallikrein-kinin system, carried out at the Escola Paulista de Medicina, is presented.

Liver participated albeit serendipitously, in the discovery of bradykinin; as reported by Rocha e Silva:

– "In 1948, Beraldo, Rosenfeld and I were interested to discover whether the venom of the *B. jararaca* liberated histamine from dog's liver, as trypsin had been shown to do. The liver was perfused with defibrinated blood through the portal vein and the perfusates collected in the inferior vena cava just above the diaphragm. Since dog's blood practically does not contain histamine or any substance stimulating the guinea-pig gut, the perfusates were assayed directly upon the gut after the muscle had been desensitized to the venom. As soon as the venom was injected into the perfusing cannula, the perfusates acquired enormous activity upon the guinea-pig ileum. This activity was obviously not due to histamine, since the type of contraction observed was entirely different from that produced by histamine. Furthermore, antihistaminics or atropine did not have the slightest effect upon it. Very puzzling was the fact that the substance disappeared very quickly from the perfusates when they were left for half an hour at room temperature; even more disturbing was the fact that even in the absence of the liver, when the venom was put directly into the blood samples, the same effect could be observed upon the gut. It was obvious that the precursor of this substance was in the blood itself and not in the liver."[(1)]

B. Kinin Catabolism by the Perfused Rat Liver

1. *Kinin-converting aminopeptidase*

The isolated, exsanguinated and perfused rat liver, converts the peptides Gly-Arg-Lys-Bk, Met-Lys-Bk and Lys-Bk, into bradykinin (BK) at a high rate[2]. A kinin- converting aminopeptidase, which had no kininase activity, was purified from human liver[3]. This chloride-independent enzyme is inhibited by puromycin and chelating agents (EDTA and 1,10-phenantroline). The activity of the 1,10-phenantroline-inhibited enzyme was restored by addition of Co^{2+}, Zn^{2+} or Mn^{2+}. These properties, as well the hydrolysis rates at L-aminoacyl-beta-naphthylamides, Met-Lys-Bk, Lys-Bk and Leu-Gly-Gly, suggested that the liver[3,4] is the source of the kinin-converting aminopeptidase purified from plasma[5]. This enzyme is possibly soluble alanyl aminopeptidase (sAAP) EC 3.4.11.14[6].

The perfused liver deactivates angiotensin II very efficiently[7]. Although the hepatic enzyme(s) responsible for this activity has(ve) not been characterized, the possibility exists that this angiotensinase activity is at least in part, also due to sAAP.

2. *Bradykinin-inactivating endopeptidase*

A rat preparation in which the perfusion route bypassed the lungs was shown to inactivate BK efficiently[2]. When the isolated and exsanguinated rat liver was perfused, we verified that following a single passage, about 90% of nanomole amounts of BK were deactivated in a dose-dependent manner. At the highest BK concentration tried (19×10^{-6} M), 1 g of liver inactivated 18 nmoles in a single passage through the organ[7]. Although the perfused liver also converts angiotensin I (AI) to AII, this conversion occurs at a much slower rate than the inactivation of BK. Indeed, BK, amides of BK and of bradykinylglycine are inactivated by the perfused liver at similar rates[8], suggesting that the inactivation of BK is not due to exopeptidases that require a free carboxyl group such as the angiotensin-converting enzyme (ACE) (EC 3.4.15.1) or plasma carboxypeptidase B (EC 3.4.17.3) [9,6].

A BK-inactivating endopeptidase, which hydrolyses the Phe^5-Ser^6 bond of BK, was purified from rat liver[10]. The fragments Arg^1-Phe^5 and Ser^6-Arg^9 may be further degraded by the perfused rat liver through the action of ACE[7]. The BK-inactivating 68 kDa, neutral serine-endopeptidase can be removed from the perfused liver by 0.05% Triton X-100; it has no angiotensinase activity[8].

Figure 1 summarizes the hypothesis that the perfused liver activates kinins/deactivates angiotensins via sAAP, and activates angiotensin I/deactivates kinins via

ACE. We postulate that the bradykinin-inactivating endopeptidase is the major kininase acting in the perfused liver.

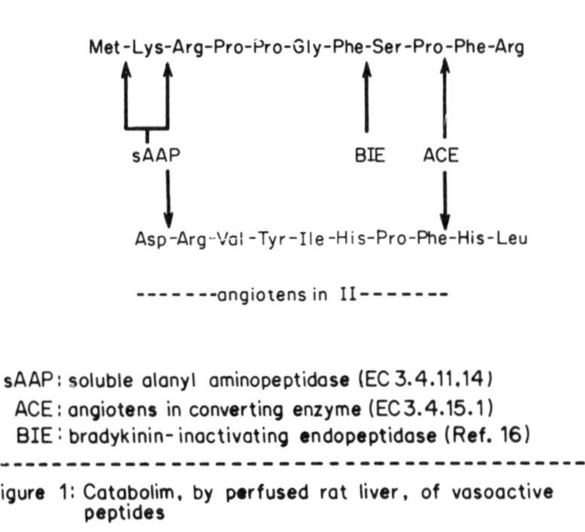

Fig. 1. Catabolism, by perfused rat liver, of vasoactive peptides.

3. *Bradykinin and portal hypertension*

Bradykinin is one of the most potent endogenous substances causing arterial/systemic hypotension. Nevertheless, BK administered as a single injection into the reservoir of the fluid perfusing the liver causes an elevation of the portal pressure, lasting about 2 minutes. A second injection, given within 5 minutes gave no response; the sensitivity was recovered within about 10 minutes(7). The molar concentrations of some vasoactive substances necessary for an equivalent increase of portal pressure of perfused rat liver are: 3×10^{-8} (angiotensin II), 5×10^{-8} (angiotensin I), 3×10^{-7} (histamine), 3×10^{-6} (bradykinin) and 5×10^{-6} (adrenaline)(7). A role for bradykinin in the pathogenesis of diseases leading to portal hypertension has not been studied.

C. Kininogen and Prokallikrein Synthesis and the Acute-Phase Response

The liver synthesizes kininogens(11) and prokallikrein(12). In humans, plasma prokallikrein concentration, is a very sensitive indicator of liver protein-synthesizing capacity(13) as well as a good prognostic indicator in chronic liver insufficiency(14). Liver synthesis of total kininogen[11] and prokallikrein[15], increases during the acute-phase response. Among the different molecular forms of kininogen, T-kininogen, found only in rats, is an acute-phase protein[16]. In the acute-phase situation in rats, the synthesis of some plasma-kallikrein inhibitors (alpha$_2$-macroglobulin, C1-esterase inhibitor) also increases.

We verified that during the acute-phase response to an inflammatory stimulus, less BK is liberated from a rat paw when heated at 45°C [15]. This result fits the counter-irritancy model, by which a reduced response to an irritant is to be expected if the recipient has already received an irritant stimulus.

D. Receptor-Mediated Endocytosis of Circulating Kallikreins by the Liver

The liver is the main organ to clear both human and rat plasma kallikreins, as well as tissue kallikreins, from rat plasma in vivo[17]. Tissue kallikreins circulating in plasma are poorly inhibited by plasma proteins. This means that an efficient mechanism, other than inhibition, is necessary to regulate plasma concentration of tissue kallikreins. We have shown that pig pancreatic and horse urinary kallikreins are endocytozed by liver cells through respectively, calcium-dependent mannosyl and galactosyl-specific lectins[18]. Rat plasma kallikrein, on the other hand, is cleared by the perfused rat liver by a calcium-independent mechanism and is metabolized by liver cell lysosomes[19]. The plasma kallikrein site binding to hepatocytes, is located on kallikrein's heavy chain; it is not exposed on prokallikrein[20]. The liver, which synthesizes the pro-enzyme and clears active kallikrein does not, per se, activate plasma kallikrein[12]. The liver receptor that binds plasma kallikrein is probably a S-type lectin[21] present in mammalian as well as in avian livers[22]. We recently verified that liver clearance rate of plasma kallikrein increases during the acute-phase response[23], and is not altered by chronic administration of ethanol[24].

In summary we can say that the liver:

1. synthesizes kininogens and prokallikrein;
2. converts precursors into bradykinin and angiotensin II;
3. deactivates kinins and angiotensins, and
4. clears circulating kallikreins through receptor-mediated mechanisms.

These liver properties are affected by the acute-phase response to inflammation, in which the kallikrein-kinin system plays a major role.

References

1. Rocha e Silva, M., Bradykinin: occurrence and properties, In: Polypeptides which stimulate plain muscle, pp. 45-57 (Ed. J.H. Gaddum). E. and S. Livingstone Ltd., Edinburgh and London 1955.

2. Prado, J.L., E.A. Limãos, J. Roblero, J.O. Freitas, E.S. Prado and A.C.M. Paiva, Recovery and conversion of kinins in exsanguinated rat preparations, Naunyn-Schmiedeberg's Arch. Pharmacol. 290, 191-205 (1975).

3. Borges, D.R., J.L. Prado and J.A. Guimarães, Characterization of a kinin-converting arylaminopeptidase from human liver, Naunyn-Schmiedeberg's Arch. Pharmacol. 281, 403-14 (1974).

4. Freitas Jr., J.O., J.A. Guimarães, D.R. Borges and J.L. Prado, Two arylamidases from human liver and their kinin-converting activity, Int. J. Biochem. 10, 81-9 (1979).

5. Guimarães, J.A., D.R. Borges, E.S. Prado and J.L. Prado, Kinin-converting aminopeptidase from human serum, Biochem. Pharmacol. 22, 3157-73 (1973).

6. McDonald, J.K. and A.J. Barrett, Mammalian Proteases, Vol. 2, Exopeptidases. Academic Press 1986.

7. Borges, D.R., E.A. Limãos, J.L. Prado and A.C.M. Camargo, Catabolism of vasoactive polypeptides by perfused rat liver, Naunyn-Schmiedeberg's Arch. Pharmacol. 295, 33-40 (1976).

8. Borges, D.R., J.A. Guimarães, E.A. Limãos, J.L. Prado and A.C.M. Camargo, Bradykinin inactivation by perfused rat liver: role of a thiol activated endopeptidase, Naunyn-Schmiedeberg's Arch. Pharmacol. 309, 197-201 (1979).

9. Erdös, E.G., Kininases, Handbook Experimental Pharmacology, In: Bradykinin, Kallidin and Kallikrein, Supplement to vol. XXV, pp. 427-487 (Ed. E.G. Erdös). Springer-Verlag, Heidelberg 1979.

10. Kouyoumdjian, M., D.R. Borges and J.L. Prado, Kinin-inactivating endopeptidase from rat liver, Int. J. Biochem. 16, 733-9 (1984).

11. Borges, D.R. and A.H. Gordon, Kininogen and kininogenase synthesis by the liver of normal and injured rats, J. Pharm Pharmacol. 28, 44-8 (1976).

12. Borges, D.R., M.E. Webster, J.A. Guimarães and J.L. Prado, Synthesis of prekallikrein and metabolism of plasma kallikrein by perfused rat liver, Biochem. Pharmacol. 30, 1065-9 (1981).

13. Manoukian, N. and D.R. Borges, Prealbumin, prekallikrein and prothrombin in hepatosplenic schistosomiasis: increased turnover of the clotting proteins?, Rev. Inst. Med. Trop. São Paulo. 26, 237-40 (1984).

14. Agnholt, J., J.H. Mikkelsen, M.I. Bud, J. Moller-Petersen, S.N. Rasmussen and J. Dyerberg, Plasma prekallikrein as a prognostic indicator in chronic liver insufficiency, Scand. J. Gastroenterol. 25, 40-4 (1990).

15. Limãos, E.A., D.R. Borges, J.C. Souza-Pinto, A.H. Gordon and J.L. Prado, Acute turpentine inflammation and kinin release in rat-paw thermic oedema, Brit. J. Exp. Pathol. 62, 591-4 (1981).

16. Greenbaum, L.M., T-kinin and T-kininogen. A historical overview, Adv. Exp. Med. Biol. 198PA, 55-9 (1986).

17. Borges, D.R., C.A.M. Sampaio, P. Llosa and J.L. Pradom, The liver is the main organ to clear plasma and tissue kallikreins from rat plasma in vivo, Adv. Exp. Med. Biol. 198A, 229-33 (1986).

18. Kouyoumdjian, M., D.R. Borges, E.S. Prado and J.L. Prado, Identification of receptors in the liver that mediate endocytosis of circulating tissue kallikreins, Biochim. Biophys. Acta. 980, 299-304 (1989).

19. Borges, D.R., A.H. Gordon, J.A. Guimarães and J.L. Prado, Rat plasma kallikrein clearance by perfused rat liver, Braz J. Med. Biol. Res. 18, 187-94 (1985).

20. Borges, D.R. and M. Kouyoumdjian, The recognition factor for clearance of plasma kallikrein is located on its heavy chain and not exposed on prokallikrein. (Submitted).

21. Borges, D.R. and M. Kouyoumdjian, The hepatocytic clearance of plasma kallikrein may be mediated by a S-type lectin, VI Congress PAABS, p. 206, N-6 (Abstr.) (1990).

22. Borges, D.R., M. Kouyoumdjian and E.A. Limãos, Native plasma kallikrein is cleared at similar rates by mammalian and avian livers, Braz. J. Med. Biol. Res. 24, 63-5 (1991).

23. Martins, B., M. Kouyoumdjian, E.A. Limãos and D.R. Borges, The hepatic clearance rate of plasma kallikrein increases during the acute-phase response, VI Congress PAABS, p. 205, N-5 (Abstr.) (1990).

24. Toledo, C.F. and D.R. Borges, Chronic administration of ethanol does not alter plasma kallikrein hepatic clearance, Braz. J. Med. Biol. Res. 23, 409-15 (1990).

AAS 36
Contributions to
Autacoid Pharmacology

THE ORIGIN OF KININ IN HUMAN URINE

V. Hial

Faculdade de Medicina do Triângulo Mineiro, Uberaba, MG, Brazil

First of all I should state that it is a great honor to be part of the group paying tribute to the memory of Prof. Mauricio Rocha e Silva in his 80º birthday.

The history of the kallikrein-kinin system began when Abelous and Bardier(1) and Frey(2) found that the intravenous injection of normal urine caused a transient fall in blood pressure in experimental animals. The presence of biologically active polypeptides in urine, which could be responsible for this effect was demonstrated by Beraldo(3). A polypeptide (substance Z) found in normal human urine lowered the blood pressure and contracted isolated smooth muscle preparations of various laboratory animals(4,5). Gomes(6) suggested the identity of this peptide with bradykinin. Gaddum and Horton(7) referred to it as urinary kinin.

More than one kinin exists in human urine. Major ones are lysil-bradykinin and bradykinin. The former is the product of the action of urinary kallikrein(8,9). Bradykinin is probably formed by an aminopeptidase which cleaves the amino-terminal lysine from lysil-bradykinin(8,10). Methionyl-lysil-bradykinin, a third kinin, was found in pooled normal urine, processed shortly after collection; it was not detected in urine stored in the frozen state. When human urine was collected into a medium of low pH, the three kinins bradykinin, lys-bradykinin and met-lys-bradykinin could be detected and separated by chromatography on SP-Sephadex C-25(11). When the pepsin inhibitor, pepstatin, was added to acidified urine, met-lys-bradykinin was either not detected or reduced by 90 percent. Addition of purified kininogen to acidified urine from a subject with congenital absence of kininogen led to the formation of met-lys-bradykinin but not bradykinin or lys-bradykinin(12,13). It is highly probable that at low pH, uropepsinogen is activated to uropepsin which acts on kininogen to produce met-lys-bradykinin. We demonstrated that met-lys-bradykinin was the kinin formed when porcine pepsin was incubated with highly purified human plasma kininogens[(14)]. Using high performance liquid chromatography for separation and radioimmunoassay for quantification, a new kinin (ala^3)-lys-bradykinin, was found in freshly voided human urine[(15)]. Low molecular weight human kininogens yielded kinins (76% lys-bradykinin, 7% bradykinin and 17% (ala^3)-lys-bradykinin, following incubation with human urinary kallikrein[(15)]. Another kinin, with hydroxyproline in position 3 has been reported[(16)]. These striking results lead to the question of how many kinin precursors exist in human urine. The story of kinins in human urine continues. Research means: to search again.

References

1. Abelous, J.E. and E. Bardier, Les substances hypotensives de l'urine humaine normale, C. R. Soc. Biol. 66, 511-512 (1909).

2. Frey, E.K., Zusammenhänge zwischen Herzarbeit und Nierentätigkeit, Arch. Klin. Chir. 142, 117-124 (1926).

3. Beraldo, W.T., Substance U- a depressor and smooth muscle stimulating principle present in urine, Am. J. Physiol. 171, 371-377 (1952).

4. Werle, E. and E.G. Erdös, XIXth International Physiological Congress, Montreal, Canada, Abstracts of Communications, p. 878.

5. Werle, E. and E.G. Erdös, Über eine neue blutdrucksenkende, darm-und uterus-erregende Substanz im menschlichen Urin, Naunyn-Schmiedeberg's Arch. Exp. Path Pharmak. 223, 234-243 (1954).

6. Gomes, F.P., A slow contracting substance in normal human urine, Br. J. Pharmac. 10, 200-207 (1955).

7. Gaddum, J. H. and E.W. Horton, The extraction of human urinary kinin (Substance Z) and its relation to the plasma kinins, Br. J. Pharmac. 14, 117-124 (1959).

8. Webster, M.E. and J.V. Pierce, The nature of the kallidins released from human plasma by kallikreins and other enzymes, Ann. N.Y. Acad. Sci. 104, 91-107 (1963).

9. Alhenc-Gelas, F., J. Marchetti, J. Allegrini, P. Corvol and J. Menard, Measurement of urinary kallikrein activity species differences in kinin production, Biochem. Biophys. Acta 677, 477-488 (1981).

10. Guimarães, J.A., D.R. Borges, E.S. Prado and J.L. Prado, Kinin-converting aminopeptidase from human serum, Biochem. Pharmac. 22, 3157-3172 (1973).

11. Miwa, I., E.G. Erdös and T. Seki, Separation of peptide components of urinary kinin (Substance Z), Proc. Soc. Exp. Biol. Med. 131, 768-772 (1969).

12. Hial, V., H.R. Keiser and J.J. Pisano, Methionyl-lysyl-bradykinin (MLBK) in human urine and the absence of kinins in subjects with congenital deficiency of kininogen, Federation Proc. 35, 692 (1976a).

13. Hial, V., H.R. Keiser and J.J. Pisano, Origin and Content of methionyl-lysyl-bradykinin and bradykinin in human urine. Biochem. Pharmac. 25, 2499-2503 (1976b).

14. Guimarães, J.A., J.V. Pierce, V. Hial and J.J. Pisano, In: Kinins: Pharmacodynamics and Biological Roles, p. 265 (Eds. F. Sicuteri, N. Back and G.L. Haberland). Plenum, New York 1976.

15. Mindroiu, T., G. Scicli, F. Perini, O.A. Carretero and A.G. Scicli, Identification of a new kinin in human urine, J. Biol. Chem. 261, 7407-7411 (1986).

16. Sasaguri, M., M. Ikeda, M. Ideishi and K. Arakawa, Identification of (hydroxiproline^3)-lysyl-bradykinin released from human plasma protein by kallikrein, Biochem. Biophys. Res. Commun. 150, 511-516 (1988).

AAS 36
Contributions to
Autacoid Pharmacology

PEPTIDES POTENTIATING KININ ACTIONS: A REVIEW

J. Assreuy, P.D. Fernandes, A.C. Resende, M.S. Rodrigues and R. Schaffel

Department of Pharmacology, ICB, Federal University of Rio de Janeiro, 21944 Rio de Janeiro, RJ, Brazil

Introduction

Quantitative and qualitative analysis of the involvement of agonists in physio-pharmacological processes usually requires the use of potent and specific antagonists. The description and synthesis of kinin receptor antagonists has only recently become available[1,2]. Although studies using antagonists rather than potentiators have been much more frequent in Pharmacology, the use of potentiators has been essential for the development of knowledge in the kinin field. Several substances, mainly peptides exhibiting differences in specificity and potency, can potentiate the actions of kinins *in vivo* and *in vitro*. In the following section these potentiators will be briefly discussed. In sequence, aspects of the pharmacology and mechanism of action of a new kinin potentiating peptide will be focussed.

Peptide Potentiators of Natural Occurrence

Peptides present in the venom of *Bothrops jararaca* were first shown to potentiate effects of kinin by Ferreira[3]. Several of these bradykinin potentiating peptides (BPP) were purified and sequenced[4]. BPPs share characteristics which include: 1) a pyroglutamyl residue in the N-terminal; 2) a high content of proline residues and 3) the tripeptide Ile-Pro-Pro in the C-terminal (Table 1). These features are responsible for the striking resistance of these compounds to enzymatic breakdown which may contribute to their relatively long-lasting effects[5].

Table 1. Bradykinin potentiating peptides of different origin.

SEQUENCE	REFERENCE
I- FROM SNAKE VENOMS	
(BPP_{9a}) pyroGLU-TRP-PRO-ARG-PRO-GLN-ILE-PRO-PRO	(25)
(BPP_{5a}) pyroGLU-LYS-TRP-ALA-PRO	(25)
pyroGLU-GLY-GLY-TRP-PRO-ARG-PRO-GLY-PRO-GLU-ILE-PRO-PRO	(25)
pyroGLU-ASN-TRP-PRO-HIS-PRO-GLN-ILE-PRO-PRO	(42)
pyroGLU-GLY-ARG-PRO-PRO-GLY-PRO-PRO-ILE-PRO-PRO	(9)
II- FROM FIBRINOGEN/FIBRIN	
ALA-ASP-SER-GLY-GLU-GLY-ASP-PHE-LEU	(10)
THR-ASP-SER-GLU-GLY-LYS-GLN-PHE-ILE	(10)
ALA-ARG-PRO-ALA-LYS	(38)
III- FROM ALBUMIN	
LEU-VAL-GLU-SER-SER-LYS	(13)
THR-PRO-VAL-SER-GLU-LYS	(13)
(A-VI-5) VAL-GLU-SER-SER-LYS	(13)
IV- FROM CASEIN	
ALA-VAL-PRO-TYR-PRO-GLN-ARG	(17,18)
PHE-PHE-VAL-ALA-PRO	(17,18)
THR-THR-MET-PRO-LEU-TRP	(17,18)

The description of BPPs has led to the publication of several reports showing potentiation of several kinin actions, including: 1) lowering of blood pressure[3]; 2) increase in vascular permeability[6]; 3) contraction of intestinal smooth muscle[7] and 4) increase in cardiac inotropism[8]. In all models studied the potentiating effect of BPPs was specific for actions induced by kinins.

BPPs have also been described in venoms of the snakes *Agkistrodon halys blomhoffi*[9] and of *A. h. pallas*[10]. The sequences of these peptides show a high degree of homology with those of *B. jararaca* venom, differences being mainly of a quantitative nature.

Peptides Potentiators Generated by Proteolytic Digestion

Peptides released by thrombin action on human fibrinogen have been found to potentiate kinin actions[11]. The active beta fibrinopeptide has 16 aminoacid residues and the fragment responsible for the potentiating effect is the N-terminal Ala-Asp-Ser-Gly-Glu- .

Aarsen[12], has shown that trypic digestion of bovine plasma or of bovine serum albumin yielded peptides which potentiated contractions of the guinea-pig ileum induced by kinins, but not contractions induced by histamine or acetylcholine. Some of these peptides have been purified and sequenced[13], the most active being peptide A-VI-5 (Val-Glu-Ser-Ser-Lys; Table 1). Further studies using this peptide showed that it was 1300-fold less potent than BPP_{5a}, a *B. jararaca* snake venom derived peptide; that the substitution of Ser^3 by Trp increased its activity 500-fold and that the potentiating effect was specific for kinins[14].

Proteolytic digestion of other proteins also led to the formation of kinin-potentiating peptides. For instance, tryptic digestion of casein released several potentiating peptides[15], whose purification and sequencing has been accomplished[16-18], (Table 1).

Mechanism of the Potentiating Effect

Inhibition of kinin metabolism by kininases was first suggested as the mechanism by which cysteine potentiates kinin effects on the guinea-pig ileum and the rat uterus[19]. The same mechanism may account for the potentiating effects of BPPs[20]. The conversion of angiotensin I into angiotensin II was also blocked by BPPs[21,22] which thus are able to inhibit kinin destruction as well as angiotensin I conversion. BPP_{5a} and BPP_{9a} are also angiotensin I converting enzyme (ACE) inhibitors. BPP_{5a} is a poor substrate and the less potent inhibitor; BPP_{9a} is completely resistant to ACE and exhibits high inhibitory potency (Ki ± 1 μM). Structure-activity studies of the interaction of peptides with ACE have shown that: 1) ACE must have a cationic site which interacts with carboxyl groups of peptides; 2) there should be a hydrogen bond-forming region adjacent to the ligand peptide C-terminal; 3) the zinc atom of ACE must coordinate with the carbonyl group of the peptide bond recognized by the active site, and 4) all active snake venom-derived peptides have a prolyl residue at the C-terminal. Taken together these informations allowed the first synthetic ACE inhibitor to be designed and produced[23,24]. Captopril (2-D-methyl-mercaptopropionyl-L-proline) is at present widely used as an antihypertensive drug. Its main characteristics are: 1) high affinity for ACE (Ki ± 5 nM) due to avid interaction through its sulphydril radical with the zinc atom present at the enzyme's active site; 2) effective absorption by the gut; 3) a 200 to 500 fold higher potency when compared to BPP_{9a} and 4) no inhibitory effect on either carboxypeptidases A or B.

That inhibition of ACE may not be the sole reason for kinin potentiation was first suggested by Ferreira(25). Several findings support this hypothesis: 1) the concentrations of peptides needed to inhibit ACE *in vitro* are higher than those required for kinin potentiation in the guinea-pig ileum(5); 2) the complete nonidentity between the aminoacid sequences of snake venom-derived and proteolytic digestion-derived peptides (Table 1); 3) the absence of an ACE inhibitory effect of some peptide potentiators(26,27); 4) the potentiating effect attained when the potentiating peptide is added to smooth muscle *after* a plateau for a given dose of kinin has been obtained(27,29); 5) potentiation of some bradykinin analogs, such as D-Pro^7-bradykinin(30), Lys-Lys-bradykinin(29), and DesArg^9-bradykinin(31), which are resistant to inactivation by ACE and 6) the ocurrence of a potentiating effect by casein-derived peptides even in the presence of chelating agents(10) or specific ACE inhibitors(15). It has been suggested that the ACE-independent mechanism of potentiation may involve a "receptor allosteric site"(25) with consequent "sensitization by an increase in receptor affinity for kinins"(27,28). Thus whichever the mechanism of potentiation, it seems to involve more than ACE inhibition. Putative ACE-independent mechanisms remain however largely unknown.

Kinin Potentiating Peptide

Background

In 1982, Guimarães and Voos(32), showed that human plasma depleted of kininogens by incubation with human urinary kallikrein and digestion with either trypsin or plasmin, generated a kinin potentiating factor called Kinin Potentiating Peptide (KPP). Such plasma proteins digests potentiated contractions of the guinea-pig ileum as well as the fall in rat blood pressure evoked by kinin. Digestion of whole plasma with trypsin and assay of released kinin on the guinea-pig ileum constitute the basis for the estimation of plasma kininogens(33). When urinary kallikrein rather than trypsin was used for this digestion, values for plasma kininogens were 3–4 times lower(34). The formation by trypsin of potentiating peptides alongside with kinins, may explain this discrepancy(34). The total potentiating activity of plasma from hypertensive subjects was 4–5 fold higher than that of normotensive subjects(35). No attempts to purify potentiating peptides from tryptic digests were made(35).

Purification of KPP

The protocol for experimental generation and purification of KPP will be briefly discussed in the following paragraphs. More detailed descriptions have been published[29,36]. Normal human plasma was incubated overnight at room temperature with human urinary kallikrein, a strategy important because urinary kallikrein specifically depletes kininogens releasing kinins. These are inactivated by plasma kininases thus avoiding both kinin interference with bioassays as well as contamination of KPP-containing fractions. The kininogen-depleted plasma was clotted, fibrinogen-free serum was separated by centrifugation and fractionated with ammonium sulphate at 30–55% saturation. The dialyzed protein solution was diluted 15-fold with ammonium bicarbonate buffer, heated to boiling, incubated with bovine trypsin and again heated to boiling. The denaturated digest was centrifuged and the supernatant ultrafiltered in a hollow fiber (3000 mol. wt. cut-off), Amicon DC-2 apparatus. The ultrafiltrate was freeze-dried, yielding crude KPP. Aliquots of this material were chromatographed on a SP-Sephadex C-25 column, equilibrated with sodium acetate buffer pH 3.5. The column was developed with a salt gradient of 0.1 to 0.42 M NaCl. Active fractions were pooled and applied to a Sep-Pak C18 cartridge. Adsorbed peptides were eluted with an acetonitrile/water mixture (40/60, v/v). The peptide material thus obtained was chromatographed on a reverse-phase HPLC column, using an acetonitrile gradient for peptide elution. The eluting peaks monitored at 214 nm, were collected and after freeze-drying, dissolved in water and assayed for potentiating activity. Active fractions were rechromatographed; only one active peptide peak was found. Analytical HPLC runs using different solvent systems confirmed the existence of only one peptide with potentiating activity. In view of the limited amount of this purified material available and considering that the partially purified preparation contained only one active peptide, this preparation was used for most of the following work, except where stated otherwise. Gel-filtration chromatography of KPP on Sephadex G-15 indicated it to have an estimated molecular weight of 1200. The amounts of KPP reported in the following sections are expressed in terms of the dry material of the active peak obtained in the second HPLC which consisted of only KPP.

KPP precursor protein

Plasma protein precursors of KPP are still unknown. Our evidence does not show fibrinogen among them since: 1) the methodology used for KPP preparation starts with fibrinogen-free serum; 2) KPP is far more active than potentiating peptides generated from fibrinogen/fibrin[32] and 3) the potentiating effect of fibrinopeptides is only seen after a preincubation period of 40–60 min with smooth muscle preparation[37,38] while the effect of KPP is immediately seen[29]. Although the sequence of KPP is not known, it is not likely to be identical with the potentiating peptide derived by tryptic digestion from albumin, since 100 μg/ml of this peptide[27], were as potent as 1 μg/ml of KPP[29]. There are as yet no clues to the nature of the protein precursor of KPP nor to the possibility of its generation to occur *in vivo*.

KPP potentiating effect

When added to the guinea-pig ileum together with bradykinin, KPP induced potentiation of the contractile effect of the kinin. The potentiating effect was inversely proportional to the kinin concentration that is, the higher the bradykinin/KPP ratio, the lower the observed potentiation. The maximal response to bradykinin was not altered by KPP[36].

KPP specifically potentiated the effects of kinin. It did not potentiate the effects of neither histamine, barium chloride, substance P or angiotensin II on the guinea-pig ileum[29] nor the edema of the rat's paw caused by histamine or serotonin[31]. The effects of all bradykinin analogs tested on the guinea-pig ileum were potentiated by KPP (Table 2). Other potentiating peptides also show this specificity towards kinin effects[25].

Table 2. Potentiation by KPP of the effect on the isolated guinea-pig ileum of different kinins.

KININ	ng/ml bath fluid	Contraction (mm)		PF[b]
		−KPP	+KPP[a]	
BK[c]	1.25	20	48	2.4
Lys-BK	7.50	23	52	2.3
Met-Lys-BK	18.0	19	40	2.1
Ile-Ser-BK	10.0	20	40	2.0
Lys-Lys-BK	7.5	20	38	1.9

(a) 10 nM in bath fluid.
(b) Potency factor: ratio between height of contractions in the presence and in the absence of KPP, respectively.
(c) Bradykinin.

Interestingly, the linear relationship between concentration and potentiating effect of KPP seems to be true only for isolated smooth muscle preparations. For instance the dose-response curve for the potentiating effect of KPP on bradykinin-induced rat paw edema is bell-shaped (Fig. 1). The reasons for this result are, as yet, unclear; it is not due to the simultaneous presence of contaminating peptides in the KPP preparation since pure

KPP (obtained in analytical HPLC runs) reproduced the same pattern of responses (Fig. 1).

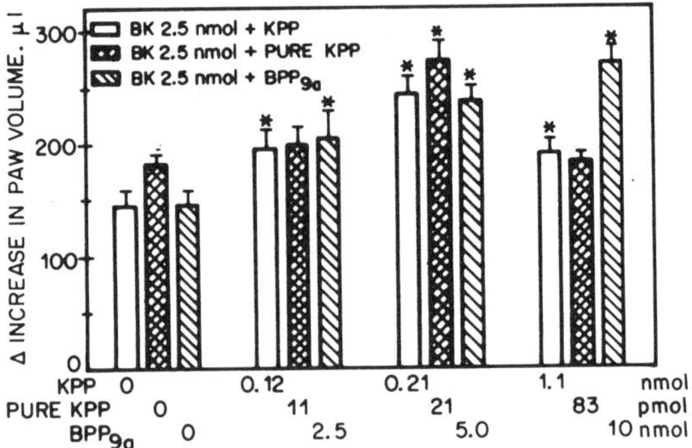

Fig. 1. Potentiation of bradykinin-induced rat paw edema by KPP, purified KPP and BPP_{9a}. The potentiating peptides were injected together with bradykinin and the edema was evaluated 30 minutes after. Note that the doses of purified KPP are expressed in pmol. *$p < 0.05$, Student's T test. Mean ± S.D. 5-6 rats for each bar.

Mechanism of the potentiating effect of KPP

A) Inhibition of angiotensin converting enzyme activity.

As mentioned above, the generally accepted explanation for the origin of peptide potentiating effects, is inhibition of ACE or kininase II. The mechanism of action of KPP is at least in part, not related to such inhibition. Evidence in favor of this hypothesis is: 1) KPP potentiated the effects of bradykinin on the rat uterus(29,36), a preparation displaying very low levels of ACE(39); 2) KPP potentiated the contractile effect of Lys-Lys-bradykinin(29), a kinin resistant to ACE(40); 3) a guinea-pig ileum already stimulated by a given amount of bradykinin, can be further stimulated by newly added KPP(29) and 4) blockade of guinea-pig ileum ACE by the ion chelator 1,10 phenanthroline did not abolish the potentiating effect of KPP(29). In addition, KPP has been shown to be an extremely weak inhibitor of ACE *in vitro* (Table 3). Also, phosphoramide, an inhibitor of neutral endopeptidases which act as kininases, failed to block kinin potentiation by KPP(29). These data clearly indicate that KPP's manner of action is unrelated to the inhibition of kinin degradation by kininases in special, ACE.

B) Arachidonic acid metabolism

In spite of several reports showing that potentiating peptides could have mechanisms of action apart from ACE inhibition, the studies on such mechanisms are scarce. Having

Table 3. Kinin potentiating and ACE-inhibitory activities of KPP, of two snake venom-derived potentiators (BPP_{9a} and BPP_{5a}) and of a peptide (A-VI-5) derived from trypsin-digested albumin.

PEPTIDE	MW	KPU/nmol	ACE INHIBITION	
			Peptide conc. M	Residual ACE %
BPP_{9a}	1101	17.0	9.1×10^{-8}	36.9
BPP_{5a}	612	0.7	4.9×10^{-7}	37.8
A-VI-5	549	0.003	1.8×10^{-4}	70.1
KPP	ca. 1200	12.0	1.3×10^{-7}	100
			1.3×10^{-4}	94.5

One KPU (kinin-potentiating unit) is the amount of peptide able to double the effect of 12.5 or 25 ng of bradykinin per 10 ml bath fluid, on the guinea-pig ileum.
ACE was a partially purified preparation from rabbit lung[(43)].

shown that KPP's potentiating effect does not seem to depend on the inhibition of kinin metabolism, we considered other possibilities to explain this effect: 1) an increase in receptor affinity for bradykinin and 2) an interference on some intracellular transductional step mediating bradykinin effects. Increased kinin receptor affinity has been suggested as the mechanism of the effect of snake venom-derived[(25)] and albumin-derived[(27)] kinin-potentiating peptides. Evidence showing that KPP does not affect bradykinin binding parameters in MDCK and rat uterus smooth muscle cells in culture has been obtained (unpublished results). Although preliminary, they suggest that increased receptor affinity for bradykinin[(1)], is not likely to explain KPP's potentiating effects. The second possibility has the following evidence in its favor: a) most of the actions of kinins are mediated by the activation of phospholipases, mainly of the A_2 type, leading to the release of arachidonic acid, which is converted to prostaglandins (PG) or leukotrienes (LT) by enzymes of the cyclo-oxygenase or lypoxygenase pathways, respectively; indomethacin, a cyclo-oxygenase inhibitor abolished the potentiation by captopril of kinin-induced bronchoconstriction in the guinea-pig[(41)]. Preliminary results from our laboratory show that cyclo-oxygenase inhibitors do not affect the potentiation of kinin effects by KPP. In contrast, drugs which interfere with the formation of leukotrienes did abolish the effect of KPP. Potentiating effects of BPP_{9a} and enalaprilate were not abolished by these drugs. Therefore, even taking the relatively low specificity of these drugs into account, our results do suggest that the mechanism of action of KPP involves leukotriene-forming pathways.

Concluding Remarks

The findings presented in this review indicate that the field of kinin potentiation still retains aspects to be discovered. The results concerning KPP raise several interesting questions. For instance, are effects of other potentiating peptides mediated by the arachidonic acid cascade? If so, how does activation of this cascade mediate kinin potentiation? Are potentiating peptides such as KPP generated *in vivo*? If so, what would be their physiological role in hypertension and inflammation? Answers to these and other questions, may provide a better understanding of the role of kinins and kinin-potentiating peptides in Physiology and Pharmacology.

References

1. Regoli, D. and J. Barabe, Pharmacology of bradykinin and related kinins, Pharmac. Rev. 32, 1-46 (1980).

2. Vavrek, R.J. and J.M. Stewart, Competitive antagonists of bradykinin, Peptides, 6, 161-164 (1985).

3. Ferreira, S.H., Bradykinin potentiating factor (BPF) present in venom of *Bothrops jararaca*, Br. J. Pharmac. 24, 163-169 (1965).

4. Ferreira, S.H., D.C. Bartelt and L.J. Greene, Isolation of bradykinin-potentiating peptides from *Bothrops jararaca* venom, Biochemistry 9, 2583-2593 (1970).

5. Stewart, J.M., Chemistry and biological activity of peptides related to bradykinin, In: Handbook of Experimental Pharmacology, vol. 25 (suppl.), pp. 227-265 (Ed. E.G. Erdös). Springer-Verlag, Berlin 1979.

6. Ferreira, S.H., Bradykinin potentiating factor, In: Hypotensive Peptides, pp. 356-367 (Ed. E.G. Erdös). Springer-Verlag, New York 1966.

7. Ferreira, S.H., Potenciação de bradicinina por um fator presente no veneno da *Bothrops jararaca*. PhD Thesis, Faculty of Medicine of Ribeirão Preto, pp. 32-34, USP, Brazil 1964.

8. Antonio, A., The coronary vasodilatador effect of bradykinin, In: Bradykinin and Related Kinins, pp. 25-29 (Eds. M. Rocha e Silva and H.A. Rothschild). Edart, São Paulo 1967.

9. Kato, H. and T. Suzuki, Bradykinin-potentiating peptides from the venom of *Agkistrodon halys blomhoffi*. Isolation of five bradykinin potentiators and the aminoacid sequence of two of them, potentiators B and C, Biochemistry 10, 972-980 (1971).

10. C.W. Chi, S.H. Wang, L.G. Xu, M.Y. Wang, S.S. Lo and W.D. Huang, Structure-function studies on the bradykinin potentiating peptides from chinese snake venom (*Agkistrodon halys pallas*), Peptides 6, 339-342 (1985).

11. Osbahr, A.J., J.A. Gladner and K. Laki, Studies on the physiological activity of the peptide released during the fibrinogen-fibrin conversion, Bioch. Bioph. Acta 86, 535-542 (1964).

12. Aarsen, P.N., Sensitization of guinea-pig ileum to the action of bradykinin by trypsin hydrolysates of ox and rabbit plasma, Br. J. Pharmac. 32, 453-465 (1968).

13. Weyers, R., P. Hagel, B.C. Das and C.van der Meer, Tryptic peptides from rabbit and bovine albumin enhancing the effect of bradykinin, Bioch. Bioph. Acta 279, 331-355 (1972).

14. Ufkes, J.G.R., B.J. Visser, G. Heuver and C. van der Meer, Structure-activity relationships of bradykinin potentiating peptides, Eur. J. Pharmac. 50, 119-122 (1978).

15. Henriques, O.B., R.B. de Deus and R.A.S. Santos, Bradykinin potentiating peptides isolated from alfa-casein tryptic hydrolysate, Bioch. Pharmac. 36, 182-184 (1987).

16. Maruyama, S., K. Nakagomi N. Tomizuka and H. Suzuki, Angiotensin I-converting enzyme inhibitor derived from an enzymatic hydrolysate of casein. II. Isolation and bradykinin-potentiating activity on the rat uterus and the ileum of rats, Agr. Biol. Chem. 49, 1405-1409 (1985).

17. Maruyama, S., M. Mitachi, J. Awaya, M. Kurowo, N. Tomizuka and H. Suzuki, Angiotensin I-converting enzyme inhibitory activity on the C-terminal hexapeptide of alfa-casein, Agr. Biol. Chem. 51, 2557-2561 (1987a).

18. Maruyama, S., M. Mitachi, H. Tanaka, N. Tomizuka and H. Suzuki, Studies on the active site and anti-hypertensive activity of angiotensin I-inhibitors derived from casein, Agr. Biol. Chem. 51, 1581-1586 (1987b).

19. Picarelli, Z., O.B. Henriques and M.C.F. Oliveira, Potentiation of bradykinin action on smooth muscle by cysteine, Experientia 18, 77-78 (1962).

20. Ferreira, S.H. and M. Rocha e Silva. Potentiation of bradykinin and eledoisin by BPF (bradykinin potentiating factor) from *Bothrops jararaca*, Experientia 21, 347-352 (1965).

21. Ng, K.K.F. and J.R. Vane, Fate of angiotensin I in the circulation, Nature 218, 144-146 (1968).

22. Ng, K.K.F. and J.R. Vane, Some properties of angiotensin converting enzyme in the lung in vivo, Nature 255, 1142-1144 (1970).

23. Ondetti, M.A., B. Rubin and D.W. Cushman, Design of specific inhibitors of angiotensin converting enzyme, Science 196, 441-443 (1977).

24. Cushman, D.W., H.S. Cheung, E.F. Sabo and M.A. Ondetti, Design of competitive inhibitors of angiotensin-converting enzyme, Biochesmistry 16, 5484-5491 (1977).

25. Ferreira, S.H., Estudos sobre o fator de potenciação da bradicinina presente no veneno da *Bothrops jararaca*. Thesis, Faculty of Medicine of Ribeirão Preto, pp. 53-56, USP, Brazil 1969.

26. Faber, D.B. and C. van der Meer, A study of some bradykinin potentiating peptides derived from plasma proteins, Arch. Int. Pharmacol. 205, 226-243 (1973).

27. Ufkes, J.G.R., P.N. Aarsen and C. van der Meer, The mechanism of action of two bradykinin-potentiating peptides on isolated smooth muscle, Eur. J. Pharmac. 44, 89-97 (1977).

28. Tewksbury, D.A., Studies on the mechanism of bradykinin potentiation, Arch. Int. Pharmacol. 173, 426-432 (1968).

29. Assreuy, J., A.A. Almeida and J.A. Guimarães, Pharmacological properties of a new kinin-potentiating peptide generated from human serum proteins, Eur. J. Pharmac. 168, 231-237 (1989).

30. Greene, L.J., A.C.M. Camargo, E.M. Krieger, J.M. Stewart and S.H. Ferreira, Inhibitors of the conversion of angiotensin I to II and potentiation of bradykinin by small peptides present in *Bothrops jararaca* venom, Circ. Res. 30, 62-71 (1972).

31. Fernandes, P.D., J.A. Guimarães and J. Assreuy, Comparative effects of two potentiating peptides (KPP and BPP_{9a}) on kinin-induced rat paw edema, Agents Actions 32(3/4), 182-187 (1991).

32. Guimarães, J.A. and A. Voos, Properties of a kinin potentiating peptide generated in kininogen-depleted human plasma, Agents Actions 9, 295-300 (1982).

33. Diniz, C.R. and I.F. Carvalho, A micromethod for determination of bradykininogen under several conditions, Annals of New York Academy of Sciences 104, 77-89 (1963).

34. Guimarães, J.A., Cininogenios do plasma humano: caracterização, preparação e propriedades funcionais. Thesis, Universidade Federal Fluminense, Rio de Janeiro, Brazil 1978.

35. Guimarães, J.A., A. Voos, G. Alves-Filho, O.L. Ramos and A.B. Ribeiro, Characterization of a bradykinin potentiating peptide generated in plasma of patients with essential hypertension, Clin. Res. 28, 331A (Abstr.) (1980).

36. Assreuy, J., A.A. Almeida and J.A. Guimarães, Characterization of a new kinin potentiating peptide obtained from human plasma proteins, Braz. J. Med. Biol. Res. 21, 452-455 (1988).

37. Blomback, B., M. Blomback, P. Edman and B. Hessel, Human fibrinopeptides: isolation, characterization and structure, Bioch. Bioph. Acta 115, 371-377 (1966).

38. Gladner, J.A., Potentiation of the effect of bradykinin, In: Hypotensive Peptides, pp. 344-355 (Eds. E.G. Erdös, N. Back and F. Sicuteri). Springer-Verlag, New York 1966.

39. Cushman, D.W. and H.S. Cheung, Concentration of angiotensin converting enzyme in tissues of the rat, Bioch. Bioph. Acta 250, 261-265 (1971).

40. Roblero, J., J.W. Ryan and J.M. Stewart, Assay of kinins by their effects on blood pressure, Res. Comm. Chem. Path. Pharmac. 6, 207-212 (1973).

41. Lau, W.A.K., M.P. Rechtman, A.L.A. Boura and R.G. King, Synergistic potentiation by captopril and propranolol of bradykinin-induced bronchoconstriction in the guinea-pig, Clin. Exper. Pharmac. Phys. 16, 849-857 (1989).

42. Ondetti, M.A, N.J. Williams, E.F. Sabo, E.F. Pluscuc, E.R. Weaver and O. Kocy, Angiotensin converting enzyme inhibitors from the venom of *Bothrops jararaca*, Biochemistry 10, 4033-4039 (1971).

43. Stewart, T.A., J.A. Weare and E.G. Erdös, Human peptidyldipeptidase (converting enzyme, kininase II), Meth. Enzym. 80 Part C, 450-460 (1981).

AAS 36
Contributions to
Autacoid Pharmacology

ACTION OF PLANT PROTEINASE INHIBITORS ON ENZYMES OF THE KALLIKREIN KININ SYSTEM

C.A.M. Sampaio, G. Motta, M.U. Sampaio, M.L.V. Oliva, M.S. Araújo, R.C.R. Stella, A.S. Tanaka and I.F.C. Batista

Department of Biochemistry, Escola Paulista de Medicina, P.O. Box 20372, 04034 São Paulo, SP, Brazil

Abstract

Serine proteinase inhibitors, in the seeds of several Leguminosae from the Pantanal region (West Brazil), were studied using bovine trypsin, Factor XIIa and human plasma kallikrein. The inhibitors were purified from *Enterolobium contortisiliquum* (Mr=23,000), *Torresea cearensis* (Mr=13,000), *Bauhinia bauhinioides* (Mr=20,000), *Bauhinia mollis* (Mr=20,000) and *Bauhinia pentandra* (Mr=20,000). *E. contortisiliquum* inhibitor inactivates all three enzymes, whereas the *T. cearensis* inhibitor inactivates trypsin and Factor XIIa, but does not affect plasma kallikrein. *B. bauhinioides* and *B. pentrandra* inhibitors, on the other hand, inactivate trypsin and plasma kallikrein but only the *B. pentandra* inhibitor affects Factor XIIa, and *B. mollis* inhibitor causes trypsin inactivation only. Calculated Ki values were between 10^{-7} and 10^{-9} M. Chymotrypsin, like trypsin, is also inhibited, but with lower affinity.

The trypsin inhibitors, isolated from *E. contortisiliquum*, *B. pentandra*, *B. bauhinioides* and *B. mollis* seem to be of the Kunitz type; the inhibitor purified from *T. cearensis* is of the Bowman-Birk type.

Introduction

Clot formation is normally the result of the convergence of two pathways, intrinsic and extrinsic. It depends on circulating zymogens, the first, which is Hageman Factor

(Factor XII), is activated to Factor XIIa when plasma kallikrein, high molecular weight kininogen and a negatively charged surface are available. In sequence, Factor XI is activated, followed by Factor IX. The extrinsic pathway is an alternative way to activate the clotting cascade when Factor X is activated by tissue factors. The subsequent steps involve prothrombin activation and, eventually, formation of the fibrin clot(1).

The early step of the intrinsic blood clotting pathway is known as the contact phase. When a small portion of Factor XII, in a given section of the vascular bed, activates prokallikrein into kallikrein, the fast activation of Factor XII by the newly-formed active kallikrein leads to the acceleration of Factor XII activation into Factor XIIa. As a consequence of this mutual activation of Factor XII and kallikrein, Factor XI activation is sped up, in an environment rendered favorable due to the presence of a negatively charged surface provided by the injured blood vessel, and also due to the presence of kininogen, which bears a prokallikrein binding region(2).

Proteinases involved in blood clotting are controlled by various mechanisms. They may undergo inactivation for example, by clearance(3) or proteolytic degradation(4). Furthermore, they can be blocked by proteinase inhibitors that display variable degrees of affinity towards the catalytic site of the enzymes(5).

Usually, most of the control of the enzymes which undergo activation from zymogens is performed by inhibitors, found in the environment where these enzymes manifest their activity(5). An example for such a situation is active plasma kallikrein and Factor XII inhibition by circulating C_1-inactivator(6). But not only animal inhibitors are suitable for the study the clotting enzymes; plant inhibitors are useful tools for the study of many properties of these proteins.

Several plants have long been known as rich sources of proteinase inhibitors, useful as model compounds for inhibition of proteolytic enzymes of animal origin(7). We report here on the isolation of plant inhibitors which inactivate trypsin and some of the serine proteinases involved in the blood clotting cascade, i.e., plasma kallikrein and Factor XII.

Material and Methods

Isolation of plant proteinase inhibitors. Over fifty Brazilian Leguminosae (Fabaceae) beans were screened; inhibitors were isolated from *Enterolobium contortisiliquum* (Mimosoideae)(8,9), *Torresea cearensis* (Papilionoideae)(10), and *Bauhinia bauhinioides*,

B. mollis and *B. pentandra* (Caesalpinoideae)[11]. These trees spread over extensive regions of Brazil; beans were harvested manually.

Reagents. Bovine trypsin and chymotrypsin were Worthington products; human plasma kallikrein was isolated as previously described[12]. Factor XIIa was a kind gift from Cuttler Laboratories. Sephadex G-150, DEAE-Sephadex A-50 and Sepharose CNBr-activated, Pharmacia; acrylamide, bis-acrylamide were from Merck Darmstadt; acetyl-phenylalanine-arginine-p-nitro-anilide (Ac-Phe-Arg-pNan) was synthesized[13]. Other chemicals were from the best quality available.

Purification. The purification procedure for all inhibitors was based upon DEAE-Sephadex chromatography (30-ml column, equilibrated with 0.05 M tris-HCl buffer, pH 8.0 and eluted with 0.05 to 0.3 M NaCl gradient), followed usually by gel-filtration on Sephadex G-150, in a 1×100 cm column, equilibrated with 0.05 M tris-HCl buffer, pH 8.0. Further purification was performed in a Superose-12 column, in 0.1 M phosphate buffer pH 8.0 and a Mono-Q column, equilibrated with 0.05 M tris-HCl, pH 8.0 initial buffer, and developed with a NaCl gradient from 0 to 0.5 M. Trypsin-Sepharose was used to purify some inhibitors; it was prepared[8], and equilibrated with 0.05 M tris-HCl buffer, pH 8.0. The adsorbed inhibitor was eluted by acidification with 0.2 M KCl/HCl, pH 2.0 .

Electrophoresis. The homogeneity and the molecular weight of the inhibitors were assessed by 10–20% SDS-polyacrylamide gel electrophoresis[14]. Proteins in solution were estimated by absorbance at 280 nm.

Inhibitory activity. Residual activity of trypsin, factor XIIa or human plasma kallikrein was measured using 1.0 mM Ac.Phe-Arg-p-Nan or H.D.Pro-Phe-Arg-p-Nan (Kabi/S-2203)[8]; trypsin residual activity was also estimated by hydrolysis of 20 mM Tos.Arg.O.Me in a pH-stat[12]. Ki and inhibitor concentration were determined using a tight binding mechanism model[15].

Results

Trypsin inhibitors (Fig. 1) were more frequently found than inhibitors directed against plasma kallikrein (Fig. 2), no major differences among the three sub-families Mimosoideae, Caesalpinoideae and Papilonoideae were noted.

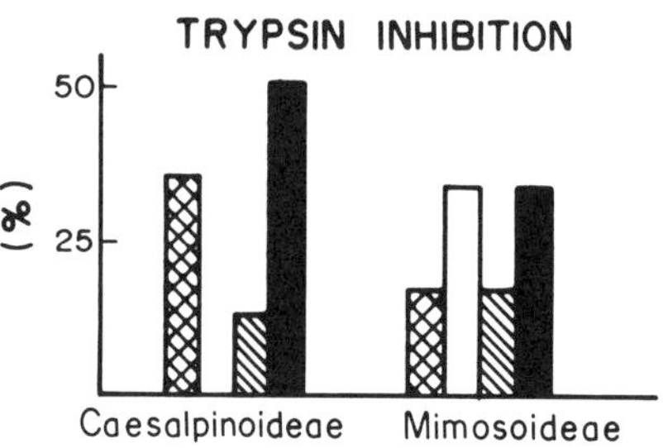

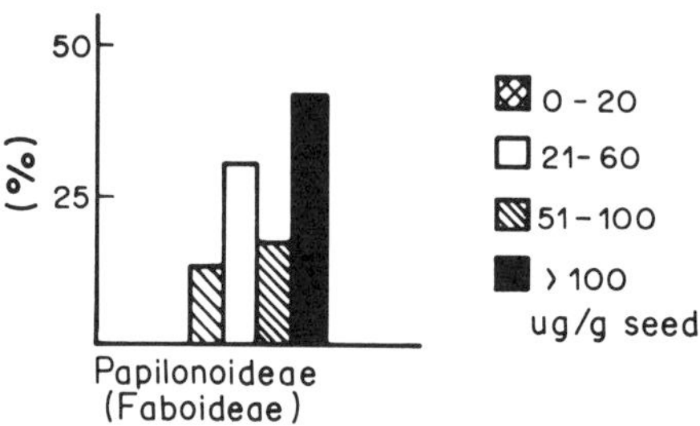

Fig. 1. Frequency of trypsin inhibitor contents in Leguminosae expressed as μg of trypsin inhibitor per gram of seeds. Inhibitor contents were divided in four groups; the Y-axis indicates the frequencies with which they were found.

The *E. contortisiliquum* trypsin inhibitor is presented as a model of this process, which with proper modifications, was applied to *Torresea* and *Bauhinia* inhibitors. Gel filtration of *E. contortisiliquum* in Superose 12 presented only one peak of inhibitory activity, having a molecular weight of around 22,000 (Fig. 3). Affinity chromatography of a preparation of *E. contortisiliquum* extracts caused specific adsortion of the inhibitor to Trypsin-Sepharose; acid stability of the inhibitor, permited elution by decreasing pH to 2.0 (Fig. 4); alternatively, the inhibitor could be eluted by a highly concentrated solution of a trypsin competitive inhibitor (1.0 M benzamidine).

A typical inhibition curve of trypsin by *T. cearensis* inhibitor can be seen in Fig. 5. The same kind of curve is defined for human plasma kallikrein and Factor XII fragment. The diversity of the inhibitor activity is indicated on Table 1 showing the Ki values for the inhibition of the enzymes studied. These were calculated from curves similar

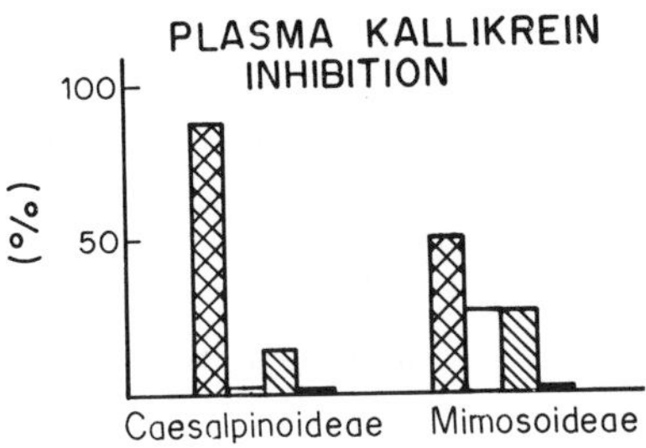

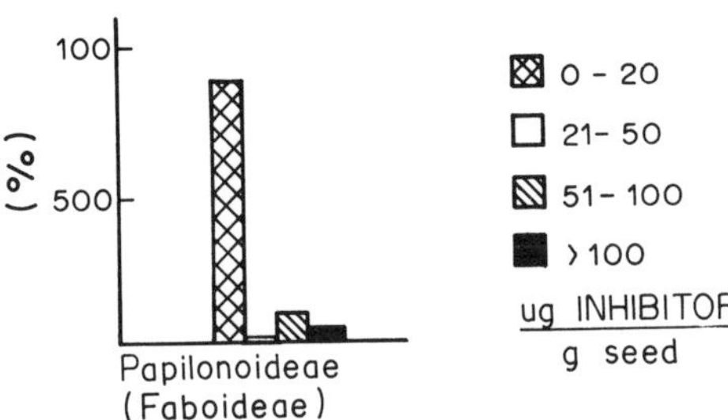

Fig. 2. Frequency of plasma kallikrein inhibitor content in Leguminosae expressed as μg of kallikrein inhibited per gram of seeds. Inhibitor contents were divided in four groups; the Y-axis indicates the frequencies with which they were found.

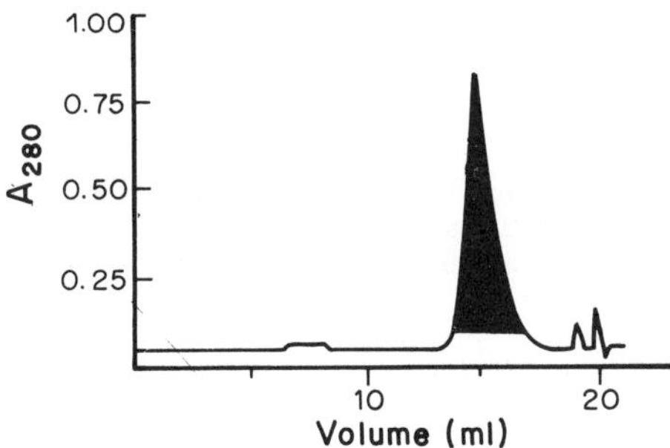

Fig. 3. Gel permeation of *E. contortisiliquum* trypsin inhibitor, Superose-12 column equilibrated and developed with 0.1 M tris-HCl buffer, 0.1 M NaCl, pH 8.0, at room temperature, 0.5 ml/min flow rate. Sample: 1.0 mg inhibitor from the DEAE-Sephadex column. Inhibitory activity (100 μl against 10 μg trypsin in 0.1 M tris-HCl buffer, 0.02 M CaCl2, pH 8.0). Remaining activity was measured by the hydrolysis of 1.0 mM Ac-Phe-Arg-p-Nan, pH 8.0, 37°C. The shadowed area indicates trypsin inhibition.

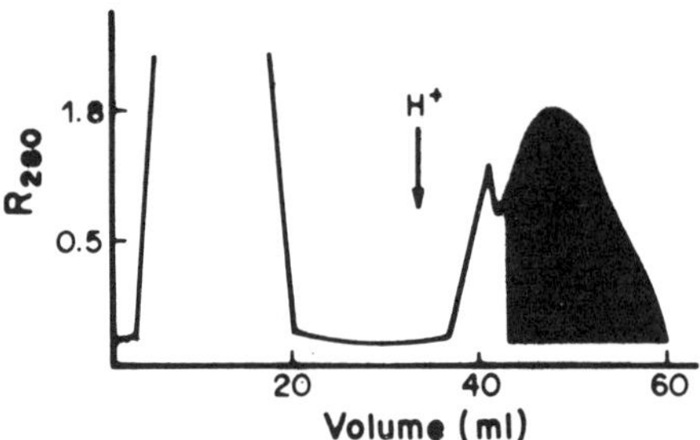

Fig. 4. Trypsin-Sepharose affinitty chromato-graphy of *E. contortisiliquum* trypsin inhibitor. Column(1 × 6 cm) equilibrated with 0.05 M tris-HCl buffer, pH 8.0. Sample: 209 mg acetone powder in 10 ml. Elution with 0.2 M KCl/HCl, pH 2.0. Inhibitory activity estimated as in Fig. 3.

to those shown in Fig. 5, by adjusting the curves to the tight binding mechanism model adapted from Morrison[15].

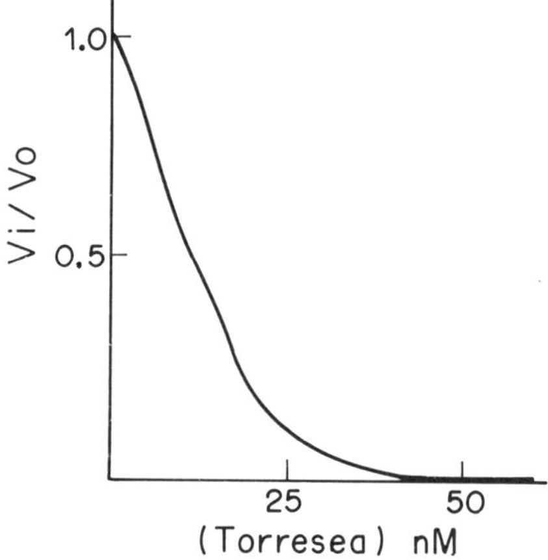

Fig. 5. Trypsin inactivation curve by *T. cearensis* inhibitor. Bovine trypsin (2.5 nM, NPGB-titrated) was pre-incubated with purified *T. cearensis* inhibitor (Io), for 10 min, at 37°C, in 1.0 ml 0.1 M tris-HCl buffer, 0.02 mM $CaCl_2$, pH 8.0 and the residual activity was followed by hydrolysis of 1.0 mM Ac-Phe-Arg-p-Nan.

SDS-polyacrylamide gel of the isolated inhibitors indicated a Mr = 13,000 for the *T. cearensis* inhibitor and a range of around 20,000 for the other inhibitors (Table 2). Only the *E. contotorsiliquum* inhibitor shows two chains after reduction.

Analysis of the elution profiles from Superose-12 column confirmed the native molecular weight 20,000 for inhibitors, but for one, from *T. cearensis*, which is eluted corresponding to a molecular weight around 12,000. In the case of *T. cearensis* is possible to isolate an enzyme-inhibitor complex corresponding to a ternary complex (one trypsin and one chymotrypsin molecules bound to one inhibitor molecule).

Table 1. Ki values (M) for serine proteinase plant inhibitors.

Inhibitor Source	Trypsin 10^{-8}	Chymotrypsin 10^{-7}	HuPK 10^{-8}	F–XII 10^{-7}
E. contortisiliquum	0.3	1.2	0.5	1.5
T. cearensis	0.1	2.4	NI	0.6
B. bauhinioides	1.8	2.9	2.3	NI
B. mollis	1.8	2.9	2.3	NI
B. pentandra	2.7	2.3	1.0	0.8

NI: no inhibition; HuPK: human plasma kallikrein;
F-XII: Factor XIIa fragment.

Table 2. Molecular weight estimation, based upon SDS-polyacrylamide gel electrophoresis (10–20 % gradient).

Inhibitor	Molecular weight Non-reduced	Reduced
E. contortisiliquum	23.000	17,000/ 8,000
T. cearensis	13,000	13,000
B. bauhinioides	21,000	21,000
B. mollis	21,000	21,000
B. pentandra	21,000	21,000

Discussion

Trypsin was inhibited by all inhibitors tested; Ki values fell within the range of 10^{-9} to 10^{-8} M. Chymotrypsin, like trypsin, was also inhibited, but with lower affinity. Human plasma kallikrein was not inhibited by *T. cearensis* inhibitor; Factor XII fragment was not inhibited by *B. bauhinioides* inhibitor. Both *Torresea* and *Bauhinia* inhibitors do not differ much in their ability to inhibit trypsin or chymotrypsin. Comparing both *Bauhinia* inhibitors, it is interesting to observe that they differ remarkably in the inhibition of Factor XII, since only that from the *B. pentandra* species affect this blood clotting enzyme.

Plant serine proteinase inhibitors are customarily divided into two major classes: of Kunitz type and of Bowman-Birk type. Kunitz type inhibitors are in the Mr range of 20,000 and contain a single inhibition center located on a single polypeptide chain. Besides molecular weight differences, these two types of inhibitors differ in some other structural aspects, including degree of homology, as well as number of disulfide bridges in their non-reduced molecules(7).

The trypsin inhibitors, isolated from *E. contortisiliquum*, *B. pentandra* and *B. bauhinioides*, belong to the Kunitz type. The inhibitor purified from *T. cearensis* (Mr = 13,000) belongs to the Bowman-Birk type since it was possible to isolate a ternary complex for this inhibitor.

References

1. Davie, E.N., K.Fujimura, M.E. Legaz and H. Kato, Role of proteases in blood clotting, In: Proteases in Biological Control (Eds. E.Reich, D.B. Rifkin and E. Shaw). Cold Spring Harbor Laboratory, New York, NY 1975.

2. Kaplan, A.P. and M. Silverberg, The coagulation-kinin pathway of human plasma, Blood 70, 1-15 (1987).

3. Borges, D., C.A.M. Sampaio, P. de la Llosa and J.L. Prado, The liver is the main organ to clear plasma and tissue kallikreins from rat plasma *in vivo*, Adv. Exp. Med. Biol. 198, 229-233 (1986).

4. Laskowski Jr., M., and I. Kato, Protein inhibitors of proteinases, Ann. Rev. Biochem. 49, 593-626 (1980).

5. Travis. J. and G. Salvesen, Human plasma inhibitor, Ann. Rev. Biochem. 52, 655-709 (1983).

6. Colman, R.W., Regulation of plasma kallikrein-kininogen system, Adv. Exp. Med. Biol. 198B, 178-183 (1986).

7. Richardson, M., Proteinase inhibitors of plants and micro-organisms, Phytochemistry 16, 159-169 (1977).

8. Oliva, M.L.V., M.U. Sampaio and C.A.M. Sampaio, Serine- and SH-proteinase inhibitors from *Enterolobium contortisiliquum* beans. Purification and preliminary characterization, Braz. J. Med. Biol. Res. 20, 767-770 (1987).

9. Oliva, M.L.V., M.U. Sampaio and C.A.M. Sampaio, Purification and partial characterization of a thiol proteinase inhibitor from *Enterolobium contortisiliquum* beans, Hoppe-Seyler Z. Biol. Chem. 369, 229-232 (1988).

10. Tanaka, A.S., M.U. Sampaio, C.A.M. Sampaio and M.L. Oliva, Purification and partial characterization of *Torresea cearensis* trypsin inhibitor, Braz. J. Med. Biol. Res. 22, 1069-1071 (1989).

11. Oliva, M.L.V., M.U. Sampaio and C.A.M. Sampaio, Isolation and characterization of plant inhibitors directed against plasma kallikrein and factor XII, Adv. Med. Exp. Biol. 247A, 467-471 (1988).

12. Oliva, M.L.V., D.M. Grisolia, M.U. Sampaio and C.A.M. Sampaio, Properties of a highly purified human plasma kallikrein, Agents Actions 9 (suppl.), 52-57 (1982).

13. Juliano, M.A. and L. Juliano, Synthesis and kinetic parameters of hydrolysis by trypsin of some acyl-arginyl-p-nitroanilides and peptides containing arginyl-nitroanilides, Braz. J. Med. Biol. Res. 18, 435-445 (1985).

14. Laemmli, U.K., Cleavage of structural proteins during the assembly of the head of bacteriophage T4, Nature 227, 680-685 (1970).

15. Knight, C.G., The characterization of enzyme inhibition, In: Proteinase Inhibitors, pp. 23-51 (Eds. A.J. Barret and G. Salvesen). Elsevier, Amsterdam 1986.

AAS 36
Contributions to
Autacoid Pharmacology

HUMAN PLASMA KALLIKREIN. IMMUNOREACTIVITY AND ACTIVITY ON NATURAL AND SYNTHETIC SUBSTRATES*

G. Motta**, C.A.M. Sampaio and M.U. Sampaio

Department of Biochemistry, Escola Paulista de Medicina, São Paulo, SP, Brazil

Abstract

Human plasma kallikrein (HuPK) is a serine protease found in mammalian plasma. Following limited proteolysis, the enzyme is activated and forms two chains. The light chain occurs with molecular weight 36,000 or 33,000 and contains the active site. The heavy chain occurs with molecular weight of 45,000 and contains the binding site for high-molecular-weight kininogen. Both chains were prepared from active HuPK, following mild reduction with dithiothreitol and carboxymethylation with iodoacetamide. The light chain was isolated in SBTI-Sepharose and its kinetic properties were determined with synthetic derivatives of arginine-p-nitroanilides, to investigate any possible alteration of the active site. These studies showed that substrate modifications affected the hydrolytic activity more than the binding capacity. The ability to cleave high-molecular-weight kininogen, as observed for intact kallikrein, was reduced in beta-kallikrein and absent in the light chain, even when equimolar amounts of both light and heavy chains were tested together. Anti-kallikrein antiserum formed immunoprecipitates not only with kallikrein itself, but also with the separated chains. The immunoreactivity of the light-chain was not identical with that of kallikrein. Immunoselected specific antibodies for both chains, depending on the selectivity, reacted with the heavy chain and kallikrein, or with the light chain and kallikrein. These antibodies were shown to be effective in binding radio-iodinated HuPK in the radioimmunoassay developed for intact kallikrein.

*Research supported by the Brazilian National Research Council (CNPq) and Financiadora de Projetos (Finep).

**Fellowship of Fundação de Amparo à Pesquisa do Estado de São Paulo (FAPESP).

Introduction

Human plasma kallikrein is an arginyl serine proteinase that activates factor XII during early stages of the intrinsic phase of blood clotting. The enzyme also releases bradykinin from high-molecular-weight kininogen[(1)]. Plasma kallikrein is present in blood as a zymogen, prokallikrein, which consists of a single polypeptide chain (Mr=90,000). The activation of the proenzyme is achieved by active Factor XII or by its low molecular weight fragment (Mr=28,000) which splits initially a single peptide bond. As further proteolysis occurs, the final product is a molecule with a heavy chain (Mr=45,000) and a light-chain (Mr=36,000 or 30,000)[(2)]. The plasma kallikrein gene was recently cloned and the primary sequence of the molecule was deduced from the nucleotide sequence of the cDNA[(3)].

Plasma kallikrein, besides being able to produce limited proteolysis of Factor XII and high-molecular-weight kininogen, also cleaves several arginine containing synthetic substrates, such as tosyl-L-arginine methyl ester, D.Pro-Phe-Arg-p-nitroanilide (S-2302, Kabi) and other related peptide derivatives[(4,5)].

Both a heavy and a light chain of kallikrein were isolated following reduction and alkylation of disulfide bridges[(6)]; the light chain retains part of the enzymatic activity and the ability to form a complex with C1-inactivator and alpha 2-macroglobulin[(7)]. Additional evidences have shown that a cleaved heavy chain alters some of kallikrein's biological properties[(8)]. Purification of the active enzyme is usually performed by specific affinity chromatography on soybean-trypsin-inhibitor-Sepharose, after acid activation of Cohn's fraction IV or using activated fresh plasma[(9,4)]. Prokallikrein is prepared after several steps involving ion-exchange chromatography and affinity adsorptions[(10)].

Enzymes related to the blood clotting system are activated by limited proteolysis, and the activation itself can produce more than one active species of enzyme, probably due to minor non-specific proteolysis. In the case of thrombin, a molecular species is known to retain the esterolytic activity but is devoid of the ability to convert fibrinogen to fibrin[(11)]. Following activation, factor XII is converted to a protein with a Mr=80,000 and by further proteolysis is transformed into a fragment of Mr=28,000, which is still able to activate plasma kallikrein but is devoid of the ability to bind to negative surfaces[(12)]. Lower molecular weight forms of factor XI and Protein C also retain part of their enzymatic activities[(13)].

The formation of lower molecular weight species might also occur with human plasma kallikrein[(14)]. Evidences that a low molecular weight form of kallikrein occurs during the purification of the active enzyme were previously reported[(4)], but no data on the immunoreactivity of these kallikrein derivatives were presented.

Materials and Methods

Human plasma kallikrein was isolated from acid-activated Cohn's fraction IV[15] or from fresh plasma, by DEAE-Sephadex chromatography (500 ml of settled gel in 0.02M sodium phosphate buffer, 5 mM NaCl, 1 mM EDTA, 2 mM EDTA, 2 mM benzamidine and 50 μg/ml Polybrene, pH 7.4, at room temperature). Prokallikrein, which is not retained by the gel under these conditions, was dialyzed against the same buffer without benzamidine and Polybrene, and the preparation was kept at 20°C for 16 hours; under these conditions, a slow activation of the enzyme is observed. Active kallikrein was adsorbed batchwise to 100 ml of SBTI-Sepharose (in 0.05 M tris-HCl, 0.3 M NaCl, pH 8.0). Kallikrein was eluted, after extensive washings, with 1.0 M benzamidine in the same buffer. Following dialysis against water and lyophilization, kallikrein was gel-filtered in a Sephadex G-150 column (2 × 90 cm) equilibrated in 0.1 M ammonium acetate buffer, pH 6.0. Two peaks of activity were eluted; they were further purified by successive gel-filtrations, under the same conditions. Heavy and light chains were also isolated by a previously described procedure[6].

Human high-molecular-weight kininogen was purified as described[16]; plasminogen was prepared by chromatography of fresh plasma on lysine-Sepharose and was activated by streptokinase (Kabi, Sweden). Bovine trypsin, obtained from Worthington, was treated with tosyl-phenylalanine-chloromethyl-ketone (TPCK). C1-inactivator was a product from Österreiches Institut für Haemoderivate, further purified in Con-A-Sepharose; human antithrombin III was from Sigma. Ala-Phe-Arg chloromethylketone was a kind gift of Dr. Elliot Shaw from Friederich Miescher Institut, Basel.

Kallikrein activity was followed photometrically by hydrolysis of a p-nitroanilide (p-Nan) peptide substrate (0.6 mM D-Pro-Phe-Arg-p-Nan) in 0.1 M tris-HCl, pH 8.0, at 37°C. The kinetic properties were measured under the same condition varying the substrate concentrations; the esterolytic activity was determined with 20 mM Tos-Arg-OMe ester in a pH-stat[15]. The hydrolysis of kininogen was followed by the release of kinin measured upon the isolated guinea-pig ileum[9].

Antibodies against kallikrein were raised in rabbits, after successive weekly subcutaneous injections of 100 μg of protein, in complete Freund's adjuvant. The antibody titers were followed by double immunodiffusion. Specific antibodies against heavy chain were immunoselected using a kallikrein-Sepharose column equilibrated with 0.05 M tris-HCl buffer, 0.15 M NaCl, pH 8.0, and eluted with 0.2 M glycine buffer, pH 2.0.

Radioimmunoassays were performed with kallikrein labeled with ^{125}I by the chloramine T procedure[17].

SDS-polyacrylamide gel electrophoresis was performed in slab gels[18], proteins were stained with 0.25% Coomassie Blue R-250. Proteins in solution were estimated by UV-absorbance at 280 nm.

Results

Plasma kallikrein partially purified on Sephadex G-150 shows a major band of activity at a molecular weight of approximately 86,000, and a second peak of activity at 36,000 (Fig. 1). When the second peak was submitted to successive chromatographies in the same column, it was possible to obtain both kallikrein and light chain (36,000)-fragments in homogeneous form (Fig. 2); eventual traces of albumin were removed by adsorption to Blue-Sepharose. The comparison of the final purification of this second activity with kallikrein shows that it represents 5.7% of the total initial activity; it presents at this stage approximately 20% of kallikrein (Table 1).

When this fragment of kallikrein was tested for its esterolytic and amidolytic activities (Table 2), no major kinetic differences were shown for these two substrates, but the fragment cleaves D-Pro-Phe-Arg-p-Nan faster than does kallikrein itself. The incubation of kallikrein with human high-molecular-weight kininogen causes release of bradykinin; no detectable kinin release was caused by the 36,000-fragment. Both preparations are able to promote unespecific cleavage of kininogen when this protein is analyzed by SDS-polyacrilamide electrophoresis (not shown).

The heavy chain and the light chains isolated from kallikrein gave cross-reactions against an anti-kallikrein serum in immunodiffusion. Identity between lines of precipitation for kallikrein and the isolated chains was observed.

Antibodies immunoselected against kallikrein heavy chain titrate native kallikrein and isolated heavy chain; curves ran parallel to that defined by normal anti-HuPK; light chain does not cross-react with heavy-chain-immunoselected antibodies (Fig. 3).

The fragment (0.8 mg/ml in 0.5 M tris-HCl, pH 8,0, 30°C), was totally inhibited by soybean trypsin inhibitor (1.5 mg/ml), aprotinin (0.8 mg/ml), C1-inhibitor (1.5 mg/ml) and alpha 2-macroglobulin (2.5 mg/ml), and Ala-Phe-Arg-CH2-Cl (0.5 mM); anti-thrombin III (2.5 mg/ml) did not cause inhibition.

Electrophoresis in SDS-polyacrylamide indicates that the fragment occurs in two forms (Mr=36,000 and 33,000); kallikrein shows a molecular weight of 86,000; when

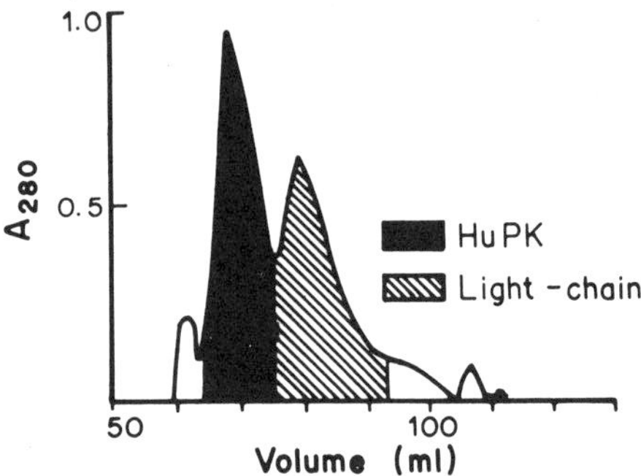

Fig. 1. Gel-filtration of plasma kallikrein (HuPK). HuPK prepared by affinity chromatography (SBTI-Sepharose) was gel filtered in a Sephadex G-150 column (1.0 × 90 cm), equilibrated with 0.1 M ammonium acetate, pH 6.0 buffer. Activity on 1.0 mM Ac.Phe-Arg-p-Nan was detected in both peaks and is indicated in the figure.

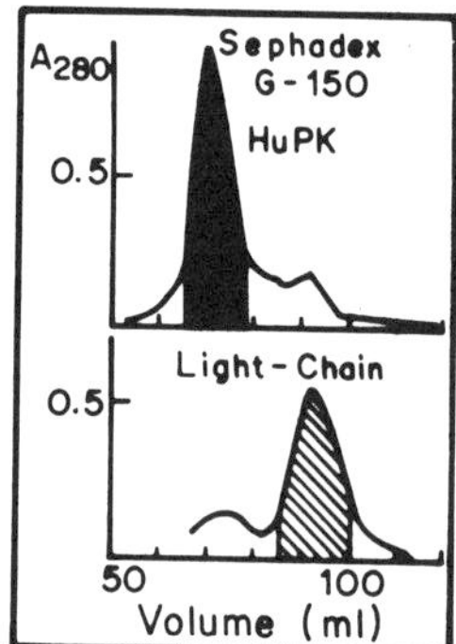

Fig. 2: Gel-filtration of kallikrein and the light chain (36,000)-fragment. Rechromatography of kallikrein and the 36,000-fragment prepared in the Sephadex G-150 column (Fig. 1). Conditions as in Fig. 1.

the samples are reduced, kallikrein forms a heavy chain (Mr=45,000) and a light chain (Mr=36,000 and 33,000). The bands corresponding to the fragment are not changed by the reduction. The electrophoresis also indicates that the fragment differs from tissue kallikrein (Fig. 4).

The evidences gathered by these experimetal data show that the original molecule of kallikrein, which contains the heavy chain and the light chain, can be split to a form corresponding to the light chain.

Table 1. Preparation of the active fragment of kallikrein from human plasma.

	Volume (ml)	Protein (mg)	Activity (Units)	Yield (%)
Plasma	300	18,000	2,800	(100)
Fragment (l.chain)	5	2.4	60	5.7
HuPK	10	10.4	785	28.0

Activity (Unit) is expressed as μmols of S-2302 hydrolyzed per minute under the conditions described in the text.

Table 2. Kinetics of hydrolysis of synthetic substrates.

	Tos-Arg.OMe		D-Pro-Phe-Arg-p-Nan	
	Km (mM)	kcat (sec-1)	Km (mM)	kcat (sec-1)
HuPK	3.4	135	0.35	71
Fragment	5.3	120	0.33	151

Incubations at pH 8.0, 30°C, as indicated in Methods.

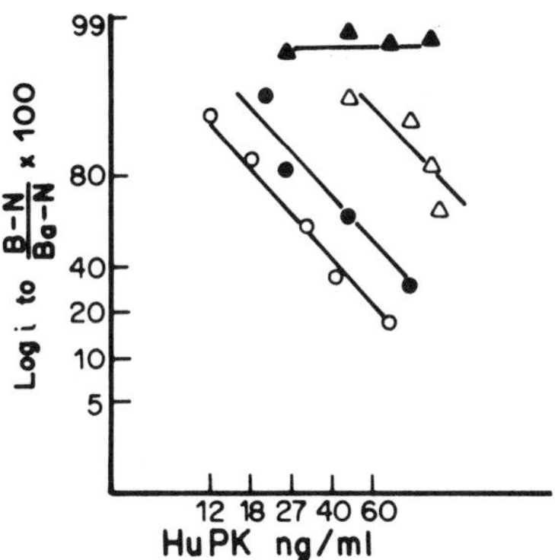

Fig. 3: Radioimmunoassay of kallikrein, heavy-chain and light chain.

(o — o) Kallikrein against normal antiserum
(•—•) Kallikrein against heavy-chain antibodies
(Δ—Δ) Heavy chain against heavy-chain antibodies
(▲—▲) Light chain against heavy-chain antibodies

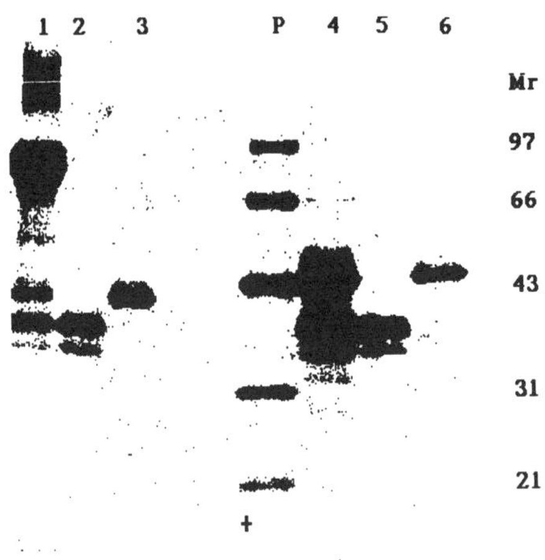

Fig. 4: SDS-polyacrylamide gel electrophoresis of kallikrein and its chains. SDS-PAGE 10–20% gel) Leemmli conditions.

1 – HuPK (14 μg)
2 – Light chain (20 μg)
3 – Heavy chain (24 μg)
P – Molecular weight standards
4 – Reduced HuPK (14 μg)
5 – Reduced light chain (20 μg)
6 – Reduced heavy chain (24 μg)

Discussion

Previous, initial results[(4)] have shown the presence in plasma of kallikrein activity with molecular weight compatible with that of several proteolytic enzymes, or their active fragments. The procedures which were described for the purification of prokallikrein, rather than of the active enzyme, failed to detect this activity because the methods used for preparation of the proenzyme require potent protease inhibitors; alternatively this fragment might be formed only during the non physiological conditions of activation of kallikrein *in vitro*. Following the activation of kallikrein, this activity can be detected when either plasma or Cohn's fraction IV are used as starting materials.

Purification from fresh plasma, yielded about 6% of the initial activity as the active fragment; recovery from Cohn's fraction IV was lower, not higher than 3–4% of the initial activity.

A similar enzyme activity had been detected previously, during gel-filtration steps of preparations from active kallikrein from different species[14]; however, there were no conclusive evidences that this material was a kallikrein fragment; experiments of immunoprecipitation with the isolated fragment and the produced light chain, confirm the nature of this fragment as part of a processed kallikrein molecule. The enzymatic activity of this fragment is somewhat different from that of native kallikrein; and some of those aspects were described previously[19].

The clearance of plasma kallikrein from plasma is attributed to its inhibition by C1-inactivator[20] and to its depuration by the liver[21]. A third possibility for the physiological removal of plasma kallikrein, after attaining its function, could be due to limited proteolysis with formation of a fragment which could still play a biological role. The heavy chain could compete with active kallikrein in its interaction with a negative surface, factor XII or high-molecular-weight kininogen, whereas the light chain could play a regulatory role by hydrolyzing other factors of the blood clotting or fibrinolytic systems.

References

1. Bouma, B.N., L.A. Miles, G. Beretta, and J.H. Griffin, Human plasma kallikrein. Studies of its activation by activated factor XII and its inactivation by diisopropyl phosphofluoridate, Biochemistry 19, 1151-1160 (1980).

2. Colman, R.W. and A. Bagdassarian, Human plasma kallikrein and prekallikrein, Methods in Enzymology 45, 303-322 (1976).

3. Chung, D.W., K. Fujikawa, A.B. McMullen and E.W. Davie, Human plasma prekallikrein, a zymogen to a serine protease that contains four tandem repeats, Biochemistry 25, 2410-2417 (1986).

4. Oliva, M.V.L., D. Grisolia, M.U. Sampaio and C.A.M. Sampaio, Properties of a highly purified human plasma kallikrein, Agents Actions 9 (Suppl.), 53-57 (1982).

5. Levinson, P.R. and G. Tomalin, The kinetics of hydrolysis of some extended N-aminoacyl-L-arginine-methyl esters by human plasma kallikrein, Biochem. J. 205, 529-534 (1982).

6. Van der Graaf, F., G. Tans, B.N. Bouma and J.H. Griffin, Isolation and functional properties of the heavy and light chains of human plasma kallikrein, J. Biol. Chem. 257, 14300-14305 (1982).

7. Van der Graaf, F., A. Rietveld, J.A. Keus and B.N. Bouma, Interaction of human plasma kallikrein and its light-chain with alpha-2-macroglobulin, Biochemistry 23, 1760-1766 (1984).

8. Colman, R.W., Y.T. Wachtfogel, V. Kunick, G. Weinbaum, S. Hahn, R.A. Riley, C.F. Scott, A. Agostini, D. Burger and M. Schapira, Effect of cleavage of the heavy-chain of human plasma kallikrein, Blood 65, 311-338 (1985).

9. Sampaio, C.A.M. and D. Grisolia, Human plasma kallikrein. Preliminary studies on hydrolysis of proteins and peptides, Agents Actions 8, 125-131 (1978).

10. Scott, C.F., E.Y. Liu and R.W. Colman, Human plasma prekallikrein. A rapid high-yield method for purification, Eur. J. Bioch. 100, 77-83 (1979).

11. Glover, G. and E. Shaw, The purification of thrombin and isolation of a peptide containing the active center histidine, J. Biol. Chem. 246, 4594-4601 (1971).

12. Fujikawa, K. and E.W. Davie, Human factor XII (Hageman Factor), Meth. Enzymology 80, 198-211 (1981).

13. Van der Graaf, F., J.S. Greengard, B.N. Bouma, D. Kerbiriou and J.H. Griffin, Isolation and functional characterization of the active light chain of the activated human blood coagulation factor XII, J. Biol. Chem. 258, 9669-9675 (1983).

14. Movat, H.Z., Plasma kallikrein kinin system and its relationship to other components of blood, In: Bradykinin, Kallidin and Kallikrein, Handb. Exp. Pharmac. 25, pp. 1-90 (Ed. E.G. Erdös). Springer-Verlag, Heidelberg 1978.

15. Sampaio, C., S.C. Wong and E. Shaw, Human plasma kallikrein. Purification and preliminary characterization, Arch. Biochem. Biophys. 165, 133-139 (1974).

16. Muller-Esterl, W., B. Dittman, H. Fritz, F. Lottspeich and A. Henschen, Structural aspects of human kininogens, Adv. Exp. Med. Biol. 156A, 157-164 (1983).

17. Greenwood, F.C., W.M. Hunter and J. Glover, The preparation of I-labelled human growth hormone of high specific activity, Biochem. J. 89, 114-123 (1963).

18. Laemmli, U.K., Cleavage of structural protein during the assembly of the head of bacteriophage T4, Nature 227, 680-685 (1970).

19. Motta, G., M.U. Sampaio and C.A.M. Sampaio, Hydrolysis of synthetic peptides and natural substrates by plasma kallikrein and its light chain, Adv. Exp. Med. Biol. 247B, 239-242 (1989).

20. Schapira, M., C.F. Scott and R.W. Colman, Contribution of plasma protease inhibitors to inactivation of kallikrein in plasma, J. Clin. Investigation 69, 462-468 (1982).

21. Borges, D.R., A.H. Gordon, J.A. Guimarães and J.L. Prado, Rat plasma kallikrein clearance by perfused rat liver, Braz. J. Med. Bio. Res. 18, 187-194 (1985).

AAS 36
Contributions to
Autacoid Pharmacology

BIOLOGICALLY ACTIVE PEPTIDES FROM *BOTHROPS JARARACUSSU* VENOM

L.A.F. Ferreira, O.B. Henriques, I. Lebrun, M.B.C. Batista, B.C. Prezoto, A.S.S. Andreoni, R. Zelnik and G. Habermehl*

Instituto Butantan, São Paulo, SP, Brazil and *Chemisches Institut, Tierärtztliche Hochschule, Hannover, Germany

Abstract

The venom of the Brazilian snake *Bothrops jararacussu*, was found to contain peptides capable of potentiating the smooth muscle contracting activity of bradykinin (BK). Chromatographic separation on Sephadex G-25 and Sephadex G-10, respectively, yielded an active peptide which at a concentration of 0.6 μg/ml doubled the effect of a single dose of BK on the isolated guinea-pig ileum. HPLC chromatography showed this material to contain one major and 4 minor components. The active peptide was 2–3 times more active than Captopril in the potentiation of the effects of BK on rat arterial blood pressure and on the isolated guinea pig ileum. It also showed marked capacity to inhibit angiotensin I-converting enzyme.

Introduction

Bradykinin is a typical plasma kinin, causing pain, contraction of smooth muscle, vasodilatation and increased vascular permeability[1]. The presence of BK potentiating peptides in snake venoms has been variously demonstrated[2,3], who isolated nine BK-potentiating peptides from *Bothrops jararaca* venom. The pharmacology of the venom of *B. jararacussu*, a related species, has been little studied. We observed this venom to contain low molecular weight peptides, one of which was found to inhibit angiotensin-converting enzyme *in vitro* and to potentiate the effects of bradykinin on rat arterial blood pressure.

Materials and Methods

Dried *B. jararacussu* venom was obtained from the Butantan Institute. Adult, 300 g male rats and 180–200 g female guinea-pigs were used. Sephadex G-25M and Sephadex G-10 were from Pharmacia, Uppsala. Bradykinin, BK potentiator B, Captopril and BPF_{5a} were from Sigma, St. Louis. Angiotensin converting enzyme (ACE) was purified from rat plasma[4].

Purification procedure. To a solution of 5 g of *B. jararacussu* venom in 100 ml of 50 mM sodium phosphate buffer pH 7.5, three volumes of boiling ethanol were added. The precipitate formed was removed by centrifugation and the ethanol in the supernate evaporated under low pressure; the remaining aqueous phase was lyophilized. 2.45 g of the dry material were dissolved in 8 ml of 50 mM ammonium acetate pH 7.7 and chromatographed at a flow rate of 40 ml/h on a 2 × 190 cm G-25 M Sephadex column. Fractions were tested on the isolated guinea-pig ileum; those exhibiting the highest BK-potentiating activity, were pooled and lyophilized. 420 mg of the dry material were dissolved in 3 ml of the same ammonium acetate buffer and rechromatographed on a Sephadex G-10, 1 × 120 cm column equilibrated with the same buffer. Active fractions were pooled. Reverse phase HPLC analytical chromatography was performed using a Waters instrument, an Ultropack TSK ODS 120 P (5 μm) 30 × 0.38 cm column and an eluting gradient system of 20% acetonitrile/80% and 15% o-phosphoric acid.

Pharmacological assays. The potentiating activity of the chromatographed fractions was measured on the isolated guinea-pig ileum[1]. One potentiating unit was defined as the amount of peptide contained in one ml of bath fluid, capable of changing the activity of a single dose of BK to that of a double one[3]. Carotid arterial blood pressure was determined in Nembutal-anesthetized rats, using a mercury manometer connected to a lever writing on a kymograph's smoked drum.

Biochemical assay. 100 μg of the ACE preparation, 100 μg of BK and 1.4 μg of the active peptide material were incubated in 600 μl of Tyrode solution at 37°C, for given time intervals. Remaining Bk activity was measured on the isolated guinea-pig ileum. Extent of hydrolysis was evaluated by reference to a standard log dose-response curve, corrected for spontaneous bradykinin hydrolysis.

Results and Discussion

Lyophilized ethanol extracts of *B. jararacussu* venom yielded peptide material capable of potentiating bradykinin effects on smooth muscle. Chromatography on a Sephadex G-25 column revealed several active venom components (Fig. 1), one of which, peak 5, following rechromatography on a Sephadex G-10 column (peak I of Fig. 2), showed an approximate 9-fold enrichment in BK-potentiating activity. When submitted to reverse phase HPLC, it yielded the pattern presented on Fig. 3. When an injection of BK into the femoral vein of the rat was preceded by the injection of the active peptide, blood pressure fell to a level approximately 5 times lower than that observed after the injection of bradykinin alone. This effect was more pronounced than that of Captopril employed at a 10-fold higher dose (Fig. 4). The comparison between the BK-potentiating action of *B. jararacussu* peptide (peak I), Captopril and BK-potentiator B on the guinea-pig ileum, showed the former to be approximately 3 times more active than the latter two compounds (Table 1). 1.4 μg of the peptide caused 50% inhibition of the bradykinin hydrolysing activity of 100 μg of the angiotensin-converting enzyme from rat plasma (Fig. 5).

References

1. Rocha e Silva, M., W.T. Beraldo and G. Rosenfeld, Bradykinin, a hypotensive smooth muscle stimulating factor released from plasma globulin by snake venoms and by trypsin, Am. J. Physiol. 156, 261-273 (1949).

2. Ferreira. S.H., A bradykinin-potentiating factor (BPF) present in the venom of *Bothrops jararaca*, Br. J. Pharmac. 24, 163-169 (1965).

3. Ferreira, S.H., D.C. Bartelt and L.J. Greene, Isolation of bradykinin-potentiating peptides from *Bothrops jararaca* venom, Biochemistry 9, 2583-2593 (1970).

4. Nishimura, K., N. Yoshida, K. Hiwada, E. Ueda and T. Kokubu, Purification of angiotensin-converting enzyme from human lung, Biochem. Biophys. Acta 483, 398-408 (1977).

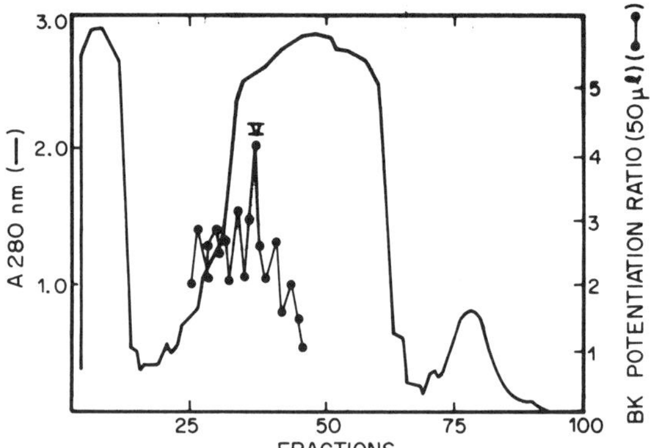

Fig. 1. Gel filtration on a Sephadex G-25M column (2 × 170 cm) of 2.45 g of a dry ethanolic extract of *B. jararacussu* venom. Eluent: 50 mM ammonium acetate, pH 4.7. Fraction volume: 3 ml. Absorbance at 280 nm (—). Bradykinin potentiation ratio (•—•).

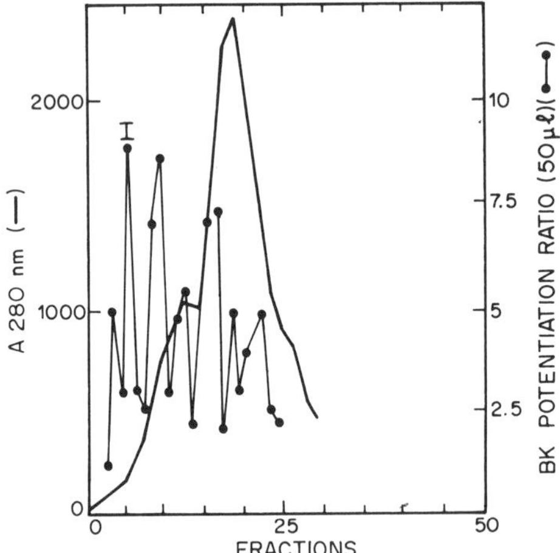

Fig. 2. Gel filtration on a Sephadex G-10 column (1 × 120 cm) of 420 mg of pooled active fractions obtained from peak V (Fig. 1). Eluent: 50 mM ammonium acetate, pH 4.7 . Fraction volume: 2 ml. Absorbance at 280 nm (—). Bradykinin potentiation ratio (•—•).

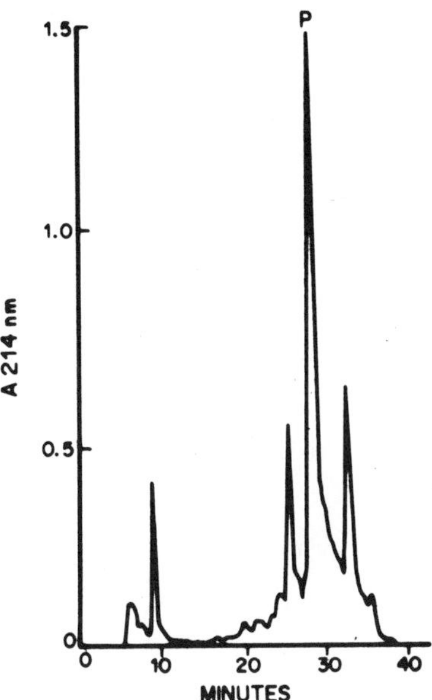

Fig. 3. Fractionation of 100 μg of the active material contained in peak I of Fig. 2, on a reverse-phase HPLC Column Ultropack ODS (5 μm), 30 × 0.38 cm. Eluent: 20% acetonitrile/ 80% and 15% ortho-phosphoric acid. Flow rate 1 ml/min.

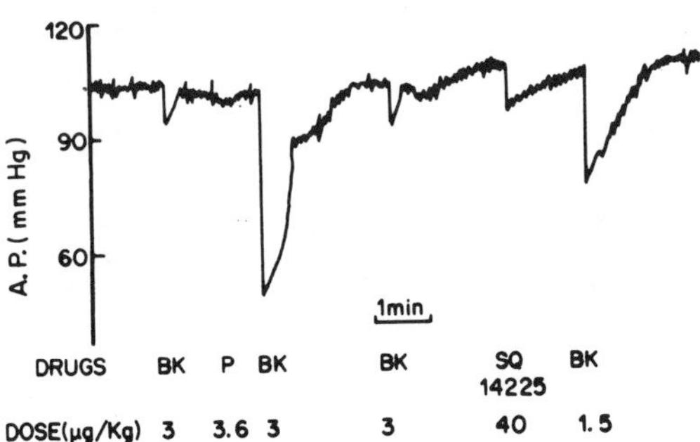

Fig. 4. Action of *B. Jararacussu* potentiating peptide (p) and of Captopril (SQ 14225) on the arterial blood pressure response of the rat to bradykinin (B). These results were confirmed by three additional experiments.

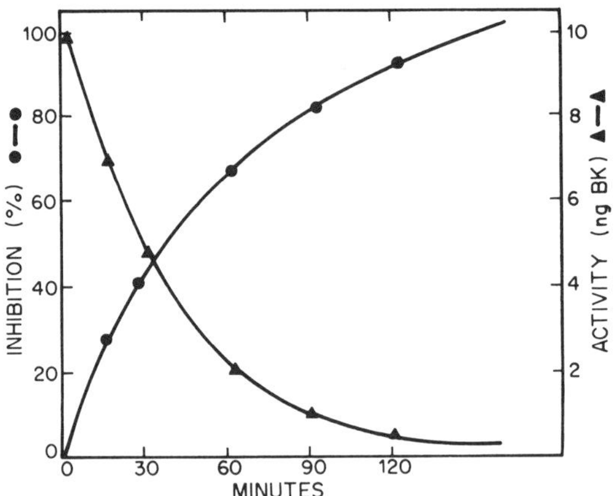

Fig. 5. Angiotensin converting-enzyme inhibition 1.4 μg of the peptide were incubated with 100 μg of angiotensin-converting enzyme (ACE) at pH 7.5 at 37°C for different times in the presence of bradykinin substrate (100 μg). Inhibition (●—●) and activity (▲—▲). Results are averages of three experimental ±SEM.

Table 1. Comparison between the potentiation by captopril, bradykinin-potentiator B, BPF 5a and *B. jararacussu* peptide (peak I, Fig. 3), of the responses of the isolated guinea-pig ileum to bradykinin.

SUBSTANCE	(μg) *PU
Captopril	2 (± 0,2)
Bradykinin-potentiator B	16×10^{-1} (± 0,3)
BPF_{5a}	8×10^{-1} (± 0,2)
Peptide	6×10^{-1} (± 0,3)

*PU - POTENTIATING UNIT: amount of peptide per ml bath fluid, capable of doubling the effect of a single dose of BK on the isolated guinea-pig ileum. Values shown represent the averaged results of three experiments, presented with their respective standard errors of the mean.

AAS 36
Contributions to
Autacoid Pharmacology

THE T-KININOGEN, T-KININ SYSTEM OF THE RAT

L.M. Greenbaum

Department of Pharmacology/Toxicology, Schools of Medicine & Graduate Studies, Medical College of Georgia, Augusta, Ga. 30912, USA

Introduction

I wish to thank Dr. Watanabe, Dr. Beraldo, and Dr. Rothschild for this splendid opportunity to return to Brazil in honor of Mauricio Rocha e Silva, the discoverer of bradykinin. Everyone in this room has been influenced by the late Dr. Rocha e Silva. I am no exception. Some 25 years ago, when I was a young assistant professor working on catheptic proteases, Dr. Rocha e Silva visited me at the Downstate Medical Center. He listened patiently to me, telling about my research, but, as was his nature, exclaimed that I was wasting my time. He said that I should be working with bradykinin! Fortunately, I took his advice. I can say to the students and young people in this room that the research adventures with kinins and proteases have been utterly fascinating. Our discovery of T-kinin and T-kininogens has to be a lesson for all researchers who have been told that kinins are no longer as exciting as other areas of research are. Research on kinins is on the upswing because of the key nature of their pharmacological properties and of recent discoveries showing that kininogens are multi-purpose proteins acting not only as precursors of kinins but also as cysteine protease inhibitors, in blood clotting and, in the case of T-kininogen, as acute phase proteins in injury and inflammation.

The Discovery of T-Kinin and T-Kininogen

In the early 1980's, Dr. Hiroshi Okamoto of Kobe, Japan, came to my laboratory in Georgia to work on leucokinins. These were long chain kinins that had never been well characterized; they are released by catheptic proteases such as cathepsin D. During his investigation using rat blood, in order to release kinins he added increasing amounts of trypsin, much more than published protocols called for. The results were astonishing: the more trypsin he added, the more kinin he obtained. The final amounts liberated were far greater than those reported in the literature. At the time we had just completed setting up a procedure for the separation of kinins by **HPLC**; one of the first laboratories to do so. After purification procedures, we applied the material to **HPLC** and discovered a new peak. We termed this peak *T-kinin* because trypsin was the liberating enzyme. Little did we know at the time that the reason we needed large amounts of trypsin was because trypsin had, uncharacteristically, to cleave a methionyl-isoleucine bond to liberate this 11 amino acid polypeptide. What was equally astonishing was that it was surprisingly simple to obtain large amounts of T-kinin from the plasma of rats that had been subjected to an inflammatory response produced by such agents as carrageenin or adjuvant arthritis(1,2,3,4). Aydin Barlas, a postdoctoral fellow from Turkey, made a very significant finding showing, for the first time, that the kininogen carrying T-kinin, termed *T-kininogen*, was an acute phase protein. While under normal conditions rat plasma contains about 70% of all kininogen, following an inflammatory response there is a *6–10 fold increase in T-kininogen* but *no* changes in HMW or LMW kininogen contents(5–6). Okamoto then went on to isolate T-kinin, whose structure is:

Ile-Ser-Arg-Pro-Pro-Gly-Phe-Ser-Pro-Phe-Arg

Rat plasma yielded *two* T-kininogens, termed T-kininogen I and II. All of this exciting work was reported starting 1983. In 1985, Nakanishi, using mRNA analysis, confirmed that there were two T-kininogens. He also showed that each was an expression of a different gene but that HMW & LMW kininogens were expressed from a single gene(7). It is the general conception that the genes of T-kininogen are exclusive to the rat. No reports of this systems in other species has been noted with one exception. Wunderer(8) has published that in a small number of cases, T-kinin is found in the ascites fluid of women afflicted with ovarian carcinoma. This unusual finding awaits confirmation.

Factors Influencing the Synthesis of T-Kininogen

The hepatic synthesis and consequently, the plasma levels of T-kininogen are rapidly accelerated, producing within hours, very high levels approaching 10X the normal level, following injury, surgery, inflammation and hormone treatment. An example of this is seen in Table 1. The adult female has about 3 times the levels of the male. As shown in several laboratories, this is clearly the result of estrogen influence. The accelerated synthesis of T-kininogen *in vitro* has been demonstrated by Dr. Lapp in our laboratory, using hepatic cells in culture treated with estrogen. Dr. Lapp has shown for the first time, that prolactin added to primary hepatocytes in culture stimulates T-kininogen synthesis. This may be the reason why lactating female rats have 2–3 times the levels of T-kininogen present in adult female rats. Newborn rats have similarly high levels. These levels of the newborn are gradually reduced to normal after about 3–4 months[(9)]. There is increasing evidence that interleukins, especially interleukin 6, may have significant influence on T-kininogen levels particularly in inflammation where leukocytes are mobilized. Since macrophages synthesize and release interleukins, there is reasonable suspicion that their presence is a major factor for the elevation of T-kininogen levels.

Table I. Differences between plasma T-kininogen levels in adult, newborn and lactating rats. Results demonstrate that normal female rats have higher plasma levels of T-kininogen than normal males. Newborn rats have very high levels as do lactating females.

AGE	T-KGN μg/ml	
	MALE	FEMALE
Adult (160 gms)	200	600
Newborn (10 days)	1150	1590
Newborn (36 days)	766	807
Lactating		1323

It is significant that anti-inflammatory drugs such as dexamethasone and indomethacin reduce the response of T-kininogen synthesis following the inflammatory response. This was first reported by our laboratory and was recently confirmed by the demonstration[(10)] that the mRNA levels for T-kininogens I and II were reduced in rats challenged with Freund's complete adjuvant and treated with dexamethasone. Further studies have revealed that the dexamethasone effect is not due to a reduction in the transcription rate of T-kininogen mRNA, but may be due to a reduction in interleukin production by white cells. The *in vivo* response is different from the response of hepatic cells actively synthesizing T-kininogen *in vitro*. In the latter case, dexamethasone *stimulates* the synthesis. Thus cytokine action would seem to be critical for the *in vivo* effect of dexamethasone.

Properties of T-Kininogen

The intense increase in the rate of transcription of T-kininogen mRNA following an inflammatory response, clearly designates T-kininogen as an acute phase protein. T-kininogens must play a very significant role in the inflammatory response; but which one? At this point we do not really know. However, judging from some of its properties, we can make some good suggestions. As a substrate, it differs considerably from HMW and LMW kininogens since kallikrein does not cleave bradykinin from it. The reason for this is that the -Ser-Arg- bond at the N-terminal portion of the bradykinin moiety is resistant to kallikrein. An enzyme termed T-kininogenase, first described by us, cleaves T-kinin from T-kininogens. However this enzyme, which we discuss later in the manuscript, is only found in the submaxillary gland, thus limiting the potential for T-kinin release. One additional significant property is that it is a thiol protease inhibitor. As noted in Table 2, it is a good inhibitor of papain-like proteases as well as of cathepsin B and Cathepsin L. We can thus imagine that as an acute phase protein, T-kininogen is synthesized and released rapidly and retards actions of cysteine proteases such as the cathepsins, thus ameliorating the potential tissue damage these enzymes inflict during inflammation. A second possibility is that T-kinin is liberated from it, thus promoting the inflammatory response.

Detection of T-Kininogen

We have been able to develop monoclonal antibodies which are specific to T-kininogen II and monoclonal antibodies which react with both T-kininogen I and II. An ELISA assay has been developed so that a minimum concentration of 20 pg may be detected. The antibodies have no cross-reactivity with HMW or LMW kininogens, T-kinin, or bradykinin[11].

Table II. Comparison of Rat T-kininogen with HMW- and LMW-kininogen.

	T-KGN I & II	HMW-KGN	LMW-KGN
Genetic	Two genes	Single gene	
M.W.	69KDa	114 KDa	68KDa
Kinin liberation			
Kallikrein	No kinin release	bradykinin	Lys-bradykinin
T-KGNase (Submax gland rat, mouse)	T-kinin	—	—
Cathepsin D	Met-T-kinin & T-kinin	No kinin released	No kinin
Cysteine Proteinase Inhibition (Ki nM)			
Papain	0.014	0.11	—
Cathepsin B	18.400	45.00	—
Cathepsin L	11.000	1.20	—
Plasma Levels			
Inflammation	increase	no change	
Estrogen	increase	no change	
Indomethacin	decrease	no change	
Dexamethasone	decrease	no change	

Properties of T-Kininogenase

Barlas in our laboratory, reported that during the inflammatory response, in addition to an increase in T-kininogen, there is an increase in free T-kinin in plasma and also in body fluids, resulting from the inflammatory response. Since kallikrein does not release T-kinin, we searched for an enzyme that did. As discussed above, we isolated it from rat submaxillary gland. A graduate student, Gao, also discovered it in the mouse submaxillary gland. The enzyme is most interesting since it requires thiol activation using T-kininogen as the substrate. It is very active at neutral pH and it is inhibited by leupeptin and by DFP-like agents. It would appear to be a molecule which has both cysteine protease and serine protease characteristics[12]. It has similar amino acids sequences as tissue kallikrein, but it is easily separated from kallikrein during purification. Additional properties are shown in Table 2.

Properties of T-Kinin

T-kinin has similar properties as bradykinin in terms of pharmacological activity causing rat uterus contraction, vascular permeability increase and depression of blood pressure. Gao in our laboratory, found that T-kinin acts through B^2 receptors in the rat uterus as demonstrated by the inhibition of its effects by B^2 antagonists and not by B^1 antagonists. The potency of T-kinin is similar to that of bradykinin. However, binding studies have shown T-kinin to have a lower affinity to the receptor than bradykinin. This implies·that there is a difference in intracellular signal transduction by the kinins. This was confirmed by findings showing that indomethacin has a greater inhibitory affect on the contraction of the rat uterus by T-kinin than by bradykinin, indicating that prostaglandin release is a greater component of T-kinin's action on the uterus than of that of bradykinin.

Summary and Conclusions

The T-kininogen-T-kinin system in the rat has to be considered one of the most dynamic systems in any animal model. The marked effort the liver performs to enhance T-kininogen synthesis immediately following injury or hormone action, forces us to probe deeper into the meaning of this. I like to think that T-kininogen is a "healing protein", produced not only to ameliorate the inflammatory response but perhaps to actually promote healing. We have at the moment not been able to prove this theory, and have to be satisfied to summarize biochemical and physiological events as shown in the accompanying figure. But this is only two dimensional and the events which occur with such speed in the T-kininogen system must have a much deeper meaning. About 25 years ago Rocha e Silva told me I should be working on bradykinin. Today, in this wonderful country, I am telling you the same thing: join the excitement and help me discover the real meaning of T-kininogen and T-kinin. Supported by grant HL 32/83.

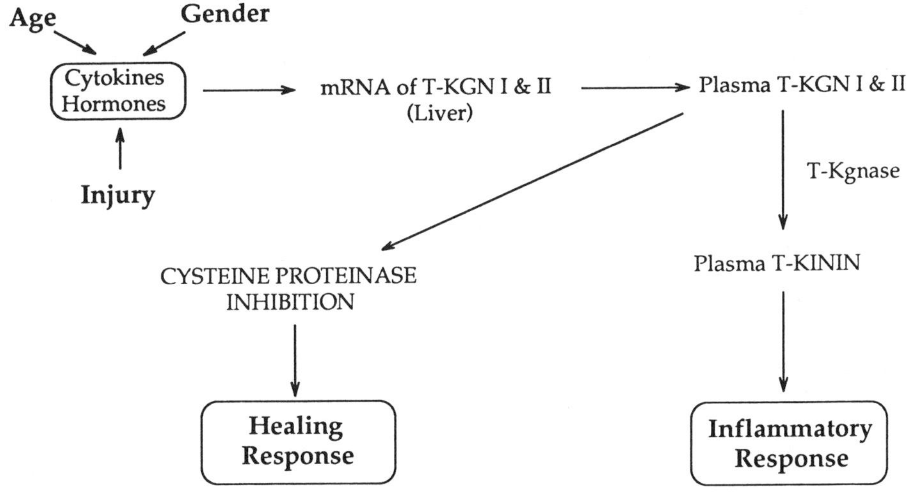

Fig 1. T-kininogen in the rat. Age, gender, and injury alter the levels of cytokines and hormones which influence the rate of transcription of T-kininogen mRNA. High levels of T-kininogens promote healing by inhibiting cysteine proteinases. T-kinin formation is a function of T-kininogenase and will enhance inflammation.

References

1. Okamoto H. and L.M. Greenbaum, Kininogen substrates for trypsin and cathepsin D in human, rabbit, and rat plasmas, Life Sciences 32, 2007-2013 (1983).

2. Okamoto, H. and L.M. Greenbaum, Isolation and structure of T-kinin, Biochem. Biophys. Res. Comm. 112, 701-708 (1983).

3. Okamoto, H. and L.M. Greenbaum, Pharmacological properties of T-kinin, Biochem. Pharmacol. 32, 2637-2638 (1983).

4. Okamoto, H. and L.M. Greenbaum, Isolation and properties of two rat plasma T-kininogens, In: (Eds. L.M. Greenbaum, H. Margolius) Kinins IV - Advances Experimental Medicine and Biology 198A, 69-75. Plenum Press, N.Y. 1986.

5. Barlas, A., H. Okamoto and L.M. Greenbaum, T-kininogen-the major plasma kininogen in rat adjuvant arthritis, Biochem. Biophys. Res. Commun. 129, 280-286 (1985).

6. Barlas, A., Okamoto, H. and L.M. Greenbaum, Release of T-kinin and bradykinin in carrageenin-induced inflammation in the rat, FEBS Lett. 190, 268-270 (1985).

7. Kitagawa H., N. Kitamura and S. Nakanishi, Differing expression patterns and evolution of the rat kininogen gene family, J. Biol. Chem. 262, 2190-2198 (1987).

8. Wunderer, G., I. Walter, E. Muller, A. Henschen, Human Ile-Ser-bradykinin, identical with rat T-kinin is a major permeability factor in ovarian carcinoma ascites, Hoppe-Seyler Zeitschr. Biol. Chem. 367, 1231-1234 (1986).

9. Cho, C. and L.M. Greenbaum, T-kininogen in lactating and normal female rats as compared to neonates, FASEB J2, A1146 (1988).

10. Howard, E.F., Y.G. Thompson, C.A. Lapp and L.M. Greenbaum, Reduction of T-kininogen messenger RNA levels by dexamethasone in the adjuvant-treated rat, Life Sciences 46, 411-417 (1990).

11. Greenbaum, L.M. and H. Okamoto, T-kinin and T-kininogen, In: (Eds. J. Abelson and M. Simon) Methods in Enzymology 163, 272-282 (1988).

12. Barlas, A., X.X. Gao, L.M. Greenbaum, Isolation of a thiol-activated T-kininogenase from the rat submandibular gland, FEBS Lett. 218, 266-270 (1987).

AAS 36
Contributions to
Autacoid Pharmacology

KININOGEN CHANGES IN THE ALLOXAN-DIABETIC RAT

M.L. Reis, R. Paschoalato and C.H.R. Serra

Department of Physics and Chemistry, School of Pharmaceutical Sciences of Ribeirão Preto, University of São Paulo, 14049 Ribeirão Preto, SP, Brazil

Abstract

Ten-day alloxan diabetic rats showed substantial increases in plasma T-kininogen, high molecular and low molecular weight kininogens, as well as significant decreases in urinary levels of kallikrein. Changes in T-kininogen were also observed following turpentine inflammatory treatment. In the diabetic rat, inflammatory responses may contribute to T-kininogen increases.

Introduction

My (M.L.R.) scientific training as a "Kininologist" started while studying kinin-forming activity of proteases from different animal species with Professor Rocha e Silva in 1965. At that time the two kininogens known, high (HKg) and low molecular weight (LKg), were only measured indirectly using the isolated guinea-pig ileum[1,2,3]. Our results showed, among other findings, that pancreatic kallikrein only generated 40–50% kinin, in comparison with kinin generated by trypsin or animal venom proteases, from rat and other animal plasmas. These results were considered to indicate differences between the structures of rat kininogen and that of other species. The discovery of T-kininogen (TKg) in rat plasma[4] confirmed this hypothesis by showing that this precursor is not sensitive to kinin-forming activity of kallikreins, but nevertheless, represents 60% of the total kininogen in rat plasma.

The involvement of the kininogen-kallikrein-kinin system (KKKS) in inflammation[5], hypertension[6] and the diabetic state[7] has been investigated by us in two different ways: by measuring alterations of kallikrein levels in plasma, kidney and urine, or, by the study of the role of kinins in glucose metabolism of skeletal muscle. However, the question of bradykinin participation in glucose uptake and protein synthesis in muscle is still controversial[8,9]. Reduction of renal and urinary kallikrein has been observed in rats with severe diabetes[10]. These alterations seem to be related to renal hemodynamic disturbances; they appear concomitantly with alterations in blood pressure. Reduction of glandular and plasma kallikrein in diabetic rats has been reported[11,12]. However, an increase in the glandular type of plasma kallikrein has been observed in human diabetes[13]. The relatively abundant amount of information on kallikrein changes in diabetes contrasts with the scarcity of studies on kinin precursor levels in this condition, both in human and animal plasma. We presently report the results of a quantitative and qualitative analysis of plasma kininogen in rats 10 and 20 days after alloxan-induced diabetes. Concomitant changes in levels of urinary kallikrein are also described.

Methods

Diabetes was induced in male 180–200 g Holtzman rats by intravenous injection of 40 mg/kg body weight of alloxan. Animals were housed in metabolic cages with free access to regular chow and water. On the 10th and 20th day after treatment, blood and urine were collected. Blood samples for kininogen determination were obtained under ether anesthesia by abdominal aorta puncture using sodium citrate (2 mg/ml) as anticoagulant. In blood samples used for plasma glucose determination, fluoride-EDTA replaced sodium citrate. Plasma was separated by centrifugation at 2000 *g* during 15 minutes, at room temperature.

Urine was collected at room temperature during 24-hour periods and centrifuged before kallikrein analysis.

Biochemical methods. Plasma glucose levels were measured according to Dubowiski[14] and expressed as mg/dl. Urinary kallikrein was determined as described by Amundsen[15], using the chromogenic substrate HD-Val-Leu-Arg-p-NA. (Kabi-Vitrum). Purified urinary kallikrein, used as standard, was a kind gift from J.P. Girolami, INSERM U-133, Toulouse, France. Results were expressed as μg/24 h.

Biological methods. Kininogen concentration in plasma was evaluated using the isolated guinea-pig ileum to assay kinin formed by trypsin from heat/acid denaturated rat plasma[2]. Kininogen is expressed in terms of μg bradykinin equivalents (BKEq) formed.

Statistical analysis. data are expressed as means ±SEM. Comparison of mean values were made by analysis of variance using Scheffé's test[16].

Results

Figure 1 shows plasma glucose and kininogen as well as urinary kallikrein changes in 10- and 20-day alloxan diabetic rats. Both groups presented a highly significant increase ($p<0.001$) in plasma kininogen concentration relative to controls. Urinary kallikrein concentration was significantly reduced in the diabetic rats, both on the 10th and the 20th day following alloxan treatment.

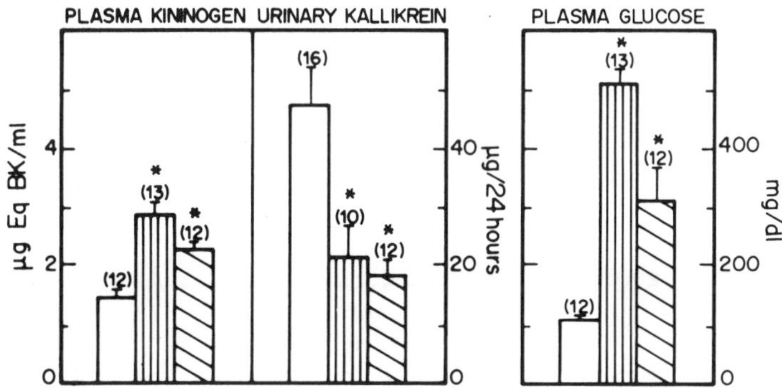

Fig. 1. Plasma kininogen (μg BKEq/ml), urinary kallikrein (μg/24 hr) and plasma glucose (mg/dl) in control ▭, 10-day diabetic ▥, and 20-day diabetic ▧, rats. $^*p \leq 0.001$.

Chromatographic separation of the different entities of plasma kininogen (manuscript in preparation) was employed to identify and quantify specific kininogen(s) in 10-day diabetic rat plasma. Figure 2 presents averaged results of three experiments in which percent increase in TKg, HKg and LKg are expressed relative to control values, considered as 100%.

Increases in TKg have been observed in inflammatory conditions[4]. The second part of Fig. 2 shows that rats responded to inflammation evoked by turpentine treatment (0.1 ml intramuscularly per 100 g body weight, 48 h prior to plasma sampling), with a large increase in TKgs (870 and 350%, respectively), but with little changes of plasma HKg and LKg.

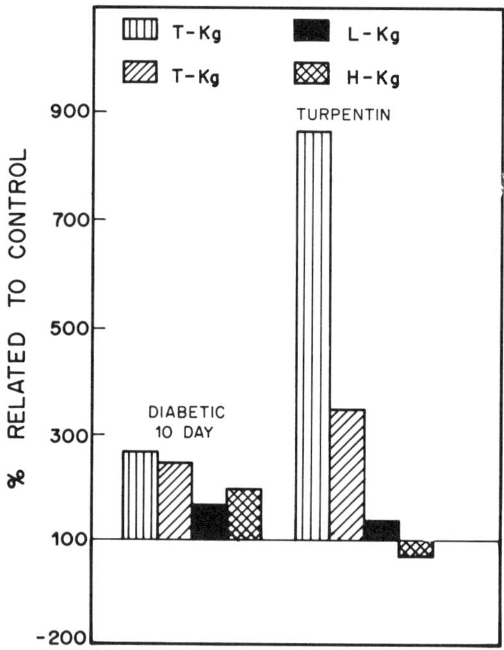

Fig. 2. Percent change of plasma TKg , LKg and HKg in 10-day diabetic rats and in turpentine-treated rats. Kininogen of control rats was assigned a value of 100%. Bars represent the means of three chromatographic analyses on DEAE-Sephacel, 1.25 × 2.5 cm columns. Kininogen fractions were eluted from the columns by a stepwise gradient containing 0.121–0.193 M Tris buffer, pH 7.7. Different Kgs were characterized by immunoreaction with HKg and TKg specific antibodies, respectively, by hydrolysis with 0.1 and 1.0 mg trypsin/ml, respectively, and by gel filtration on Sephacryl S-200.

Discussion

The present results demonstrate that alloxan diabetic rats show significant increases in plasma kininogen as well as a significant reduction in urinary kallikrein on days 10 and 20 following the diabetogenic stimulus. Similar changes have been observed in urinary, renal and plasma glandular kallikrein levels of streptozotocin-diabetic rats[10,11]. Changes in renal kallikrein concentration were considered to be related to altered renal plasma flow and glomerular filtration rate in these rats[17]. Arteriolar dilatation produced by kinins infused into the kidney and/or applied to the luminal or anti-luminal side of isolated perfused glomerular arterioles has been described[18,19]. These reports, in addition to pointing towards the localization of kallikrein and kininogen within connecting tubules and principal cells respectively, reinforce the concept of a relevant role of the KKKS in renal hemodynamic control[20]. Insulin replacement in experimental diabetic rats effectively raised renal kallikrein synthesis to normal values, a result suggesting that insulin may act as a hormonal regulator of kallikrein synthesis[10,21]. Nevertheless, the significant increase in plasma kininogen presently observed in diabetic rats cannot be explained solely as a consequence of the reduction of urinary kallikrein levels. It is known that the submandibular gland is the major source of plasma glandular kallikrein[22]. Diabetic rats produced less submandibular kallikrein than their controls when examined fourteen days after alloxan or streptozocin treatment[11]. High levels of plasma kininogen could therefore be partly due to a reduction of plasma glandular kallikrein. Studies on glandular and plasma kallikrein changes in 10- and 20-day alloxan-diabetic rats are presently in progress in our laboratory.

Although in our research, all forms of kininogen were increased in diabetic rats, it is known that LKg and HKg, but not TKgs, are substrates for the kinin-generating action of plasma glandular kallikrein[23]. The large increase of TKg in diabetic rats may be a consequence of a residual inflammatory reaction evoked by alloxan. It could be associated with cysteine proteinase inhibitor functions of TKgs[24], not yet described in the diabetic state. It may be worth emphasizing that TKg, while acting as a substrate for cysteine proteinases like cathepsin D and E, generates T-kinin[25,26].

The high HKg concentration in diabetic rats could, in part, contribute towards the hypercoagulability associated with this condition. In addition to pre-kallikrein, factors XI and XII, HKg is known to be an important co-factor of the intrinsic blood coagulation process[27].

References

1. Jacobsen, S., Substrates for plasma kinin forming enzymes in human, dog and rabbit plasma, Brit. J. Pharmac. 26, 403-411 (1966).

2. Diniz, C.R. and I.F. Carvalho, A micromethod for determination of bradykininogen under several conditions, Ann. N.Y. Acad. Sci. 104, 77-89 (1963).

3. Rocha e Silva, M., Bradykininogen and the release of kinins, In: Kinin Hormones, pp. 107-117. Charles C. Thomas Springfield 1970.

4. Barlas, A., H. Okamoto and L.M. Greenbaum, T-kininogen – the major plasma kininogen in rat adjuvant arthritis, Biochem. Res. Comm. 129, 280-286 (1985).

5. Reis, M.L., J. Garcia Leme and L.S. Sudo, Plasma kininogen levels in rats with adjuvant arthritis, Agents Actions (Suppl.) 9, 368-377 (1982).

6. Reis, M.L., W.D.P. Jesus, L.M.B. Sabbag, E.M. Krieger and J.L. Greene, Increased levels of new spasmogenic substances released by trypsin from plasma of hypertensive rats, Hypertension. 6, 255-261 (1984).

7. Reis, M.L., C.H.R. Serra, M.J.F. Ribeiro, C.A.A. Silva and A.C.C. Spadaro, Kininogens in alloxan diabetic rats, Eur. J. Pharmacol. 183, 658 (1990).

8. Dietze, G., E. Maerker, C. Lodri, R. Schifman, M. Wicklmayr, R. Geiger, E. Fink, I. Boettger, H. Fritz and H. Mehnert, Possible involvement of kinins in muscle energy metabolism, Adv. Exp. Med. Biol. 167, 63-71 (1984).

9. Wicklmayr, M., K. Rett, E. Fink, W. Tschollar, H. Baldermann, M. Tymiec and H. Mehnert, Bradykinin is not liberated by working skeletal muscle in diabetes type II, Horm. Metab. Res. 21, 222-223 (1989).

10. Mayfield, R.K., H.S. Margolius, G.S. Bailey, D.H. Miller, D.A. Sens, J. Squires and D.H. Mamm, Urinary and renal tissue kallikrein in streptozotocin diabetic rats, Diabetes 34, 22-28 (1984).

11. Jaffa, A.A., J. Pratt, A. Ashford and G.S. Bailey, A study of glandular kallikrein in experimental diabetes, Adv. Exp. Med. Biol. 198B, 367-371 (1986).

12. Sulaiman, M.I. and Saud, Relevance of plasma glandular and urinary kallikrein in renal hypertrophy in streptozotocin diabetic rats, Acta Diabetol. Lat. 23, 253-259 (1986).

13. Federspil, G., R. Veltor, E. De Palo, D. Padovan, N. Sicolo and C. Scandellari, Plasma kallikrein activity in human diabetes mellitus, Metabolism. 32, 540-542 (1983).

14. Dubowski, K.M., An o-toluidine method for body fluid glucose determination, Clin. Chem. 8, 215-235 (1962).

15. Amundsen, E., Y. Putter, P. Faibergen, M. Larsbraten and G. Glaeson, Methods for the determination of glandular kallikrein by means of a chromogenic tripeptide substrate. Adv. Exp. Med. Biol. 120A, 83-95 (1979).

16. Hays, W.L., In: Statistics of Social Sciences, pp. 605-607 (Eds. R. Hold and H. Winston). Academic Press, N.Y. 1973.

17. Harvey, J.N., A.A. Jaffa, H.S. Margolius and R.K. Mayfield, Renal kallikrein and hemodynamic abnormalities of diabetic kidney, Diabetes 39, 299-304 (1990).

18. Edwards, R.M., Responses of isolated renal arterioles to acetylcholine, dopamine and bradykinin, Am. J. Physiol. 248, F. 183-189 (1985).

19. Baylis, C., W.M. Deen, B.D. Meyers, B.M. Brenner, Effects of some vasodilator drugs on transcapillary fluid exchange in renal cortex, Am. J. Physiol. 230, 1148-1158 (1976).

20. Figueroa, C.D., A.G. Maclver, J.C. Mackenzie and K.D. Bhoola, Localization of immunoreactive kininogen and tissue kallikrein in the human nephron, Histochemistry 89, 437-442 (1988).

21. Jaffa, A.A., D.H. Miller, G.S. Bailey, J. Chao, H.S. Margolius, R.K. Mayfield, Abnormal regulation of renal kallikrein in experimental diabetes: effects of insulin on pro-kallikrein synthesis and activation, J. Clin. Invest. 80, 1651-1659 (1987).

22. Lawton, W.J., D. Proud, M.G. Warner, J.V. Pierce, H.R. Keiser and J.J. Pisano, Characterization and origin of immunoreactive glandular kallikrein in rat plasma, Biochem. Pharmacol. 30, 1731-1737 (1981).

23. Alhenc Gelás, F., J. Marchetti, J. Allegrini, P. Corvol and J. Ménard, Measurements of urinary kallikrein activity: species differences in kinin production, Biochem. Biophys. Acta 677, 477-488 (1981).

24. Moreau, T., N. Gutman, A.E. Moyahed, F. Esnard and F. Gauthier, Relationship between the cysteine-proteinase-inhibitory function of rat T-kininogen and the release of immunoreactive kinin upon trypsin treatment, Eur. J. Biochem. 159, 341-346 (1986).

25. Okamoto, H. and L.M. Greenbaum, Kininogen substrates for trypsin and cathepsin D in human and rat plasmas, Life Sciences 32, 2007-2013 (1983).

26. Sakamoto, W., K. Yoshikawa, A. Yokoyama and M. Kohri, T-kinin is released from T-kininogen by consecutive changes by cathepsin E-like proteinase and 72KDa proteinase, Biochim. Biophys. Acta. 884, 607-609 (1986).

27. Damas, J. and V. Bourdon, The significance of high molecular weight kininogen for contact activation of rat blood coagulation, *in vitro*, Arch. Intern. Physiol. Biochem. 98, 67-73 (1989).

Acknowledgements

We thank Dra. Ana Isabel de Assis for her helpful discussion of the manuscript.
We also acknowledge the support for this study, received from CNPq (GRANT 401052.87-7).

AAS 36
Contributions to
Autacoid Pharmacology

KININOGEN CHANGES EVOKED IN PLASMA BY FEEDING, PSEUDO-ALIMENTARY, VAGAL AND CARBAMYLCHOLINE STIMULATION OF THE RAT

A.M. Rothschild, I.C. Fortunato and E.L.T. Gomes

Department of Pharmacology, School of Medicine of Ribeirão Preto, University of São Paulo, 14049 Ribeirão Preto, SP, Brazil

Abstract

Changes in plasma total (BKg), low (LKg), or high (HKg) molecular weight kininogens are indirect means of studying the participation of kinins in biological processes. To investigate kinin involvement in digestive activity, rats fasted overnight, but given access to water, were allowed to feed for one hour. BKg levels increased by 18% ($p<0.001$); LKg by 29% ($p<0.01$); HKg remained apparently unchanged. Changes were reversed after 120 min. Decreases in circulatory HKg are probably masked by a compensatory response of the organism aimed at rapidly re-establishing kinin precursor levels in the circulation following their consumption by parasympathetic activity accompanying feeding. This conclusion is based on observations showing that fasted rats submitted to sham-feeding caused by visual/olfactory stimulation by food, present extensive (61%) reduction ($p<0.001$) of HKg, but not of LKg. It is further supported by results demonstrating that electrical stimulation of the distal stump of the cut left abdominal vagus nerve, as well as intravenous administration of carbamylcholine, a parasympathomimetic drug, also produce these changes, all of which were prevented by prior atropinization of the experimental animals. These results open the way for investigations on a possible role of kinins in the control of post-prandial vascular changes.

Introduction

The search for the pathological and physiological significance of endogenous, highly active substances is never-ending. Kininogens, like angiotensinogen for the angiotensins, are ever-available protein storehouses of kinins, functionally comparable to mast cells storing histamine, cholinergic nerve terminals storing acetylcholine and chromaffin granules storing catecholamines. The study of changes in such circulatory or cellular precursors of biological mediators has often been a way to elucidate mediator function.

Little is known about the role of kinins in the control of vascular changes[1] associated with normal digestive activity. In an attempt to fill this gap, we have studied plasma kininogen changes occurring during digestive activity evoked by feeding and related stimuli in the healthy rat.

Material and Methods

Male 180–250 g, Wistar rats were used. All animals had undergone an overnight fast with free access to water. Following Nembutal (80 mg/kg, subcutaneously) anesthesia or, in some instances, ethyl ether anesthesia, a maximal 2-ml sample of oxalated blood was drawn from their hearts and plasma was separated. Following a one hour rest period, the fasted rats were submitted to experimental treatment; a second blood sample was then withdrawn, again under anesthesia. Preliminary trials established that such double bleeding did not change circulatory kininogen of the animal; the first plasma samples could thus be used to accompany changes caused by experimentation. To determine total bradykininogen (BKg), plasma samples were processed[2] using trypsin for kinin release and the isolated guinea pig ileum as test preparation. To determine low molecular weight (LKg), fresh, control or experimental samples of plasma, were incubated for 15 min at 37°C, with 500 mg/ml finely powdered Pyrex laboratory glassware. Following centrifugation, plasma was processed for remaining bradykininogen[2]. High molecular weight kininogen (HKg), was obtained by subtracting LKg values from BKg values in each plasma sample.

Fed animals were prepared by allowing access to their pelleted ration (CIZIP, Brazil) for one h, in a darkened room, between 8:00 and 10:00 A.M. Fasted rats received visual/olfactory stimulation from their customary ration kept in a partially perforated plastic bag, suspended above their cages. To enhance dissemination of the odour of food, a gently blowing fan was placed at approximately 2 m from the cage. Preparation of the animals was conducted in a darkened room, at 22 ± 2°C, between 8:00 and 10:00 A.M.

Drugs. Carbamylcholine hydrochloride, bradykinin triacetate, atropine sulfate, DPCC – treated trypsin were from Sigma Chemical Co., USA.

Results

Figure 1 shows circulatory total kininogen changes occurring immediately after feeding. A maximal increase was observed after 60 min; it was maintained for another 30 min and fell to pre-feeding values within 2 h. Gel electrophoresis (results not shown), did not reveal any changes in total plasma protein or in levels of major serum proteins after feeding. Thus, increases in circulatory kininogen are not a result of a generalized change in plasma protein. Figure 1 also shows that kininogen changes were not observed in rats which had

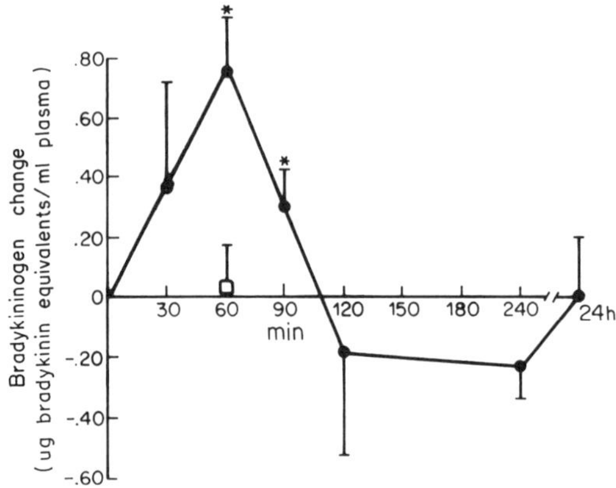

Fig. 1. Changes in total circulatory kininogen (BKg) caused by feeding rats following an overnight fast. Results express differences between plasma BKg levels obtained from rats prior to and at different times following a one-hour feeding period. BKg returned to pre-feeding values after 120 min; it did not change during a renewed fast. Note the lack of effect of feeding on BKg of animals administered 1 mg/kg atropine sulfate, i.p., 1 h prior to feeding ( ). Each figure represents the average of five experiments ± standard error of the mean. Statistical comparisons (*$p<0.05$), performed by Student's t test for paired samples.

been atropinized prior to feeding; preliminary experiments had shown that such treatment did not change the amount of food ingested by the experimental animals. By virtue of its muscarinic effects, atropine may be expected to interfere with the effects of parasympathetic vagal activity, which normally modulates the digestive process in mammals(3). That such activity may control, at least in part, levels of kininogen and free kinin in the blood had been suspected ever since it was demonstrated that cholinergic stimulation by intravenously administered carbamylcholine lowers bradykininogen and transiently raises free kinin in the blood of the rat(4). However, an apparent contradiction between this outcome and the results presented in Fig. 1, should be noted. Why should feeding cause an increase in circulatory kininogen, while a parasympathetic stimulant like carbamylcholine caused lowering of this precursor? An answer to this question to be discussed below, emerges from the examination of results shown in Fig. 2. In the first column, changes in total (HKg+LKg) bradykininogen in the plasma of rats are shown following respectively, feeding after a fast, a pseudo-alimentary (sham-feeding) stimulus evoked by exposing a fasted rat to the odour and sight of its customary ration, electrical

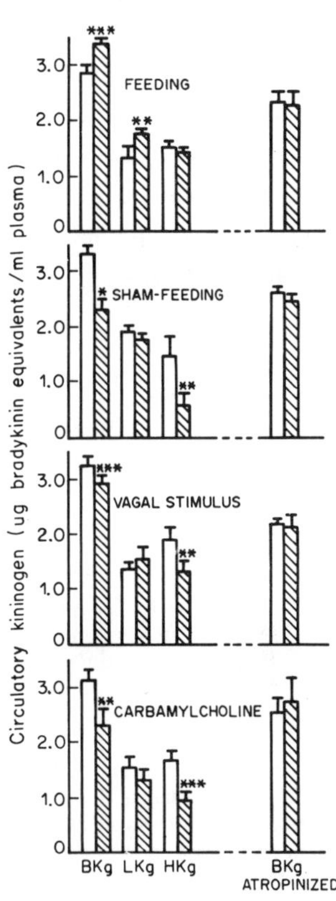

Fig. 2. Changes in circulatory total bradykininogen (BKg), low molecular weight kininogen (LKg), and high molecular weight kininogen (HKg) caused by feeding (1 h), sham-feeding (10 min exposure to the smell of food), stimulation (6 min, at 4V, 10 ms, $5s^{-1}$) of the abdominal vagus nerve, or intravenous administration of 5 µg/kg carbamylcholine. Animals were sacrificed immediately following treatment; they served as their own controls. *Atropinization:* the two last columns to the far left show that responses were abolished in animals atropinized 1 h prior to treatment. Values presented are averages ±SEM of the results of 5 experiments. Statistical significance of comparisons between paired samples: $^{*}p<0.05$; $^{**}p<0.01$; $^{***}p<0.001$.

stimulation of the cut abdominal branch of the vagus nerve or intravenous administration of carbamylcholine. The first of these treatments led to an increase of 0.49 µg of total kininogen per ml of plasma when expressed in terms of bradykinin equivalents. The other three treatments caused significant decreases of circulatory kininogen. The second column of Fig. 2 shows that a significant increase in LKg occurred in animals submitted to feeding; changes in this protein were inconspicuous following the other three treatments. An opposite picture was observed for HKg: insignificant changes were noted in fed rats, but very large decreases, amounting to 0.88 μg/ml (61%), were noted in the sham-fed animals. In the case of vagal stimulation losses were 0.60 μg/ml (31%), and following carbamylcholine treatment, 0.69 μg/ml (42%). The right side of Fig. 2, shows that changes in total BKg levels evoked by any of the experimental treatments tested could be prevented by prior atropinization of the animals. Changes in LKg or HKg were not studied after atropine. It should be noted that changes in circulatory kininogen evoked by these treatments are not the result of eventual alterations in the capacity of rat plasma hydrolysates to potentiate kinin responses of the guinea-pig ileum[5]. The results shown in Fig. 3, indicate that the kinin-potentiating activity of trypsin hydrolysates obtained from plasma of control (fasted) rats, was not different from the potentiating activity of plasma hydrolysates obtained from the same animals after experimental treatment. Values of kininogen levels reported in this study were therefore not corrected for the effects of potentiating factors.

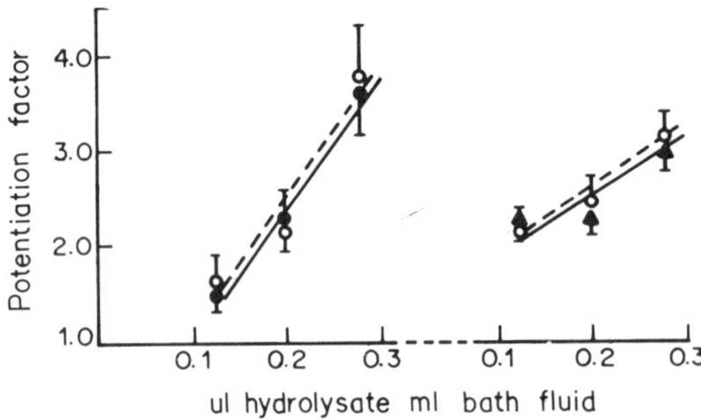

Fig. 3. Absence of changes in bradykinin-potentiating capacity of trypsin hydrolysates of rat plasma following feeding or sham-feeding of the donor rat. The potentiating factor expresses the ratio between the height in cm of the responses of the isolated guinea-pig ileum to the same concentration of bradykinin in the presence or the absence, respectively, of increasing amounts of trypsin hydrolysates of plasma. (o — o), Plasma from control (fasted) rats. (•—•), Plasma from 1 h fed rats. ▲—▲, Plasma from sham-fed rats. Each sample of plasma submitted to hydrolysis represents a pool of plasma obtained from 3 rats.

Discussion

Little is known about fluctuations of plasma kininogen levels during normal daily life. The present results suggest the existence of a link between feeding and an upsurge of total bradykininogen in rat plasma. This effect should be considered a specific response:

electrophoretic determinations (not shown), revealed changes in total protein, albumin or major plasma globulins due to feeding, to be insignificant and nowhere near the 28.8±6.6% ($p<0.001$), increase of BKg observed following such treatment.

Increased release of kininogen from tissue stores or, alternatively, decreased turnover in the circulation of the fed rat could lie at the root of this effect. Decreased consumption of kininogen, possibly resulting from an inhibition of cleavage by plasma and/or tissue kallikrein, although not directly denied by the present results, is unlikely. It has been shown[(6)] that in the rat the combined high and low molecular weight kininogens make up the circulatory reserves of kallikrein-sensitive kininogen. LKg, which is sensitive to tissue kallikrein, was increased as a result of feeding by the same relative extent as total BKg. This outcome, of course, implies that HKg should change little or not at all as a consequence of feeding. At first glance, our results corroborate this conclusion (Fig. 2), suggesting that circulatory HKg is practically unaffected by the passage of the rat from the fasted to the fed condition. By implication, plasma kallikrein, the major enzyme cleaving this substrate, should also remain unaltered during feeding. Direct evidence for or against this assumption is lacking; however, it appears unlikely for the following reasons. Feeding is a coordinated activity, which starts with the sighting and smelling of prospective food[(7)]. In the present study, we submitted fasted rats to this form of stimulation, refraining them from actual access to food. This situation constitutes pseudo or sham-feeding. Its consequences are part of the naturally conditioned response of the rat to food ingestion. Efferent vagal and, in part, sympathetic stimuli subsequently activate salivation, flow of gastric juice, gastric motility and other responses required for digestion[(3)]. Plasma kininogen changes evoked by sham-feeding were different from those evoked by full feeding: the observed marked decreased of HKg suggests that increased cleavage of this protein does occur during sham-feeding and presumably, the early phase of true digestion. Sensitivity to atropine characterizes this response as a parasympathetically-mediated event. Results show that when the peripheral stump of the left abdominal vagus nerve was electrically stimulated, a significant, again atropine-sensitive lowering of both total and HKg occurred, confirming this conclusion, as does the finding that identical effects are observed following the administration of carbamylcholine, a parasympathomimetic drug. Taken together, these findings suggest that while early during the feeding period extensive consumption of HKg occurs as a consequence of parasympathetic activity, additional stimulation, perhaps arising as a consequence of the actual presence of food in the digestive tract, may lead to the reposition, and even overshooting of the basal, fasting levels of kininogen in plasma. As shown by the present experiments, this effect would be reflected mainly by raised LKg levels. This precursor, by being resistant to the action of plasma kallikrein, would tend to temporarily accumulate in the circulation of the fed rat. The possibility that plasma kallikrein causes parasympathetic system-mediated consumption of HKg has been demonstrated in earlier research[4,8]; it has been shown that carbamylcholine causes rapid consumption of HKg in rat blood *in vitro* as well as *in vivo*. Plasma kallikrein would be the major, if not sole, kininogenase responsible for this effect. Further research will be required to extend this conclusion to HKg-consumption occurring in the circulation of the fed or sham-fed rat. There is evidence that glandular kallikrein emanating from buccal digestive glands is mobilized to release kinin during electrical stimulation of nerve structures supplying this region[9]. The question as to whether such an enzyme outpouring also occurs during normal digestive activity or sham-feeding and if so, could be responsible for the considerable reduction of circulatory kininogen observed in our experiments, deserves experimental consideration. It appears, however, that other sites, for instance blood itself[4,8], may also act as suppliers of kallikrein(s) involved in kininogen consumption during digestion. Transient increases of free kinin have been detected in the plasma of the carbamylcholine-treated rat[4]. In the present work, sham-fed, vagally- or carbamylcholine-stimulated rats presented, within 3–10 min, a lowering of circulatory HKg equivalent to the release of between 0.5 and 1.0 μg bradykinin per ml plasma. This indicates that 20–40 μg kinin per kg rat may become available in the body during digestion or related stimuli. These estimates are probably too high, because, although not changed by feeding or sham-feeding (present work), bradykinin-potentiating factors in trypsin hydrolysates of plasma would nevertheless artificially enlarge existing differences between kininogen levels in the plasma of experimental and control animals, respectively. Even bearing this restriction in mind, it is clear that amounts of kinin released from kininogen consumed during digestion could exert significant vasodilatory activity in the organism. One site of such action could be post-prandial vasodilatation in the splanchnic area, a process whose mediators are still controversial[1].

Large reservoirs of the T-kinin precursor T-kininogen exist in rat blood[10]. Since this protein is insensitive to cleavage by either plasma or tissue kallikrein[10], it is unlikely to play a role as a kinin supplier during the digestive process. Nevertheless, the ease with which the rat responds to certain pathological stimuli with increased levels of T-kininogen[10] would make the study of changes in this protein during digestion worth following.

References

1. Tepperman, B.L. and E.D. Jacobson, Mesenteric circulation, In: Physiology of the Gastrointestinal Tract, pp. 1317-1336 (Ed. L.R. Johnson). Raven Press, New York 1981.

2. Diniz, C.R. and I.F. Carvalho, A micro-method for determination of bradykininogen under several conditions, Ann. N.J. Acad. Sci. 104, 77-89 (1963).

3. Shepherd, G.M., Visceral Brain: Feeding, In: Neurobiology, pp. 539-549. Oxford University Press, New York 1988.

4. Rothschild, A.M. and A. Castania, Sensitivity to cyclic nucleotides and to aspirin of the kininogen-consuming system activated by adrenaline or carbamylcholine in rat blood, Agents Actions 8, 132-138 (1978).

5. Arsen, P.N., Sensibilization of the guinea pig ileum to the action of bradykinin by trypsin hydrolysate of ox and rabbit plasma, Br. J. Pharmac. 32, 453-465 (1968).

6. Jacobsen, S., Substrates for plasma kinin forming enzymes in rat and guinea-pig plasma, Br. J. Pharmac. 28, 64-72 (1966).

7. Ladd Prosser, E., Feeding and digestion, In: Comparative Animal Physiology, pp. 144-186. Saunders, Philadelphia 1952.

8. Rothschild, A.M., J.C. Gomes and A. Castania, Adrenergic and cholinergic control of the activity of the kallikrein-kinin system in rat blood, Adv. Exp. Biol. Med. 70, pp. 197-199 (Ed. F. Sicuteri; N. Back, G.L. Haberland). Plenum Press, New York 1976.

9. Sicli, A.G., T.B. Orstavik, S.F. Rabito, R.D. Murray, O.A. Carretero, Blood kinins after sympathetic nerve stimulation of the rat submandibular gland, Hypertension 5 (Suppl. I, 2), L-101-106 (1983).

10. Greenbaum, L.M., T-kinin and T-kininogen – An Historical Overview, Adv. Exp. Med. Biol. 198A, pp. 55-75 (Ed. L.M. Geenbaum and H.S. Margolius). Plenum Press, New York 1986.

AAS 36
Contributions to
Autacoid Pharmacology

IS GUANYLATE CYCLASE ACTIVATION THROUGH THE RELEASE OF NITRIC OXIDE OR A RELATED COMPOUND INVOLVED IN BRADYKININ-INDUCED PERIVASCULAR PRIMARY AFFERENT EXCITATION?

A.P. Corrado and G. Ballejo

Department of Pharmacology, School of Medicine of Ribeirão Preto, University of São Paulo, 14049 Ribeirão Preto, SP, Brazil

Abstract

In dogs under light thiopentobarbital anesthesia, intracarotid injection of bradykinin (BK) causes a dose-dependent "pain response" represented by hyperpnea, bradycardia, vocalization and ipsilateral contraction of the sternocephalic muscle. These events result from the activation of primary afferent nerves located in the wall of the carotid vessels distributed mainly in occipital artery territory. We present evidence indicating that these BK-induced reflex phenomena are 1) mediated by the activation of B_2 receptors; 2) potentiated by prostaglandin E_2 (PGE_2) and serotonin (5-HT) the latter acting via sub-type 5-HT_3 receptors; 3) reduced by indomethacin and/or N^G-nitroarginine, and 4) abolished by methylene blue. These results suggest that 5-HT plays a modulatory role on BK action; the latter depends on the release of prostaglandins and nitric oxide or a related compound and includes the activation of guanylate cyclase which appears to be involved in primary afferent excitation.

Introduction

Since this Symposium is dedicated to Professor Rocha e Silva, we present the current status of our research on the mechanisms by which bradykinin (BK), when injected in the carotid artery, triggers several reflexes. Our investigations of this problem resulted in several publications, the first one of which in collaboration with Professor Rocha e Silva[1] with whom one of us (A.P.C.) had the pleasure of working for more than 2 decades.

In these early papers, we described that BK, injected counter-current into the carotid artery through the lingual artery (Fig. 1) in dogs under deep anesthesia, caused salivation, apnea, bradycardia, hypotension and contraction of the homolateral neck muscles. The sialogogic effect exhibited tachyphylaxis and involved the synthesis of prostaglandins[2]. When the maxillary arteries were occluded (number 1 in Fig. 1), the sialogogic effect of BK disappeared while its cardiovascular, respiratory and muscular effects became more evident (Fig. 2, panel B).

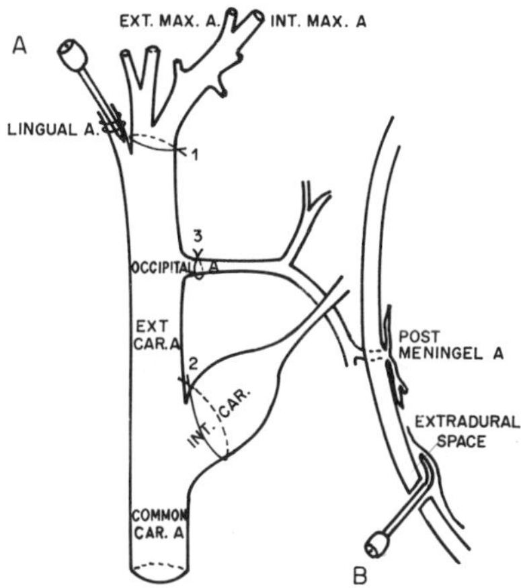

Fig. 1. *Carotid vascular tree:* One or more of the following vessels were occluded (see text): Trunk of maxillary (1), internal carotid (2), occipital (3) arteries. With the exception of methysergide, ketanserine and indomethacin, all other drugs were injected into the lingual artery at A. In some experiments, bradykinin was also injected in the extradural space (B).

BK-induced apnea and bradycardia have been described in anesthetized rabbits and dogs[3,4] and were attributed to a direct action of BK on the central nervous system (CNS). BK-induced contraction of the neck muscles has not been described; it probably corresponds to the BK-induced head movement described in the rat[5]. In our experiments we recorded only the contractions of the sternocephalic muscle; it is representative of other neck muscles, which acting together, are responsible for ipsilateral flexion of the head to the injected side (Fig. 3).

Evidence[1,6] indicating that BK-induced responses were reflexes elicited by the activation of primary afferent nerves located in the wall of vessels irrigating the territory of the occipital artery and not the result of a direct action of BK on the CNS or on

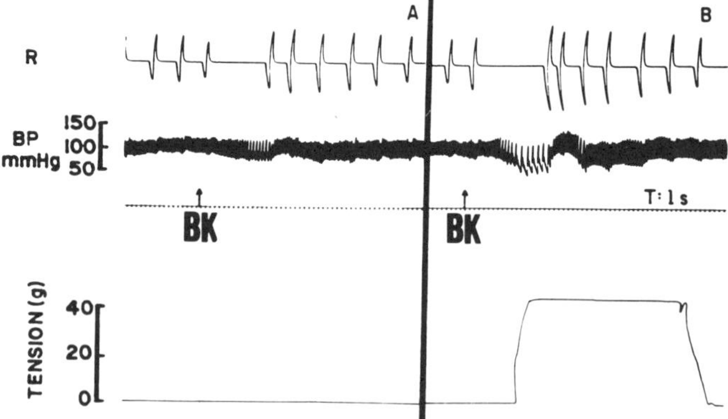

Fig. 2. *Apnea, bradycardia and ipsilateral muscle contraction induced by the injection of bradykinin* (BK) into a 12-kg dog under deep pentobarbital anesthesia (30 mg/kg i.v.). From top to bottom: Simultaneous recording of respiration (R), femoral blood pressure (BP) and sternocephalic muscle contraction. At arrows, BK (1.0 μg/kg) was injected into the lingual artery. Note that after the maxillary arteries were occluded (between Panels A and B), responses become particularly evident. In the following related experiments, the trunk of the maxillary arteries was occluded.

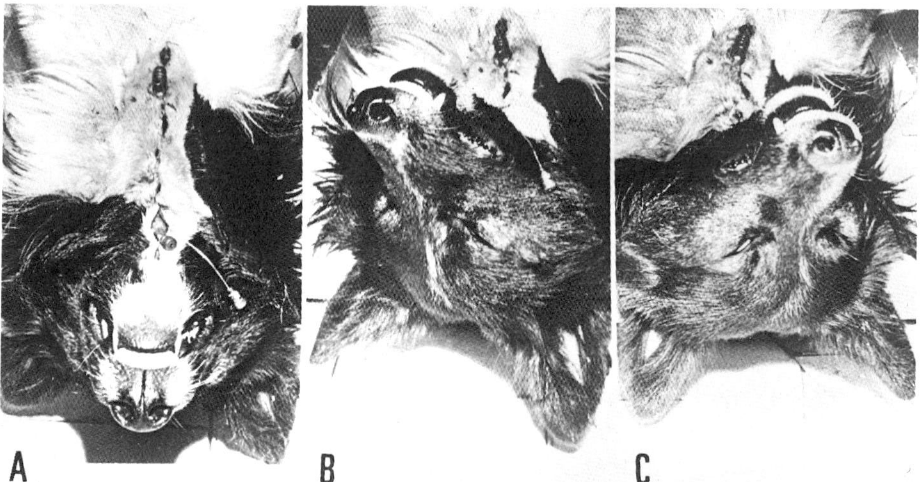

Fig. 3. *Ipsilateral head flexion induced by intracarotid injection of bradykinin* in a 11.5 kg dog under deep pentobarbital anesthesia (30 mg/kg i.v.). Panel A, control. Panels B and C, 20 seconds after bradykinin administration at the left and right intracarotid artery, respectively. Note the flexion of the head ipsilaterally to the side of injection.

effector tissues were as follows: 1) phrenic nerve action potentials disappeared during the period of apnea; 2) the bradycardic response was abolished by bilateral vagotomy; 3) muscular contractions were abolished by sectioning the ipsilateral accessory nerve; 4) a marked decrease in splanchnic nerve discharge was observed during the hypotensive effect; 5) the responses persisted after the occlusion of the internal carotid artery but were significantly reduced after the occlusion of the occipital artery which does not directly irrigate the CNS[(7)]; 6) potentiation of the bradykinin-induced effects was obtained by previous or simultaneous intracarotid injection of serotonin (5-HT), a substance which does not cross the blood-brain barrier[(8)]; its potentiating effect was peculiar in that, when unilaterally administered in small doses (5 μg/kg), it influenced only the effects of ipsilaterally injected bradykinin; larger doses (25–100 μg/kg) had to be used to potentiate events induced by contralaterally injected bradykinin as well; 5-HT-induced potentiation lasted for 30–60 min and could be reproduced at will throughout the experiment. It is worth noting that intravenous injection of bradykinin did not reproduce these events; instead, it promoted a positive chronotropic effect[(9,10,11)] and an increase in respiratory rate and amplitude[(3,12,13)]; 7) capsaicin, an agent that initially stimulates and latter desensitizes pain receptors [(14,15)] was able to block BK-induced responses; this blockade was ipsilateral, demonstrating that nervous centers, acting as probable integrators of the reflex phenomena, were not directly affected by the polypeptide; 8) finally, it could be shown that direct application of BK to the surface of the dura mater (Fig. 1), at the meningeal territory of the occipital artery, was followed by apnea, bradycardia, hypotension and muscular contraction.

These findings led us to suggest that reflexes involved in these actions of BK were probably due to stimulation of perivascular nerve endings distributed along the territory of the occipital artery. Such nerve endings could be similar to those described in the vessels of the knee, spleen, intestine and meninges by Lim *et al.*[(16)], who observed "pseudoaffective" responses, characterized by hyperpnea, vocalization and hypertension after intra-arterial (femural, splenic, coronary or internal carotid) administration of BK to conscious or lightly anesthetized dogs. Indeed, in dogs under light thiopentobarbital anesthesia, we observed that BK injection into the external carotid artery caused a "pain response" characterized by hyperpnea, gasping and vocalization, in addition to bradycardia and neck muscle contraction[(1,17)].

In this communication we present and discuss our more recent findings dealing with the mechanisms involved in BK-induced nociceptive response in animals under light anesthesia; in addition we describe the modulation of this response by serotonin and prostaglandin.

Material and Methods

Mongrel dogs of both sexes, lightly anesthetized with sodium thiopentobarbital (12.5 mg/kg, i.v.), were prepared for the simultaneous recording of femoral blood pressure, respiratory movements and sternocephalic muscle contractions, using a Grass Model 5D Polygraph[1]. With the exception of ketanserin, methysergide and indomethacin which were injected intravenously, all other drugs were injected through a polyethylene tube (PE 20) introduced into the lingual artery with the tip placed in the direction of the carotid artery (Fig. 1). The maxillary arteries were occluded in all experiments, thus leading to the enhancement of bradykinin effects (Fig. 2).

Results

Bradykinin-induced nociceptive responses. In all 29 animals studied, BK (0.1 to 1.0 μg/kg) triggered a pain response characterized by hyperpnea, gasping, vocalization, bradycardia and contraction of the sternocephalic muscle. All events were dose-dependent, although vocalization and gasping only appeared after higher doses of BK (Fig. 4, Panels A, B and C).

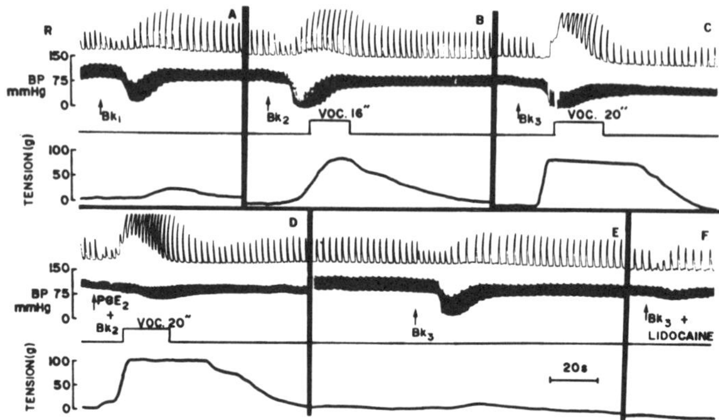

Fig. 4. *Hyperpnea, bradycardia, vocalization and neck muscle contraction induced by intracarotid injection of bradykinin* in a 10-kg dog under light thiopentobarbital anesthesia. From top to bottom, as indicated in Fig. 2. The nociceptive responses are dose-related (BK_1, BK_2 and BK_3: 0.25, 0.5 and 1.0 μ/kg of bradykinin, respectively). Note that vocalization and gasping denoted by a sustained inspiratory effect appear only after higher doses of the polypeptide. Combined injection of BK with prostaglandin E_2 resulted in the potentiation of BK-induced effects (compare Panel B with D). BK effects were blocked by indomethacin (4 mg/kg i.v., injected between Panels D and E), as well as by simultaneously administered 2% lidocaine (0.05 ml/kg intracarotideally, Panel F).

Receptors involved (6 dogs). Nociceptive responses were selectively induced by BK-like peptides, such as T-kinin and kallidin; tachykinins (substance P and neurokinin-A) caused only hypotension, without the appearance of bradycardia or muscle contraction (Fig. 5). The responses induced by BK-like peptides were competitively blocked by the synthetic BK-analog B-4307[18] in a dose-dependent manner (Fig. 6). Spantide, a selective antagonist of substance P, did not affect BK-induced responses at doses that abolished hypotension caused by substance P (data not shown); the specific B_2 BK-antagonist, B-4307, failed to alter the hypotensive response to substance P (Fig. 5 Panel E).

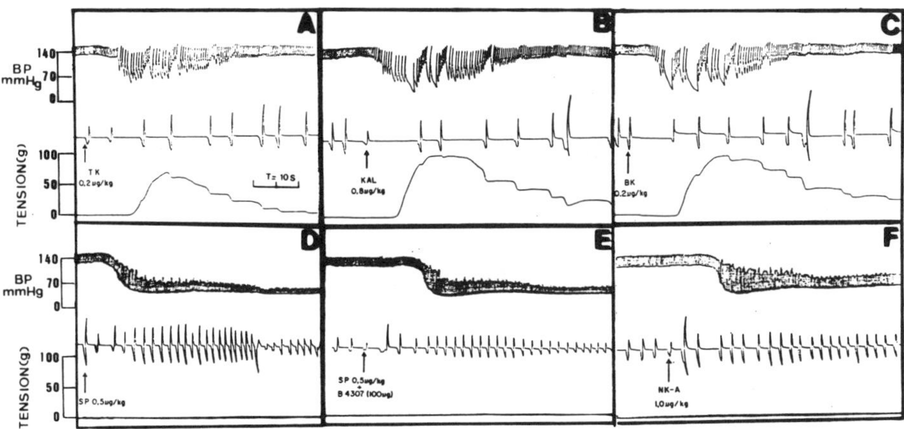

Fig. 5. *Nociceptive responses induced by bradykinin-like peptides* in a 12.8-kg dog under light thiopentobarbital anesthesia. From top to bottom, simultaneous recording of femoral blood pressure, respiration and tension of the sternocephalic muscle. T-kinin and kallidin (Panels A and B) were able to mimic BK-induced effects (Panel C), while tachykinins (substance P (SP), Panel D, and neurokinin-A (NK-A) Panel F) caused only hypotension. The BK antagonist, B-4307, failed to alter the response to SP (Panel E).

Potentiation of BK-induced pain response (15 dogs). Prostaglandin E_2 (PGE_2) and serotonin (5-HT) induced pain responses only after administration of doses 10 times higher than effective doses of BK (data not shown). At lower doses (2.5 to 5.0 µg/kg), however, both autacoids potentiated BK-induced nociceptive responses (Fig. 4, Panel D for PGE_2, and Fig. 7, Panels B and C for 5-HT). The potentiating effect of 5-HT was dose-dependent (data not shown), and appears to result from the activation of $5\text{-}HT_3$ receptors, since it was not blocked by methysergide (1 mg/kg i.v.) or ketanserin (1 mg/kg i.v.) but was totally inhibited by ICS-205930, a selective antagonist of such 5-HT receptor (Fig. 7, Panel D).

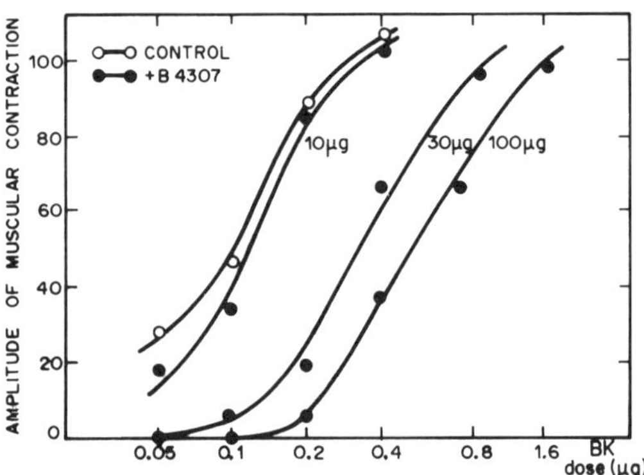

Fig. 6. *Dose-response curves to intracarotid bradykinin (BK) injection* in the absence (Control) and in the presence of increasing doses (10, 30 and 100 μg) of intracarotid injected B-4307, in a 10-kg dog under light thiopentobarbital anesthesia. The response to BK measured was the amplitude of the contraction of the sternocephalic muscle, expressed as tension, in g.

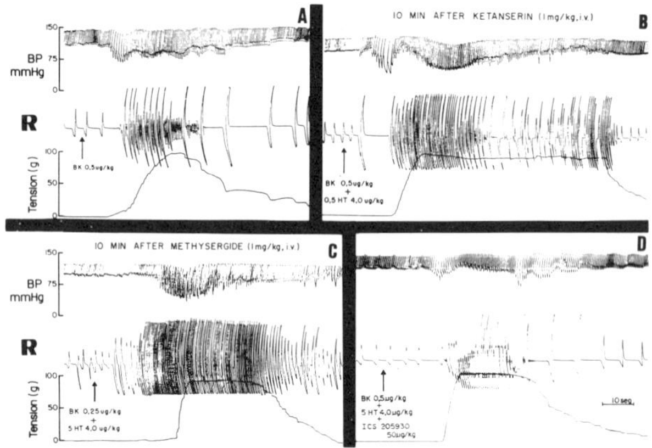

Fig. 7. *Blockade of 5-HT-evoked potentiation of BK-induced nociceptive response* in a 11.5-kg dog under light thiopentobarbital anesthesia. From top to bottom as indicated in Fig. 5. Neither intravenously injected ketanserin (Panel B) nor methysergide (Panel C) could block the potentiation caused by 5-HT, which was, however, abolished by ICS-205930, a selective antagonist of 5-HT_3 receptors (Panel D).

Desensitization of BK-induced nociceptive responses (4 dogs). Capsaicin (1.0 to 5.0 μg/kg) triggered an intense pain response similar to that caused by BK (Fig. 8). Repeated ipsilateral injections of capsaicin (4 to 6) blocked the capacity of BK to trigger the pain response (Fig. 9).

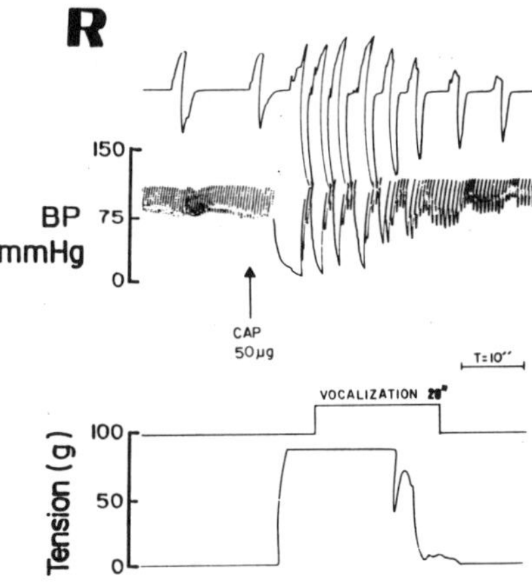

Fig. 8. *Capsaicin-induced BK-like nociceptive responses* in a 15-kg dog under light thiopentobarbital anesthesia. From top to bottom as indicated in Fig. 2.

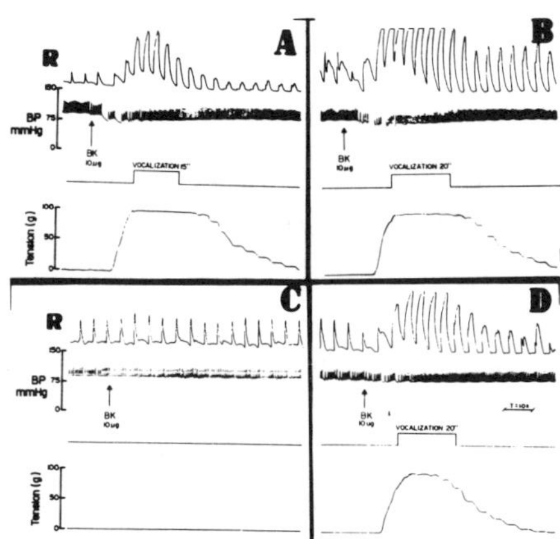

Fig. 9. *Desensitization of BK-induced nociceptive responses* in a 10-kg dog under light thiopentobarbital anesthesia. From top to bottom as indicated in Fig. 2. Panels A and B, injections of BK (10 μg) in the left and right carotid arteries, respectively; between Panels B and C, desensitization by means of six successive injections of capsaicin (5.0 μg/kg each), in the left carotid artery. Panels C and D, injection of BK (10 μg) in the left (desensitized) and right (untreated) side, respectively.

Inhibition of BK-induced pain response (4 dogs). Previous administration of N^G-nitroarginine (20 mg/kg) caused a slight increase in arterial blood pressure and partly blocked BK-induced nociceptive responses; these were abolished by previous administration of methylene blue (40 μg/kg) (Fig. 10).

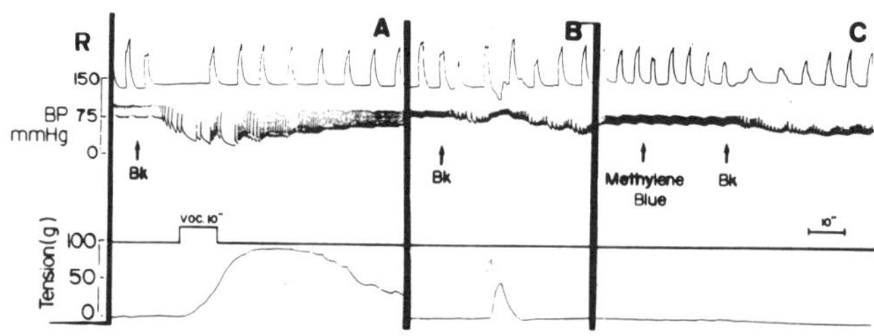

Fig. 10. *Blockade of BK-induced pain responses* in a 11.3-kg dog under light thiopentobarbital anesthesia. From top to bottom as indicated in Fig. 2. Previous administration of N^G-nitroarginine (20 mg/kg - between Panels A and B) causes a slight increase in arterial blood pressure and a partial blockade of BK-induced nociceptive responses; the intracarotid injection of methylene blue (40 μg/kg, Panel C) fully abolished rèsponses to BK. At BK, intracarotid injection of bradykinin (BK) (0.25 μg/kg).

4. Discussion

The intracarotid injection of bradykinin in dogs under light anesthesia caused hyperpnea, vocalization, bradycardia and contractions of the homolateral sternocephalic muscle. It was previously shown in dogs under deep anesthesia that the bradycardia and the contractions of neck muscles induced by similar administration of bradykinin are reflex responses triggered by the activation of perivascular primary afferents located mainly in the territory of the occipital artery(1). The responses observed in animals under light anesthesia also seem to be reflex since similar responses were evoked by the intracarotid injection of capsaicin, a selective activator of a population of primary afferent fibers(19). The observation that responses to high doses of BK included vocalization indicates that BK may be activating perivascular polymodal receptors; the finding that serotonin and PGE_2 potentiate BK action gives support to this assumption, since both agents were shown to enhance responses of polymodal receptors to bradykinin(20).

Bradykinin could activate perivascular primary afferents by a direct action on nerve fibers or, alternatively, since it was injected intravascularly, through the release of an intermediate substance from the endothelium. Although the ability of bradykinin to directly stimulate afferent fibers has been repeatedly reported(21,22), the second possibility should also be considered since we observed that previous administration of N^G-nitroarginine which blocks nitric oxide synthesis from 1-arginine(23) greatly reduced reflexes and pain caused by intracarotid injection of bradykinin. This observation indicates that nitric oxide or a related compound is an activator of primary afferents, a suggestion consistent with recent observations(24) showing that intravenous administration of S-nitrosocysteine, a putative endothelium-dependent relaxing factor (EDRF)(25), is able to activate vagal afferents. S-nitrosocysteine, but not the nitric oxide-liberating compound sodium nitroprusside, is also able to cause a BK-like pain response in dogs (A.P. Corrado, unpublished data). Prostaglandins released by BK could also contribute to the stimulation of primary afferents since we observed that indomethacin reduced BK-induced nociceptive responses.

Interestingly, BK-induced responses were abolished by the previous intracarotid injection of methylene blue. Since methylene blue inhibits guanylate cyclase activation by nitric oxide(26), this finding could indicate the participation of the nitric oxide-guanylate cyclase system in the activation of perivascular polymodal receptors by BK. This system could also be involved in the serotoninergic potentiation of bradykinin effects. Indeed, our findings indicate that 5-HT_3 receptors are likely to mediate this potentiation since it was blocked by ICI-205930 but not by ketanserin or methysergide. This interpretation is consistent with the observation that 5-HT activates vagal and cutaneous afferents through 5-HT_3 receptors(27). Furthermore, as recently reported(28), serotonin stimulates the accumulation of cyclic GMP in mouse neuroblastoma-rat glioma hybrid cells by acting, in part, via nitric oxide or a related nitroso compound.

In conclusion, our results could fit the scheme shown in Fig. 11. Thus, intracarotid injection of bradykinin could activate perivascular primary afferents of the occipital territory by direct action upon nerve fibers and/or through the release of nitric oxide from the endothelium. In either case, the stimulation of the primary afferents seems to involve the activity of guanylate cyclase, since responses were blocked by methylene blue. The activation of primary afferents by BK seems to be modulated by prostaglandins and serotonin.

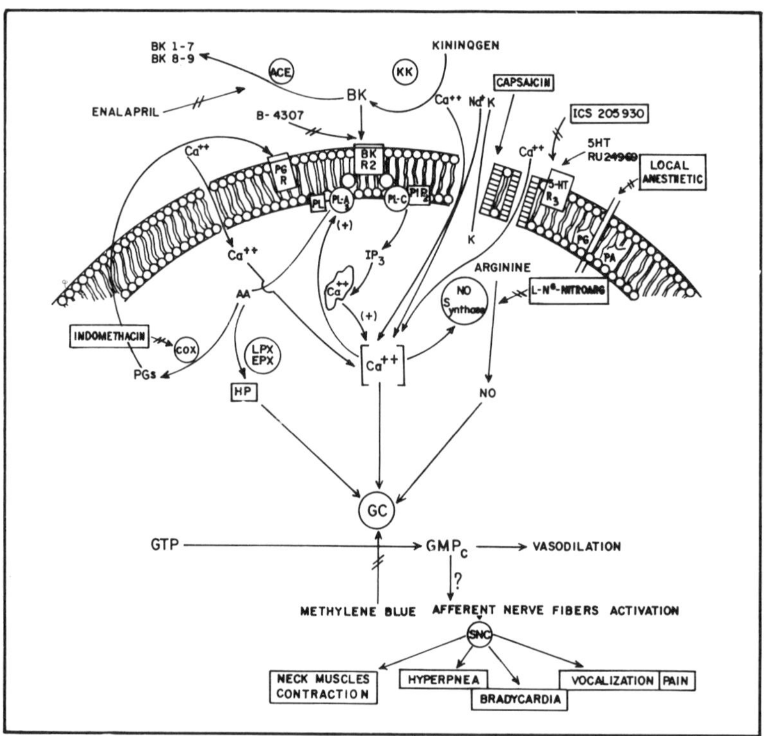

Fig. 11. *Model proposed for the pathway by which BK activates primary perivascular afferents and for the manner of its modulation by 5-HT and prostaglandins.* Bradykinin acting at B_2 receptors (R-2) activates phospholipase A_2 (PL-A_2) and phospholipase C (PL-C). The latter leads to an increase in intracellular calcium [Ca^{++}], which, in turn, activates nitric oxide synthase and cooperates in the activation of guanylate cyclase (GC) and of PL-A_2. The resultant increase in cyclic GMP (GMPc) is responsible for vasodilatation and, probably, afferent nerve depolarization, which will trigger observed bradycardia, neck muscle contraction, hyperpnea and pain. All responses are blocked by local anesthetic agents. Broken arrows indicate inhibition. Double lines crossing arrows indicate probable sites of inhibitory effects of indomethacin, compounds B-4307, ICS 205930, local anesthetics, L-N^G-nitroaginine and methylene blue. COX: cyclo oxygenase; AA: arachidonic acid; LPX: lipoxygenase; EPX: epoxide oxygenase; HP: hydroperoxides; IP_3: inositol triphosphate.

Acknowledgements

We are grateful to Drs. J.M. Stewart, G. Engel and G. De Nucci for their kind gifts of B-4307 (D-ARG$_0$-Hyp$_3$-Thy$_{5,7}$-D-Phe$_8$-BK), ICS- 205930 and N^G-Nitroarginine, respectively. We also thank Mr. D.S. Reis for excellent technical assistance, Miss I.D. Scatena for secretarial assistance and Miss F.H. Ferreira for typing this manuscript.

References

1. Riccioppo-Neto, F., A.P. Corrado and M. Rocha e Silva, Apnea, bradycardia, hypotension and muscular contractions induced by intracarotid injection of bradykinin, J. Pharmacol. Exp. Ther. 190, 316-326 (1974).

2. Corrado, A.P. and M. Grellet, Mechanisms of the sialagogic effect induced by bradykinin in dogs; possible mediation by endogenous prostaglandins, In: Kinins: Pharmacodynamic and Biological Role, pp. 81-95 (Eds. F. Sicuteri and N. Back). Plenum Press, New York 1976.

3. Gjuris, V., B. Heicke and E. Westermann, Apnea nach Bradykinin und Kallidin, Naunyn-Schmiedebergs Arch. Exp. Pathol. Pharmakol. 248, 540-551 (1964).

4. Buckley, J.P., R.K. Bickerton, R.P. Halliday and H. Kato, Central effects of peptides on the cardiovascular system, Ann. N.Y. Acad. Sci. 104, 299-311 (1963).

5. Defenu, G., L. Pegrassi and B. Lumachi, The use of bradykinin-induced effects in rats as an assay for analgesic drugs, J. Pharm. Pharmac. 18, 135 (1966).

6. Riccioppo-Neto, F., D.S. Reis and A.P. Corrado, Stimulation of perivascular intracranial receptors by bradykinin and kallidin, In: Bradykinin and Related Kinins, Cardiovascular, Biochemical and Neural Actions, pp. 548-554 (Eds. F. Sicuteri and N. Back). Plenum Press, New York 1970.

7. Bradley, O.C. Topographical Anatomy of the Dog, 5th Ed., p. 156. The MacMillan Company, New York 1948.

8. Udenfried, S., H. Weisbach and D.F. Bogdanski, Increase in tissue serotonin following administration of its precursor 5-hydroxytryptophan, J. Biol. Chem. 224, 803-810 (1957).

9. Maxwell, G.M., R.B. Elliot and G.M. Kneebone, Effects of bradykinin on the systemic and coronary vascular bed of the intact dog, Circ. Res. 10, 359-363 (1962).

10. Montague, D., R. Rosas and D.F. Bohr, Bradykinin: vascular relaxant cardiac stimulant, Science. 141, 907-908 (1963).

11. Nakano, J., Effects of synthetic bradykinin on the cardiovascular system, Arch. Int. Pharmacodyn. Ther. 157, 1-13 (1965).

12. Rocha e Silva, M., A.P. Corrado and A.O. Ramos, Potentiation of duration of the vasodilatador effects of bradykinin by sympatholytic drugs and by reserpine, J. Pharmacol. Exp. Ther. 128, 217-226 (1960).

13. Westermann, E., Vagal reflex influence of breathing through plasma kinins, Acta Neurochir, 28, 319-338 (1966).

14. Keele, C.A. and D. Armostrong, Substances producing pain and itch, p. 249. Edward Arnold, London 1964.

15. Jancso, N., Desensitization with capsaicin and related acylamides as a tool for studying the function of pain receptors, In: Pharmacology of Pain, pp. 33-55 (Eds. R.K.S. Lim, D. Armstrong and E.G. Pardo). Pergamon Press, Oxford 1968.

16. Lim, R.K.S., N.C. Lim, F. Guzman and C. Braun, Visceral receptors concerned in visceral pain and the pseudo affective response to intra-arterial injections of bradykinin and other algesic agents, J. Comp. Neurol. 118, 269-193 (1962).

17. Corrado, A.P. and G. Ballejo, Algogenic receptors in the carotid vascular bed, In: Recent Advances in Pharmacology and Therapeutics, pp. 37-42 (Eds. M. Velasco, A. Israel, E. Romero, H. Silva). Elsevier Science Publ., Amsterdam 1989.

18. Vavrek, R.J. and J.M. Stewart, Competitive antagonists of bradykinin, Peptides 6, 161-164 (1985).

19. Buck, S.H. and T.F. Burks, The neuropharmacology of capsaicin: review of some recent observations, Pharmac. Rev. 38, 179-226 (1986).

20. Mizumura, K., J. Sato and T. Kumazawa, A. Effects of prostaglandins and other putative chemical intermediaries on the activity of canine testicular polymodal receptors studied in vitro, Pflügers Arch. Physiol. 408, 565-572 (1987).

21. Steranka, L.R., D.C. Manning, C.J. Dehaas, J.W. Ferkany, S.A. Borosky, J.R. Connor, R.J. Vavrek and J.M. Stewart, Bradykinin as a pain mediator: Receptors are localized to sensory neurons and antagonists have analgesic actions, Proc. Natl Acad. Sci. USA 85, 3245-3249 (1988).

22. Mizumura, K., M. Minagawa, Y. Tsujii and T. Kumazawa, The effects of bradykinin agonists and antagonists on visceral polymodal receptors activities, Pain 40, 221-227 (1990).

23. Moore, P.K., O.A. Al-Swayeh, N.W.S. Chong, R.A. Evans and A. Gibson, L-N^G-Nitroarginine (L-NORAG), a novel L-arginine-reversible inhibitor of endothelium-dependent vasodilatation in vitro, Br. J. Pharmacol. 99, 408-412 (1990).

24. Meller, S.T., S.J. Lewis, J.N. Bates, M.J. Brody and G.F. Gebhart, Is there a role for an endothelium-derived relaxing factor in nociception?, Brain Res. 531, 342-345 (1990).

25. Myers, P.R., R.L. Minor, R. Guerra, J.N. Bates and D.D. Harrison, Vasorelaxant properties of the endothelium-derived relaxing factor more closely resemble S-Nitrosoysteine than nitric oxide, Nature 345, 161-163 (1990).

26. Waldman, S.A. and F. Murad, Cyclic GMP synthesis and function, Pharmacol. Rev. 39, 163-196 (1987).

27. B.P. Richardson and G. Engel, The pharmacology and function of 5-HT_3 receptors, Trends in Neurosci. 9, 424-428 (1986).

28. G. Reiser, Mechanism of stimulation of cyclic GMP level in a neuronal cell line mediated by (5-HT_3) receptors, Eur. J. Biochem. 189, 547-551 (1990).

AAS 36
Contributions to
Autacoid Pharmacology

BRADYKININ MODULATION OF THE HYDROOSMOTIC EFFECT OF THE ANTI-DIURETIC HORMONE IN WATER-TRANSPORTING EPITHELIA

M.R. Furtado

Laboratory of Kidney and Biomembranes, School of Medicine of Ribeirão Preto, University of São Paulo, 14049 Ribeirão Preto, SP, Brazil

Abstract

Rocha e Silva's utmost contribution to science was the isolation of **bradykinin**, a naturally occurring nonapeptide known to have a broad spectrum of actions. Amongst them, considerable evidence suggests that the diuretic effects of endogenous bradykinin are, in part, mediated by inhibition of vasopressin-stimulated water transport. This is true for both the mammalian renal cortical collecting tubule and the urinary bladder of the toad (functionally analogous to the tubule). A review of the main contributions that led to that knowledge is presented.

Terrestrial adaptation conditioned animals to the need of permanently conserving body fluids to survive. This was achieved by means of a homeostatic mechanism involving the secretion of anti-diuretic hormone (ADH) by the neurohypophysis, and the responses of the target-organs.

In mammals, vasopressin (ADH) plays an important role in the renal machinery that concentrates urine, thus economizing water for the body. In amphibians, this pivotal role is played by vasotocin, which acts on the kidneys reducing urine formation(1), on the skin where it promotes an increase in the tissue permeability to water(2), and also on the urinary bladder where it favors water reabsorption thus increasing urine concentration(3). This behavior of the urinary bladder of amphibians has made it a functional analogue of the mammalian collecting tubules with which it is phylogenetically homologous. This is why observations carried out with one of these structures can usually be replicated on the other.

Two facts induced us to work with kinins expecting them to interact with ADH on transporting epithelia. First, knowledge that isolated toad bladders when repetitively stimulated with neurohypophyseal hormones, exhibited progressive inhibition of the hydroosmotic responses. This phenomenon has been known as "intrinsic inhibition", "refractoriness" or "desensitization"[4]. Second, the fact that bradykinin (BK), when directly infused into the renal artery of the dog, was capable of increasing urine flow (and free-water clearance) even in the presence of vasopressin[5,6]. These two facts, taken together, suggested that kinins could well function as inhibitors of ADH. Moreover, it also implied that the "intrinsic inhibition" could be due to the occurrence of an intrinsic (or endogenous) inhibitor in the bladder tissue. These two possibilities were analyzed.

I. Kinin Action on the Urinary Bladder Isolated from Toads

The *in vitro* preparation of the isolated urinary bladder of the toad *Bufo marinus paracnemis* Lutz was used[7]. The bladder was suspended in a Ringer's solution that bathed the serosal surface of a hemi-bladder sac preparation which contained a diluted Ringer's solution in its mucosal side. This assembly allows the measurement of net osmotic water movement across the wall of the bladder by weighing the vesical assembly *before* and *after* a given period of time. It is well known that the addition of ADH (vasopressin or oxytocin) to the serosal side increases the bladder permeability to water[7]. The addition of BK to the serosal (or even to the mucosal) bladder solution did not affect the basal osmotic water flow across the bladder[8]. Although lacking intrinsic activity on the bladder, bradykinin when added to the preparation together with ADH, reversibly inhibited the permeability effects of the ADH (Fig. 1). Kallidin, eledoisin, and physalaemin also inhibited ADH action on the bladder[9]. Antagonism between these kinins and ADH was surmountable, and apparently competitive (Fig. 2). Thus, though lacking intrinsic activity, kinins show affinity for receptor sites also common to ADH, causing a parallel shift of the log-dose/response curves for ADH.

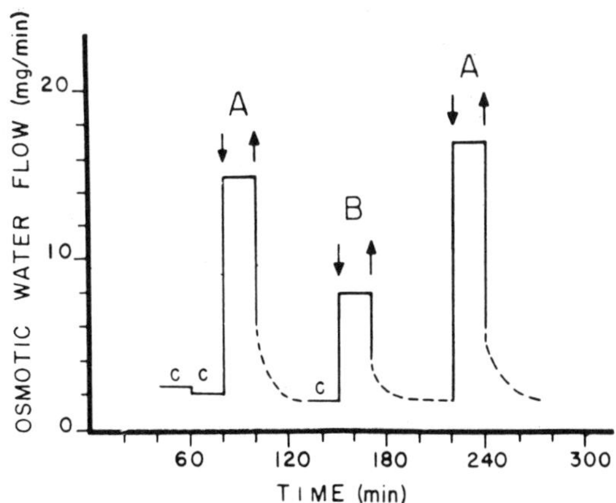

Fig. 1. Responses of one hemi-bladder to three separate additions of 1.3×10^{-8} M vasopressin (*A*). In *B*, the hormone was added together with bradykinin (9.5×10^{-7} M). Drugs were applied (↓) to the serosal Ringer's solution for a period of 20 min. (↑) = washouts. C = basal osmotic water flow.

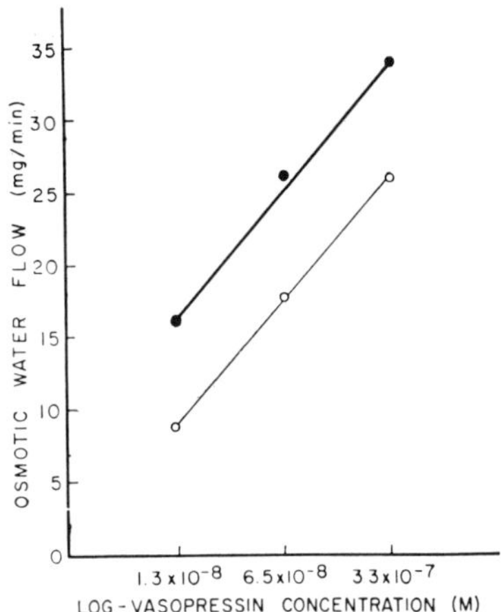

Fig. 2. Log-dose/response relationship for the effects of vasopressin on the permeability to water of the toad bladder in the absence (•) and in the presence (o) of 9.5×10^{-7} M bradykinin. Each point is the mean of five determinations.

II. Occurrence of a Kinin System in the Toad Bladder

While working on ADH antagonism by kinins, it occurred to us that at least part of the phenomenon of "refractoriness" of the bladder to the action of ADH, could be due to the intrinsic generation of kinins in the bladder tissue. A first approach to this question was as follows: hemibladders were mounted as for water transport experiments, except that they were filled with complete Ringer's solution, the same Ringer's bathing the bladder sacs, leading therefore to the absence of an osmotic gradient. One of the bladders (*A*), was incubated for 60 min under these conditions. The other halfbladder (*B*), had its serosal Ringer's changed every 15 min during 60 min. The mucosal solutions bathing the mucosal side were then changed to diluted (1:5) Ringer's; hemibladder *A* kept its original serosal Ringer's, but halfbladder *B* had its serosal Ringer's changed once more. 2 mU/ml oxytocin (Oxy) were then added to the serosal solutions bathing bladders *A* and *B*. Bladder sacs were weighed at the beginning and after each of three additional 20-min periods of incubation. The pH of the serosal Ringer's was maintained at 8.0 throughout the experiment. Table 1 shows that hemibladder *B* responses to Oxy were much smaller than those of bladder *A*, suggesting that an intrinsic inhibitor had been liberated from bladder tissue into the serosal bathing medium during the initial 60-min incubation period.

Table 1. Influence of a 60-min incubated serosal solution on the hydroosmotic response to oxytocin of the isolated toad bladder*. All values are expressed as percentages of period I of bladders A (mean ± SEM). N = 6 experiments.

	Period I	Period II	Period III
Bladder A	100	106.0 ± 23.1[a]	135.2 ± 30.0[a]
Bladder B	42.4 ± 4.1[b]	44.6 ± 3.5[b]	48.2 ± 6.7[b]

[a]Statistically not different from the value of period I (bladder A).
[b]Statistically significant difference ($p > 0.01$) from value of period I (A).

**Experimental Protocol:*

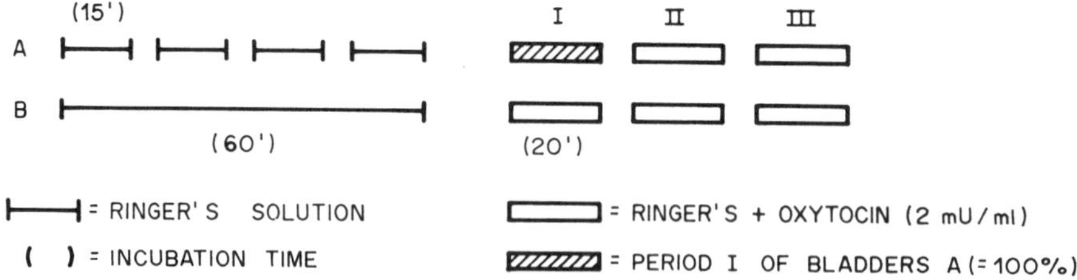

These results led to a preliminary pharmacological characterization of the active principle derived from the bladder. Again, hemibladders were mounted as for the water transport experiments. Three sets of experiments were carried out: a) the serosal Ringer's solution had a pH of 6.5; b) serosal pH was 7.5; c) external pH was adjusted to 8.3–8.5. Bladders, filled with external 1:5 diluted Ringer's, were incubated for 40 min, at 25°C. Aliquots of the bath fluid were applied to a coupled preparation of isolated guinea-pig ileum and rat duodenum conveniently mounted in a single organ chamber containing Tyrode's solution, atropine and diphenhydramine. Fig. 3 shows that, like BK, bladder perfusates (A,B,C) contracted the ileum preparation and relaxed the rat duodenum. These

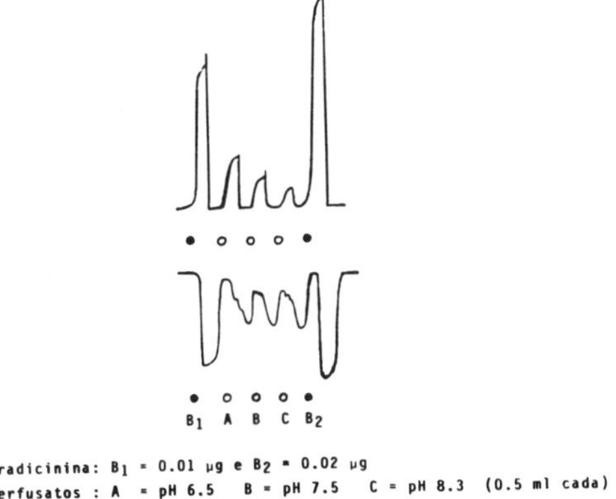

Bradicinina: B_1 = 0.01 µg e B_2 = 0.02 µg
Perfusatos : A = pH 6.5 B = pH 7.5 C = pH 8.3 (0.5 ml cada)

Fig. 3. Toad bladders were mounted in Tyrode's solution of varying pH and incubated at 25°C. pH: A, 6.5; B, 7.5; C, 8.3. After a 40-min incubation, a 0.5 ml aliquot of each incubate was applied to an organ bath containing both a fragment of guinea-pig ileum, and of rat duodenum; the bath fluid contained atropine sulphate and diphenhydramine. A total of five experiments was performed.

results stimulated us to attempt the extraction of similar material from bladder tissue with methanol[10]. Defatted and deproteinized methanol extracts of toad bladders were partially purified by chromatography on Sephadex G-25 and gel filtration with Bio-Gel P-2. The material obtained was assayed on isolated smooth muscle preparations where it behaved, in part, like BK (Table 2). It also produced hypotension following injection into the dog or cat[10]. The isolated toad bladder preparation was singularly sensitive to the bladder extract, as compared to BK, as far as the inhibition of the hydroosmotic effects of ADH was considered[10]. Like BK, the principle in bladder extracts was resistant to trypsin but destroyed by chymotrypsin, suggesting a polypeptide structure. However, paper electrophoresis showed it to be strongly anionic, contrasting with the cationic character of

BK. The comparison between the elution patterns of BK and the bladder peptide on a Bio-Gel P-2 column established the molecular weight of the active substance from the bladder as being slightly above 1000 Da, i.e., close to that of BK. Although its structure has not as yet been elucidated, a proper name for this substance would be *bufokinin*(10). Other components of the kinin system also occur in the toad bladder. It is rich in kinin-forming and kinin destroying enzymes. Kallikrein activity became apparent following acid (pH 5.0) treatment and dilution. Bladder tissue displayed esterase activity on benzoyl arginine methyl ester (BAME). Bladder kininase was inhibited by EDTA, 1,10-phenanthroline, and *a,a'*- dipyridyl(10).

Table 2. Characterization of the toad bladder extract.
[a]Response to the bladder extract. *Symbols:* Λ = spasmogenic responses; V = depressant effects (myorelaxant, hypotensive); ↓ = inhibitory effect.
[b]*in-vitro* preparation of the toad bladder stimulated by neurohypophyseal hormone. The inhibitory response refers to the inhibition of the pituitary hormone effects upon the bladder's permeability to water.

Assay organ	Response[a]
Guinea-pig ileum	Λ
Rat uterus	Λ
Cat jejunum	Λ
Rat duodenum	V
Rat stomach	Λ
Rabbit duodenum	Λ
Dog arterial pressure	V
Cat arterial pressure	V
Toad bladder[b]	↓

No great interest on this subject was shown in the literature up to 1980. Recently, several papers confirmed our findings on the antagonism by kinins, of the hydroosmotic response to ADH. This was confirmed both in the toad bladder(11,12), and in isolated mammalian collecting tubule preparations(13-18). Some of these reports also showed antagonism and therefore modulation of ADH effects by endogenous kinin.

III. Possible Mechanisms of Action of Bradykinin (BK)

Because of the apparently competitive character of its antagonism of water transport, an action of BK on V_2 receptors of the toad bladder cell membrane cannot be dismissed. Probably important is the action of BK on receptors causing activation of membrane phosphodiesterase (phospholipase C) leading to: a) generation of inositol triphosphate (IP_3) which stimulates an increase in intracellular calcium, $[Ca^{2+}]i$,[17,19]; b) generation of diacylglycerol (DAG) which activates protein kinase C[18], an inhibitor of ADH-stimulated formation of cyclic adenosine monophosphate; c) activation of phospholipase A by DAG, thus increasing formation of prostaglandins which are known to inhibit the hydroosmotic response to ADH[20,21]. Vasopressin (ADH) itself has been shown to stimulate V_1 receptors present in collecting tubule and toad bladder cells, causing increases in $[Ca^{2+}]i$ [21] and formation of prostaglandins[22,23]. Whether and how bradykinin interferes with the terminal exocytotic insertion of water channels into the luminal membrane of the cell is not known. Whatever the mechanism involved, the above mentioned activation of membrane phospholipase C by bradykinin, ultimately leads to inhibition of the ADH-induced increase in permeability to water. A schematic model showing bradykinin acting as a modulator of the anti-diuretic action of vasopressin is illustrated in Fig. 4.

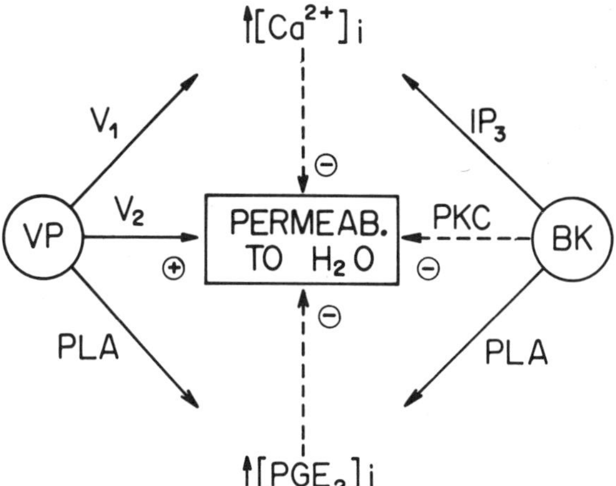

Fig. 4. Diagrammatic representation of a conceptual model for the homeostatic interplay of neurohypophyseal hormone and bradykinin. **Abbreviations:** VP = vasopressin; BK = bradykinin; V_1 = V_1 receptors; V_2 = V_2 receptors; $[Ca^{2+}]i$ = intracellular Ca^{2+} concentration; $[PGE_2]i$ intracellular PGE_2 concentration; PKC = protein kinase C; IP_3 = inositol triphosphate; PLA = phospholipase A.

Teleologically, one may expect that the tendency to compensate for the distortions of fluid homeostasis acted to provoke kinin formation. It is pertinent to recall that the kallikrein-forming site in the nephron, the cortical connecting tubule[24], where urine arrives diluted and water is reabsorbed in the presence of ADH (collecting tubule), presents the characteristics of a site where dilution could activate kallikrein. The physiological role of bradykinin as a possible homeostatic inhibitor of the hydroosmotic effects of ADH is now well documented; it is therefore possible to envisage the participation of kinin in pathological conditions such as nephrogenic diabetes insipidus.

Acknowledgements

I am indebted to Ester G. Silva for help in the technical work, and to Regina H. Bertoli, Ednéia F. Verceze, and Rodolfo S. Campanini for the preparation of this paper. The original research was supported by FAPESP.

References

1. Sawyer, W.H., Increased renal reabsorption of osmotically free water by the toad (*Bufo marinus*) in response to neurohypophyseal hormones, Am. J. Physiol. 189, 564-568 (1957).

2. Adolph, E.P. The skin and kidneys as regulators of the body volume of frogs, J. Exp. Zool. 47, 1-30 (1927).

3. Sawyer, W.H. and R.M. Schisgall, Increased permeability of the frog bladder in response to dehydration and neurohypophyseal extracts, Am. J. Physiol. 187, 312-314 (1956).

4. Goldberg, D.C., M.A. Schoessler and I.L. Schwartz, Intrinsic and extrinsic inhibition of the reactivity of the toad bladder to vasopressin, Physiologist 6, 188 (1963).

5. Heidenreich, O., P. Koller and Y. Kook, Die Wirkungen von Bradykinin und Kallidin auf die Nierenfunktion des Hundes, Arch. Exp. Path. Pharmak. 247, 243-2537 (1964).

6. Barraclough, M.A. and I.H. Mills, Effect of bradykinin on renal function, Clin. Sci. 28, 69-74 (1965).

7. Bentley, P.J., The effect of neurohypophyseal extracts on water transfer across the wall of the isolated urinary bladder of the toad *Bufo marinus*, J. Endocrin. 17, 201-209 (1958).

8. Furtado, M.R. and M.M. Machado, Effects of bradykinin on the movement of water and sodium in some isolated living membranes, Acta Physiol. Lat. Am. 16,63-65 (1966).

9. Furtado, M.R., Inhibition of the permeability response to vasopressin and oxytocin in the toad bladder: effects of bradykinin, kallidin, eledoisin, and physalaemin, J. Membrane Biol. 4, 165-178 (1971).

10. Furtado, M.R., Occurrence of a kinin-like peptide in the urinary bladder of the toad *Bufo marinus paracnemis* Lutz, Biochem. Pharmac. 21, 118-124 (1972).

11. Carvounis, C.P., G. Carvounis and L.A. Arbeit, Role of the endogeneous kallikrein-kinin system in modulating vasopressin-stimulated water flow and urea permeability in the toad urinary bladder, J. Clin. Invest. 67, 1792-1796 (1981).

12. G. Carvounis, C.P. Carvounis and L.A. Arbeit, Independent action of prostaglandins and kinins on vasopressin-stimulated water flow, Kidney Int. 27, 512-516 (1985).

13. Fejes-Tóth, G., T. Zahjszky and J. Filep, Effect of vasopressin on renal kallikrein excretion, Am. J. Physiol. 239, F388-F392 (1980).

14. Schuster, V.L., J.P. Kokko and H.R. Jacobson, Interactions of lysyl-bradykinin and anti-diuretic hormone in the rabbit cortical collecting tubule, J. Clin. Invest. 73, 1659-1667 (1984).

15. Rouse, D., W. Dalmeida, F.C. Williamson and W.N. Suki, Captopril inhibits the hydroosmotic effect of ADH in the cortical collecting tubule, Kidney Int. 32, 845-850 (1987).

16. Shayman, J.A., K.A. Hruska and A.R. Morrison, Bradykinin stimulates increased intracellular calcium in papillary collecting tubules of the rabbit, Biochem. Biophys. Res. Comm. 134, 299-304 (1986).

17. Shayman, J.A. and A.R. Morrison, Bradykinin-induced changes in phosphatidyl inositol turnover in cultured rabbit papillary collecting tubule cells, J. Clin. Invest. 76, 978-984 (1986).

18. Dixon, B.S., R. Breckon and J. Fortune, Bradykinin activates protein kinase C in cultured cortical collecting tubular cells, Am. J. Physiol. 257, F808-F817 (1989).

19. Fasolato, C., A. Pandiela, J. Meldolesi and T. Pozzan, Generation of inositol phosphates, cytosolic Ca^{2+}, and ionic fluxes in PC12 cells treated with bradykinin, J. Biol. Chem. 263, 17350-17359 (1988).

20. Grantham, J.J. and J. Orloff, Effect of prostaglandin E_1 on the permeability response of the isolated collecting tubule to vasopressin, adenosine-3', 5'-monophosphate and theophyline, J. Clin. Invest. 47, 1154-1161 (1968).

21. Schlondorff, D. and J.A. Satriano, Interactions of vasopressin, cAMP, and prostaglandins in toad urinary bladder, Am. J. Physiol. 248, F454-F458 (1985).

22. Wuthrich, R.P. and M.B. Vallotton, Prostaglandin E_2 and cyclic AMP response to vasopressin in renal medullary tubular cells, Am. J. Physiol. 251, F499-F505 (1986).

23. Burnatowska-Hledin, M. and W.S. Spielman, Vasopressin increases cytosolic free calcium in LLC-PK_1 cells through a V_1 receptor, Am. J. Physiol. 253, F328-F332 (1987).

24. Proud, D., M.A. Knepper and J.J. Pisano, Distribution of immunoreactive kallikrein along the rat nephron, Am. J. Physiol. 244, F510-F515 (1983).

AAS 36
Contributions to
Autacoid Pharmacology

THE BRADYKININ RECEPTOR OF THE RAT UTERUS AFFECTS THE LIGAND PROPERTIES OF CHARGED MERCURIALS

A.L. Silva, J.A.A. Rodrigues and I.F. Heneine

Department of Physiology and Biophysics, Institute of Biological Sciences, Federal University of Minas Gerais, 31270 Belo Horizonte, MG, Brazil

Abstract

Using monovalent organic mercurials to modify the response to the oxytocic action of bradykinin (BK) on the rat uterus, a charge effect, related to the reagent applied, was noted. With neutral, and positively charged mercurials, a bimodal pattern of activity, causing stimulation of BK contraction at lower, and inhibition at higher concentrations was observed. With negatively charged mercurials transient stimulation occurred, inhibition only appearing after very large doses and long periods of incubation. Anionic charges of the bradykinin receptor affect the ligand properties of mercurials, repelling negative charges. By themselves, mercurials did not cause any response.

Introduction

The affinity of sulphydryl reagents to superficial sulphydryl (SH) groups on the cell membrane, has been shown to be dependent on a combination of various factors, including size, charge and chemical character of the reagent itself, as well as others related to the SH group, e.g. accessibility and influence of vicinal residues[1,2,3]. Acting by mercaptide formation, monovalent organic mercurials are well known modifiers of membrane-dependent processes, giving a bimodal pattern with stimulation at lower, and inhibition at higher concentrations[1,2]. By using charged mercurials, it has been possible to explore the electrical environment provided by ionized residues close to the SH groups[1,2,4].

Since the bradykinin receptor is known to contain both SH groups and anionic sites[5] we decided to test its responsiveness to charged mercurials. We describe modifications of the response to BK of the rat uterus after contact with organic monovalent mercurials. For comparison, acetylcholine (Ach) was tested under the same conditions. A brief report of this work has been presented[6].

Materials and Methods

Chemicals. The mercurials used were neutral p-phenylmercury-acetate (PMA^o) from Sigma, positively charged p-aminophenylmercury (PAM+) (Aldrich), negatively charged p-hydroximercury benzoate (PMB–) (Sigma) and p-phenylmercury sulfonate (PMS–) having a strong negative charge, (Sigma). Mercurial solutions were prepared as described[8]. Bradykinin and acetylcholine were from Sigma, oestradiol valerianate from Berlimed.

Biossay. Female Wistar rats (170 to 200 g), were ovariectomized and after 12 days, injected with 5 μg/g of oestradiol valerianate. They were killed by decapitation 48 h later and the isolated uterus mounted in a 10 ml bath in Tyrode solution (mol $\times l^{-1}$: NaCl, 1.4×10^{-1}; KCl, 2.7×10^{-3}; $NaHCO_3$, 1.2×10^{-2}; NaH_2PO_4, 4.2×10^{-4}; $CaCl_2$, 7.2×10^{-4}; $MgCl_2$, 2.1×10^{-3} and glucose 5.6×10^{-3}), at 37°C, pH 7.4, aerated with atmospheric air. The auxotonic lever[7] employed exerted a tension on the uterus of 1 g.cm^{-1}, and was adjusted to give a 1 cm displacement with a 0.1 g mass (work equal to 1×10^{-5} J). After a period of accommodation, the organ was challenged with BK or Ach in increasing concentrations; responses to 6×10^{-9} M (BK), and 4×10^{-5} M (Ach) were considered as unitary references. After incubation with the mercurials for times and at concentrations indicated, the preparation was washed, agonists were added, and responses registered. Washing was repeated at the end of each response. The statistical significance of differences between means was evaluated according to Student's t distribution. Each experiment was repeated on at least 5 different uterine horn preparations.

Result

Control Responses. Lever displacement caused by control 6×10^{-9} M BK, varied between 3.5 to 4.5 cm; experimental responses were given positive percentage values when stimulation occurred; negative percentage values were attributed to responses showing inhibition. Ach (4×10^{-5} M), gave responses of a similar amplitude. No spontaneous contractions occurred during the testing periods, the preparation remaining in its initial state for as long as 2 h. Observed changes were always significant at $p < 0.05$.

The response to BK. The response elicited by BK after mercurial treatment of uterine horns are represented in Fig. 1. PMA^{o} or PAM+, acting for 90 sec at 2×10^{-5} M, stimulated contraction (A). The stimulated state could be detected for as long as 40 min, by

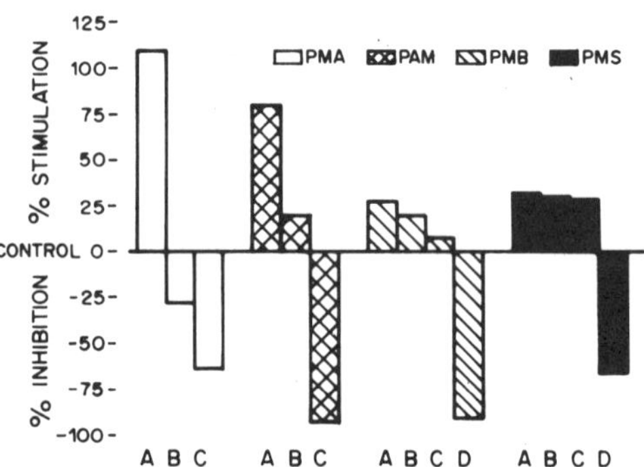

Fig. 1. Response of the rat uterine horn preparation to BK after incubation with organic mercurials at different concentrations and for different times. A, 2×10^{-5} M, 90 sec; B, 4×10^{-5} M, 90 sec; C, 6×10^{-5} M, 90 sec; D, 18×10^{-5} M, 270 sec. Results are presented in terms of percent change of control responses.

applying repeated doses of BK during this period. Following a second incubation, now with 4×10^{-5} M of either mercurial, contractions (B) returned to near control values. 6×10^{-5} M of the compound caused definite inhibition (C), more pronounced with PAM+; PMB– and PMS– caused transient stimulation at these concentrations. Increasing doses of PMB– caused progressively diminished responses of the uterine horn, not observed with PMS–. Inhibition by PMB– or PMS– appeared only at higher concentrations and after a longer period of action of the mercurials (D); this effect was more intense with PMB–.

In all experiments, the return from stimulated to control states could be accelerated by repeated washing of the uterine preparations; this return could be further accelerated by the addition of free-thiol compounds (N-acetylcysteine or dithiothreitol, 2×10^{-4} M) to the washing fluid.

Response to Ach. Response to Ach of the rat uterus was inhibited by mercurials at all concentrations tested. Preparations treated with mercurials at 2×10^{-5} M, although inhibited in their responsiveness to Ach, maintained their increased responsiveness to BK.

Inhibition by mercurials of responses to either BK or Ach was irreversible; it resisted washing of the preparations with either N-acetyl cysteine or dithiothreitol.

Discussion

Bradykinin has an isoelectric point of 10 to 10.5[9,10]; at physiological pH, this confers it a cationic character which participates in the binding of the peptide to anionic charges on its receptor. The results of the present investigation confirm and extend results on the bimodal pattern of stimulation at lower, and inhibition at higher concentration, of responses of the rat uterus to BK modified by organic mercurials. Stimulation by neutral and positively-charged mercurials suggests that no charge barrier interferes with their action. In contrast, anionic charges on the BK receptor probably interfere with the ligand abilities of the negatively-charged mercurials by repelling their approach to active receptor sites. This repulsion would clearly be more intense with PMS− than with the less charged PMB−. The transience of stimulation by the negative mercurials could be due to electric repulsion reinforcing mercaptide rupture by intrinsic thiols. This charge effect may be operative in ligand properties of BK analogs and antagonists.

Acknowledgements

This work was supported by CNPq, CAPES, PRP-UFMG and FAPEMIG. We acknowledge the advice of Professor W.T. Beraldo. The technical assistance of Mercia de Paula Lima is recognized.

References

1. Rothstein, S., Sulfhydryl groups in membrane structure and function, In: Current Topics in Membrane and Transport, vol. 1., pp. 135-176 (Eds. F. Bronner and A. Kleinzeller). Academic Press, New York 1970.

2. Strauss, W.L., Sulfhydryl and disulfide bonds: modification of amino acid residues in studies of receptor structure and function, In: Receptor Biochemistry and Methodology, vol. 1., pp. 85-97 (Ed. J. Craig Venter and Len C. Harrison). Alan C. Liss, Inc., New York 1984.

3. Mann, K., F. Bachhuber, H. Kather and B. Simmon, Amplification of the bradykinin response in rat uterus by PCMB-dextran T 10, Agents Actions 5, 236-238 (1975).

4. Nunes, P.H.M. and I.F. Heneine, Propriedades dos grupos sulfidrila da lisozima da *Carica papaya*, 1º Congresso da Sociedade Brasileira de Biofísica, Academia Brasileira de Ciências, Rio de Janeiro, pp. 6, Abstr. 2. (1976).

5. Odya, C.E. and T.L. Goodfriend, Bradykinin receptors, In: Bradykinin, Kallidin and Kallikrein, pp. 287-300 (Ed. E.G. Erdös). Springer-Verlag, Berlin 1979.

6. Silva, A.L., I.F. Heneine e J.A.A. Rodrigues, Estudo da influência de mercuriais orgânicos sobre as ações da bradicinina e acetilcolina no útero de rata, XVIII Congresso da Sociedade Brasileira de Fisiologia, pp. 286, Abstr. G24 (1983).

7. Paton, W.D.M., A pendulum auxotonic lever, J. Physiol. 137, 35-37 (1957).

8. Oliveira, Z.E.G., I.F. Heneine and M.V. Gomez, The effect of sulfhydryl reagents on the tityustoxin-induced acethylcholine release in rat brain slices, J. Neurochem. 27, 43-46 (1976).

9. Walaszek, E.J. and D.C. Dyer, Polypeptide receptors mechanisms: influence of pH, In: Hypotensive Peptides, pp. 329-339 (Eds. E.G. Erdös, N. Back and F. Sicuteri). Springer-Verlag, Berlin 1966.

10. Wiegershausen, B., I. Paegelow, H. Arold and S. Reissman, The problem of latency at bradykinin and some analogues, In: Vasopeptides, pp. 325-330 (Eds. N. Back and F. Sicuteri). Pergamon Press, New York 1972.

AAS 36
Contributions to
Autacoid Pharmacology

THE ACTION OF IODINATED KALLIKREIN ON THE RAT UTERUS

M.H. Feitosa, J.L. Pesquero, G.M.R. Oliveira, W.T. Beraldo and I.F. Heneine

Department of Physiology and Biophysics, Institute of Biological Sciences, Federal University of Minas Gerais, 31270 Belo Horizonte, MG, Brazil

Abstract

Iodinated kallikrein appeared inactive on synthetic substrates, was unable to liberate kinins from rat plasma, did not cause contraction of the rat uterus and did not potentiate bradykinin activity. After several doses of iodinated kallikrein were applied to the muscle, the contraction caused by kallikrein was blocked, but the response of the preparation to bradykinin was unaltered. If a double dose of kallikrein was applied, the contraction appeared again, and the response to bradykinin was also potentiated. These results support a kinin-mediated oxytocic action of kallikrein, and suggest a new interpretation for the mechanism of kallikrein desensitization in this preparation.

Introduction

Rat kallikrein elicited contraction of the rat uterus; when the addition of the same dose of the enzyme was repeated several times, responses were abolished. However, when a double dose of kallikrein was applied, the contraction reappeared(1). When several uterine horns were placed in an organ bath containing an uterine preparation previously desensitized by repeated treatment with large doses of kallikrein, the preparation again responded to kallikrein. It was concluded that the oxytocic action of kallikrein depended on kinin release from fresh uteri and that desensitization to kallikrein was due to uterine kininogen exhaustion by the enzyme(2). These findings suggested that kallikrein may bind to receptors in the uterus after liberating kinin, there remaining in an enzymatically inactive form capable of blocking responses of the organ to further additions of the enzyme. The concept of an inactive form of kallikrein occupying receptor sites, could bring a new light to the problem of the mechanism of the oxytocic action of kallikrein.

Iodination is a widely used procedure to prepare derivatives of tyrosine and/or histidine containing proteins(3), whose properties are modified by the gradual incorporation of iodine into their structures. This procedure has been used to detoxify venoms and toxins(4-7), and to deactivate insulin's capacity to cause hypoglycemia(8). The present paper describes the results of experiments designed to test whether iodination would change the biological activity of kallikrein on the rat uterus.

Materials and Methods

Kallikrein purification. Glandular kallikrein was fractioned by DEAE-cellulose chromatography(9).

Iodination of kallikrein. 1 ml of a solution of kallikrein in sodium phosphate buffer 0.1 M, pH 8.0, having an A_{280} of 0.270 A cm^{-1}, was treated at 0°C, with 10 μl of a 2×10^{-2} M ICl solution(10). Mock-iodinated and untreated samples served as controls.

Chemicals. Bradykinin was synthesized and supplied by the Escola Paulista de Medicina, São Paulo, Brazil. 17 β-estradiol and APApNA (Acetyl-phenylalanyl-α-arginyl-p-nitroanalide) were purchased from Sigma Co.

Amidase Activity and Kinin Liberation from Rat Plasma. The hydrolysis of APApNA was followed as previously described(11); kinin liberation was assayed by incubating samples with rat plasma(1).

Bioassay. Virgin female Wistar rats weighing 80 to 100g, were injected intramuscularly with 5 mg/kg 17 β-estradiol 72 h before use. One uterine horn freed from fat was suspended at 37°C in 5 ml of modified Tyrode solution containing ($mol.l^{-1}$): NaCl, 1.4×10^{-1}; KCl 2.7×10^{-3}; $NaHCO_3$, 1.2×10^{-2}; NaH_2PO_4, 4.2×10^{-4}; $CaCl_2$, 7.2 10^{-4}; $MgCl_2$, 2.1×10^{-3}; glucose 5.6×10^{-3} at pH 7.4 . Air was continuously bubbled through the bath fluid. Isotonic contractions were recorded with a frontal writing lever at ten-fold magnification. The sensitivity of this recording was similar to that of the Grass force displacement transducer (FDT 3C). Agonists were left for 2 min in contact with the preparation; the bath fluid was changed twice after each agonist addition, which was repeated after a 5 min period of rest.

Results

Kallikrein amidase activity was abolished by iodination. No contractions of the uterine preparation was elicited by rat plasma incubated with iodinated kallikrein, indicating loss of kinin liberating activity.

Figure 1 represents responses of uterine horns to bradykinin (BK), kallikrein (K), and iodinated kallikrein (KIo). The control response to bradykinin is shown at (BK_1). Following application of kallikrein (K_1), this response (BK_2) was potentiated. Iodinated kallikrein did not contract the uterus (KIo_1), and did not affect the response to bradykinin (BK_3). Renewed addition of kallikrein evoked a contraction (K_2) and the expected potentiation of bradykinin (BK_4). A renewed cycle of additions (KIo, K and BK), caused early desensitization to kallikrein. Repeated additions of iodinated kallikrein to the bath caused desensitization of the uterus to native kallikrein (Fig. 2) K_1 and K_2 are responses to the same dose of active kallikrein, applied prior and after the additions of iodinated kallikrein (KIo), respectively. It can be seen that inhibition began to appear after 9 to 10 doses of KIo (A and B), reaching about 90% after 13 doses (C), and becoming complete after 15 doses of KIo (D). After complete inhibition, the preparation still responded to bradykinin (result not shown).

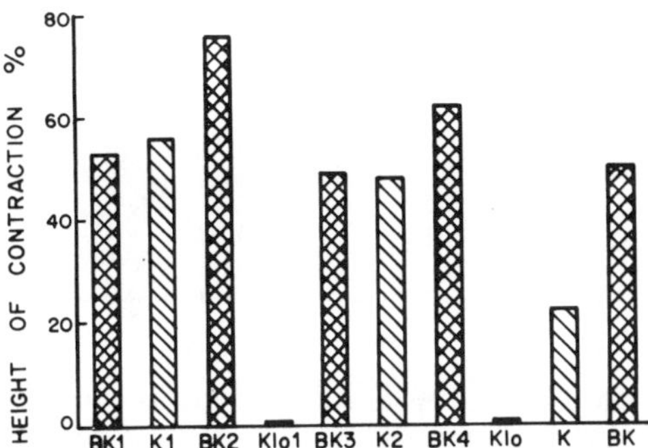

Fig. 1. Response of the rat uterus to kallikrein, bradykinin and iodinated kallikrein. BK_1 to BK_4 = bradykinin, 4 ng; K_1, K_2 and K = kallikrein, 350 ng; KIo = iodinated kallikrein, 350 ng (n=3). BK, bradykinin, 4 ng, normalized as 50% height of contraction.

In another series of experiments, as shown in Fig. 3, the preparation became completely refractory to native kallikrein (K) after application of 15 doses of iodinated kallikrein (KIo 15 ×). Response to bradykinin (BK) was unaltered. A double dose of kallikrein ($2 \times K$), caused a contraction after which the effect of bradykinin (BK) was potentiated.

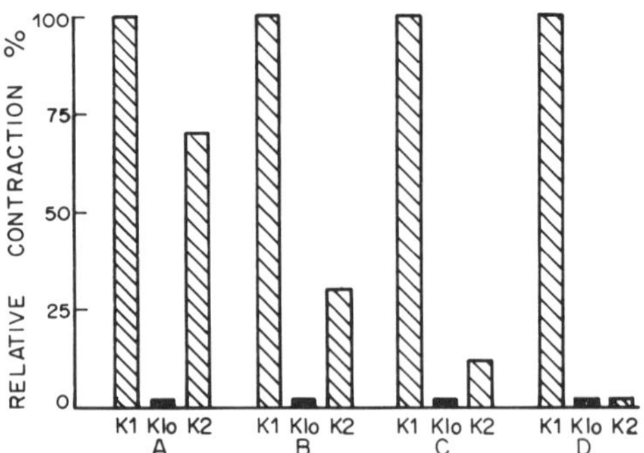

Fig. 2. Influence of previous additions of iodinated kallikrein on the response of the rat uterus to native kallikrein. K_1 = kallikrein, (350 ng), normalized as 100%; K_2 = kallikrein (350 ng), response after iodinated kallikrein additions; KIo = iodinated kallikrein, (350 ng). Number of additions of KIo: A=9, B=10, C=13 and D=15 (n=3).

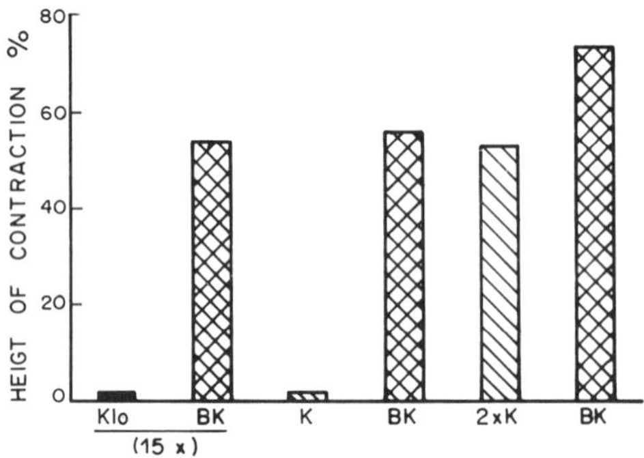

Fig. 3. Reversal of kallikrein inhibition caused by the action of iodinated kallikrein. BK = bradykinin, 4ng; KIo = iodinated kallikrein, 350 ng; K = kallikrein, 350 ng; $2 \times K$ = kallikrein, 700 ng.

Discussion

The present results indicate that iodinated kallikrein when applied in sufficient amounts, can occupy the sites of kallikrein binding to the rat uterus without interfering with sites of bradykinin action. These findings speak in favour of a kinin-mediated mechanism for the oxytocic action of kallikrein. They furthermore suggest that bradykinin action occurs without steric hindrance by kallikrein. Iodinated kallikrein can apparently be removed by a double, competitive dose of kallikrein, causing the muscle to show a renewed contraction to this enzyme(1).

These results suggest that kallikrein desensitization, can occur by two different mechanisms: 1) Occupancy of receptor sites by inactive kallikrein molecules, when a *physiological* amount of kallikrein is applied to the uterine horn(1). 2) Depletion of kininogen and possible damage to its synthesis mechanisms, when *excessive* doses of kallikrein are left to act for a long time on the uterine tissue(2). The first mechanism may be active in modulating the physiological role of kallikrein.

Acknowledgements

Supported by grants and fellowships from CNPq, and grants from FAPEMIG and FINEP. We acknowledge the technical assistance of Mercia de Paula Lima.

References

1. Beraldo, W.T., N.S. Lauar, G. Siqueira, I.F. Heneine and O.L. Catanzaro, Peculiarities of the oxytocic action of rat urinary kallikrein, In: Chemistry and Biology of the Kallikrein-Kinin System in Health and Disease, Fogarty Int. Cent. Proc. 27, 375-378 (1974).

2. Figueiredo, A.F.S., A.H.I. Salgado, G.R.T. Siqueira, C.R. Veloso and W.T. Beraldo, Rat uterine contraction by kallikrein and its dependence on uterine kininogen, Biochem. Pharmacol. 39, 763-769 (1990).

3. Ramachandran, L.K., Protein-Iodine interaction, Chem. Revs., 56, 199-218 (1956).

4. Heneine, L.G.D., V.N. Cardoso, J.P. Daniel and I.F. Heneine, Detoxification of the T2 fraction from a scorpion (*Tityus serrulatus*, Lutz and Mello) venom by iodination and some properties of the derivatives, Toxicon, 24, 501-505 (1986).

5. Daniel, J.P., L.G.D. Heneine, C.A.P. Tavares, M.C.S. Nascimento and I.F. Heneine, Generation of protective immunesera by *Crotalus durissus terrificus* venom detoxified by controlled iodination, Braz. J. Med. Biol. Res. 20, 713-720 (1987).

6. Heneine, I.F., L.G.D. Heneine, J.P. Daniel, M.C.S. Nascimento and O.A. Rocha, Properties of proteins toxins and venoms modified by controlled iodination, Rep. Acad. Sci., St. S. Paulo, 57-II, 55-66 (1987).

7. Bicalho, R.X., O.A. Rocha, L.G.D Heneine, A. Magalhães and I.F. Heneine, The effect of stepwise iodination on the biological properties of *Bothrops jararaca* venom, Toxicon 28, 171-179 (1990).

8. Nascimento,M.C.S. e I.F. Heneine, Iodação controlada de insulina, Proc. First Meeting Fed. Braz. Soc. Exp. Biol. (Abstr.), R-12.17 (1986).

9. Araujo, G.W., J.B. Pesquero, C.J. Lindsay, A.C.M. Paiva and J.L. Pesquero, Identification of serine proteases with tonin-like activity in the rat submandibular and prostate glands, Biochim. Biophys. Acta, in press.

10. Contreras, M.A., W.F. Bale and I.L. Spar, Iodine monochloride (ICI) iodination techniques, Meth. Enzymol. 92, 277-292 (1983).

11. Oliveira, L., M.S. Araujo-Viel, L. Juliano and E.S. Prado, Substrate activation of porcine pancreatic kallikrein by N-a derivatives of arginine 4-nitroanilides, Biochemistry 26, 5032-5035 (1987).

AAS 36
Contributions to
Autacoid Pharmacology

KALLIKREIN-KININ SYSTEM IN THE PLASMA OF SNAKES

Z.P. Picarelli, B.C. Prezoto, E. Hiraichi and F.M.F Abdalla.

Serviço de Farmacologia, Instituto Butantan, C.P. 65, 05504, São Paulo, SP, Brazil

Abstract

Using pharmacological preparations suitable for assay of mammalian kinins, it was shown that *Bothrops jararaca* (Bj) venom and other kininogenases were unable to release kinins from snake plasma. The kallikrein-kinin system presents species-specificity in birds. In order to detect such a specificity in snakes, the effects of Bj venom on snake blood pressure and the effect of incubates of snake plasma with trypsin, on snake blood pressure and snake uterus, were studied. The possibility of activating snake plasma kallikrein with ellagic acid, glass beads or kaolin was also investigated. Whereas plasma of the snakes *Waglerophis merremii* (Wm) and *Crotalus durissus* (Cd), were shown to contain factor XII, prekallikrein, kininogen, kininases and to present a low but definite activation rate of the kinin system, the plasmas of Bj, *Bothrops mojeni* (Bm) and *Oxyrophus trigeminus* (Ot), yielded only kininogen and kininases. Activation of the system was not even detected by the sensitive substrate Ac-Phe-Arg-Nan (acetyl-phenylalanyl-arginyl-4nitro-anilide), indicating that the plasma of these species does not possess either factor XII and/or prekallikrein. Snake plasma may constitute an interesting model for the study of blood clotting, fibrinolytic and complement systems.

Introduction

Bj venom produces hypotension in several mammalian species. This effect was attributed to the release of histamine as well as of bradykinin[1,2] because it was partially antagonized by antihistaminic drugs and because bradykinin was released during incubation of mammalian plasma with Bj venom. The peptide resulted from the action of a kininogenase present in the snake venom upon plasma kininogen, a component of the plasma kallikrein-kinin system.

Experiments using pharmacological preparations suitable for the assay of mammalian kinins have shown that Bj venom, trypsin and some other kininogenases active on mammalian plasma, were unable to release kinins from Bj plasma. Only two components of the kallikrein-kinin system have been detected in this plasma: kininases and inhibitors of kininogenases; no evidence that it contained either active factor XII, prekallikrein or kininogen could be found(3).

Like snake plasma, avian plasma has been shown to be free of factor XII(4) a principle involved in the activation of blood clotting, as well as of the fibrinolytic, the C_1 complement and the kallikrein-kinin systems. However, avian plasma presented all other components of the kallikrein-kinin system, since a kinin was released when it was shaken with glass beads containing adsorbed mammalian or alligator factor XII(5,6). In addition, it was demonstrated(6-8) that a kinin, different from mammalian kinins in terms of structure and pharmacological activity, was also liberated from chicken plasma by pancreatic kallikrein of birds. Ornithokininogen has been purified from chicken plasma and the structure of the kinin released from this substrate by bovine plasma kallikrein, determined(9). This peptide induced contractions of chicken smooth muscle and had a strong hypotensive effect in the chicken; however, it did not contract the rat isolated uterus.

It was considered of interest to investigate whether snake plasma contains a specific kallikrein-kinin system not detected by pharmacological preparations responsive to mammalian kinins. This was done either by testing the effects of Bj venom on this animal's carotid artery blood préssure, or by incubating snake plasma with snake venom or trypsin and assaying released substance(s) on snake blood pressure and snake isolated uterus.

In mammals, the active form of prekallikrein, a plasma protease zymogen activated by factor XII(10), is capable of cleaving kinin from kininogen and of releasing p-nitroaniline from chromogenic p-nitroanilide-derived substrates(11). We presently report results of experiments in which the activation of the kallikrein-kinin system of snake plasma was examined by determining whether a substance, or substances active on snake blood pressure, snake uterus or a chromogenic substrate was, or were released from such plasma by ellagic acid, glass bead or kaolin treatments, all known to evoke the release of kinin from mammalian plasma.

Material and Methods

The animals used in these experiments were adult male rats (200–300 g), adult pigeons and male or female snakes (100–500 g) of three venomous (*Bothrops jararaca*-10 specimens; *Crotalus durissus*-4 specimens; *Bothrops moojeni*-2 specimens) and two non-venomous (*Waglerophis merremii*-7 specimens and *Oxyrophus trigeminus*-1 specimen), species. Snakes were collected from nature and classified by the Herpetology sector of the Butantan Institute. After an observation period of at least 15 days, the snakes were kept under controlled environmental conditions (12 hrs light/12 hrs darkness, 26°C and 65% air humidity).

Descriptions of the preparation of rat, pigeon, snake and human plasma[12,13], of drugs used[12,13], of the procedures employed for the recording of rat and snake blood pressure[12] and of the responses of isolated smooth muscle preparations[13], have been published. Methods used for the follow-up of the release of pharmacologically active substances have been described[14,15], as have methods for the study of the activation of the plasma kallikrein-kinin system by glass beads[12] and other means[16-18].

Results

Effect of Bj venom on this snake's blood pressure. Bj venom caused a fall in the carotid artery blood pressure of anesthetized Bj. This effect was tachyphylactic and potentiated by captopril (Fig. 1); it was partially antagonized by promethazine plus cimetidine but was not affected by atropine (Fig. 2).

Release of active(s) substance(s) from snake plasma by trypsin. Incubation of Bj plasma with trypsin released a substance(s) that produced hypotension in the snake itself but not in the rat (Fig. 3). This effect was potentiated by captopril. Trypsinized Bj plasma contracted the Bj isolated uterùs, but did not act on pigeon oviduct and rat uterus (Fig. 4), though it displayed a weak action on guinea-pig ileum (not shown).

Similar results (not shown) were obtained with the plasma of Wm, Cd, Bm and Ot, excluding the result showing that the substance released from Ot plasma contracted the rat uterus.

Properties of the released substance(s). Like mammalian kinins, the released substance(s) was (were) dialysable, thermostable in acid but not in alkaline pH and inactivated by

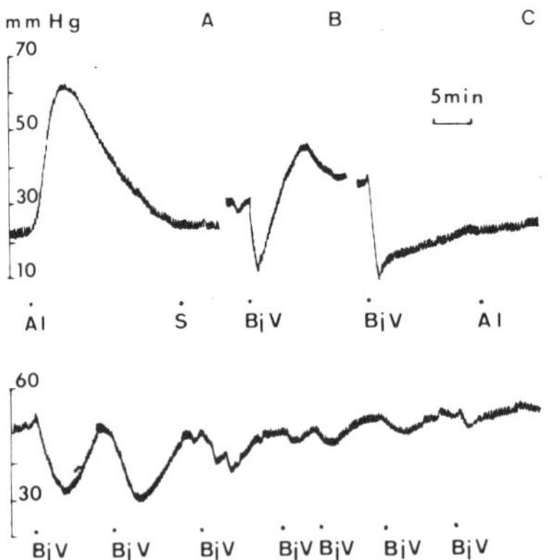

Fig. 1. Effect of *Bothrops jararaca* venom on the snake carotidean blood pressure – Female snakes (above – 170 g, below – 140 g) anesthetized with pentobarbital (30 mg/kg, i.p.) and heparinized (400 iu/kg). AI-angiotensin I (0.44 μg/kg); S-NaCl 0.9% (2.35 ml/kg); BjV-*Bothrops jararaca* venom (30 mg/kg). Between B and C, captopril (0.1 mg/kg) was administered. The tachyphylactic hypotensive effect of BjV is potentiated by captopril.

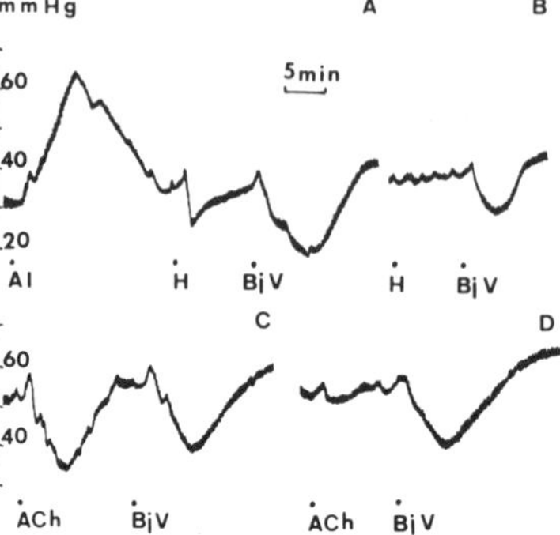

Fig. 2. Effect of antihistaminic drugs or atropine on the hypotension caused by *Bothrops jararaca* venom on the same species of snake – female (130 g, above) and male (120 g, below). Same conditions and same symbols as in Fig. 1. H-histamine; ACh-acetylcholine. Doses administered AI (0.1 μg/kg), H (60 μg/kg), BjV (above, 30 and below, 15mg/kg), ACh (100 μg/kg). Between A and B, promethazine (4 mg/kg) + cimetidine (15 mg/kg) and between C and D, atropine (1 mg/kg s.c. and 1 mg/kg i.v.) were administered. Whereas the antihistaminic drugs diminished the hypotension produced by BjV, atropine did not affect it.

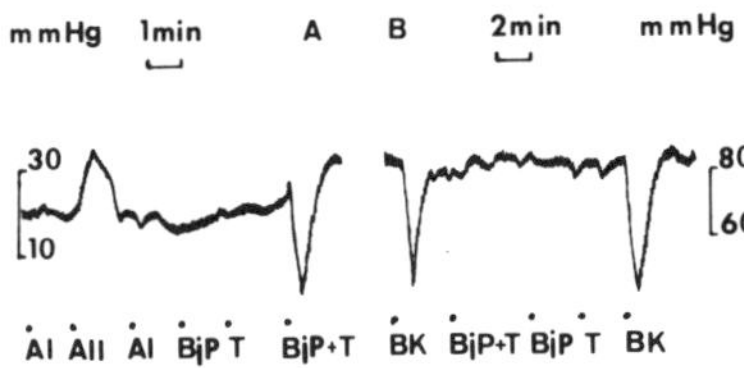

Fig. 3. Effect of the substance(s) released by trypsin from the plasma of *Bothrops jararaca* on the same species of snake (A) and the rat (B) blood pressure – Female snake (150 g), previously treated with captopril (0.5 mg/kg); male rat (300 g). AI-angiotensin I (0.14 μg/kg); AII-angiotensin II (0.10 μg/kg); BjP, T or BjP + T – 0,3 ml of incubates (37°C, pH 7.6) of *Bothrops jararaca* plasma, trypsin or both; BK-synthetic bradykinin (3.0 μg/kg). The substance(s) released by trypsin from *Bothrops jararaca* plasma is (are) inactive on rat blood pressure but produces hypotension in the snake itself.

Fig. 4. Effect of the substance(s) released by trypsin from the plasma of *Bothrops jararaca* upon *Bothrops jararaca* or rat uterus and pigeon oviduct- Isolated preparations suspended in 10 ml of Ringer solution for snakes (snake uterus), Jalon solution (rat uterus) and Ringer-Locke solution (pigeon oviduct). ACh-acetylcholine (0.5 μg on snake uterus and 5 μg on pigeon oviduct); BK-bradykinin (15 ng on rat uterus and 5 μg on pigeon oviduct); BjP, T or BjP + T – incubates of snake plasma, trypsin or both at 37°C, pH 7.6; PP, T or PP + T – incubates of pigeon plasma, trypsin or both at 37°C pH 7.6. The released substance(s) was(were) dried and diluted in 2 ml 0.9% NaCl. Volumes of incubates tested: snake uterus – 0.2 ml; rat uterus – 0.28 ml; pigeon oviduct – 0.1 (for PP, T or PP + T) and 0.2 (for BjP + T)ml. Whereas the substance(s) released by trypsin from the plasma of *Bothrops jararaca* contracted the own snake uterus, it(they) did not affect rat uterus or pigeon oviduct.

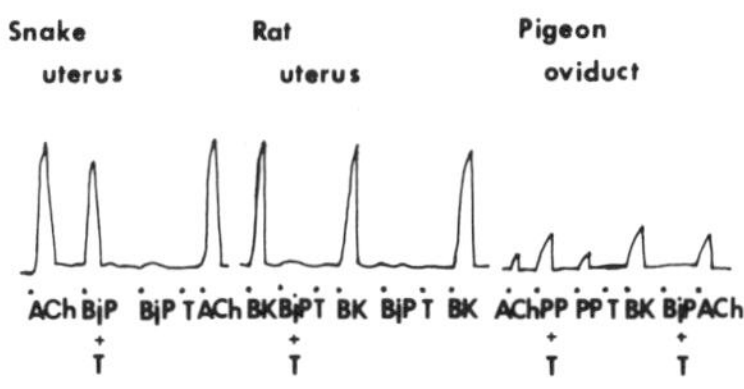

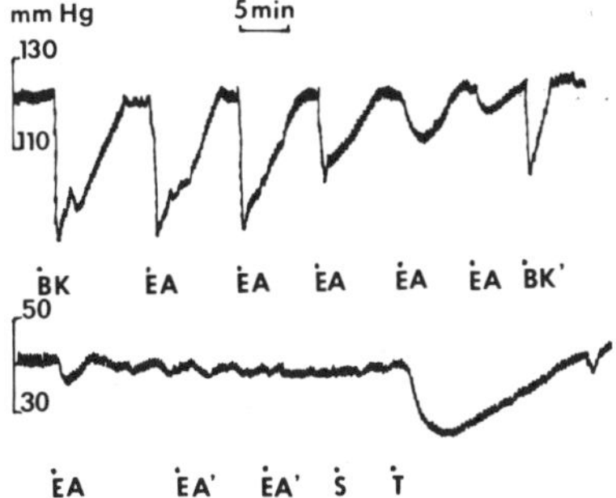

Fig. 5. Effect of repeated injections of ellagic acid on rat (above) and *Bothrops jararaca* (below) blood pressure. BK and BK' – 1.0 and 0.5 μg synthetic bradykinin; EA and EA' – 0.22 and 2.2 mg/kg ellagic acid; S – 0.9% NaCl. T – 8.0 mg/kg trypsin. The snake was previously treated with 0.5 mg/kg captopril. EA did not produce the hypotension and tachyphylaxis in *Bothrops jararaca* observed in the rat.

chymotrypsin but not by trypsin; its (their) inactivation by Bj kininase II was inhibited by captopril (Table 1).

Activation of the snake plasma kallikrein-kinin system. As may be seen in Fig. 5, doses of ellagic acid ten times greater than those producing a tachyphylactic hypotensive effect in rats, did not alter Bj (and also Wm) blood pressure. In addition, contrary to the decrease in kininogen observed in mammalian plasma after contact with glass, the kininogen content of snake plasma rotated with glass beads in glass vessels was found to be similar to that of the corresponding plasma kept in polyethylene vessels (Fig. 6). Furthermore, no substance with activity on Bj uterus was detected after treatment of Bj or Wm plasma with chloroform and kaolin (Fig. 7).

However, whereas Wm plasma was shown to be free of inhibitors of the contact system since its addition to rat plasma did not affect the kininogen decrease observed after contact of such plasma with glass, Bj plasma was shown to possess a high concentration of such inhibitors (Fig. 6).

On the other hand, incubation of Wm or Cd plasma with kaolin generated significant activity on the chromogenic substrate (Table 2). In contrast, Bj, Ot, and Bm, plasma did not hydrolyse this substrate even when previously treated with chloroform under conditions necessary to inhibit prekallikrein and factor XII inhibitors. The activity upon the chromogenic substrate Ac-Phe-Arg-Nan generated by contact of Wm or Cd plasma with kaolin is pH, time and temperature dependent. Whereas at 37°C this activity was 12.27 ± 0.37 (n=4) and 12.65 ± 0.8 (n=3) nmoles/ml for Wm and Cd plasma respectively, at 1°C, these values changed to 0.76 ± 0.42 (n=4) and 0.63 ± 0.26 (n=5) nmoles/ml. At pH 5.60 or 9.60, activities changed to 2.71 ± 0.18 (n=2) and 4.73 ± 0.22 (n=3) for Wm plasma, and to 2.70 ± 0.25 (n=4) and 1.72 ± 0.37 (n=4) nmoles/ml for Cd plasma.

The amidolytic activity exhibited by Wm or Cd plasma following contact with kaolin was blocked by hexadimethrine as well as by Trasylol (Fig. 8).

Discussion

The data show that the hypotension observed in Bj after administration of its own venom or trypsin, is tachyphylactic, partly antagonized by antihistaminic drugs, not affected by atropine and potentiated by captopril. These findings strongly suggest that, besides releasing histamine, Bj venom or trypsin release a kinin-like substance from the snake plasma. This is supported by the results of the *in vitro* experiments in which incubates of the

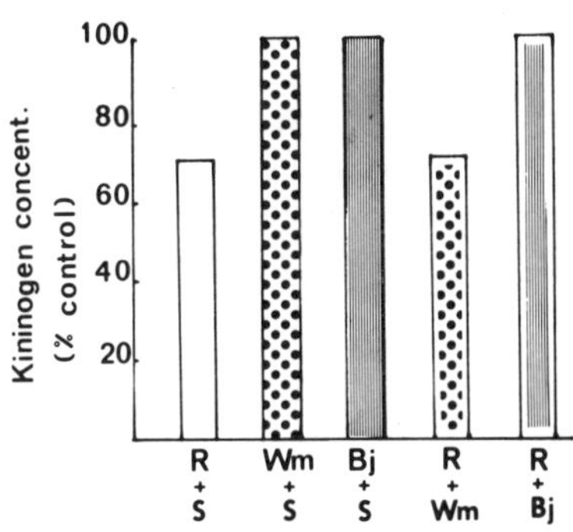

Fig. 6. Kininogen concentration of rat (R), *Waglerophis merremii* (Wm) or *Bothrops jararaca* (Bj) plasma, shaken with glass beads in glass vessels for 180 minutes. S–0.9% NaCl. Kininogen was quantified by the method of Diniz and Carvalho(15), the resulting kinin being assayed on the isolated rat uterus for R plasma and on the Bj isolated uterus for snake plasma. Controls were the respective plasmas maintained in polyethylene vessels. Whereas a 30% decrease in kininogen concentration was observed in R plasma, the kininogen concentrations of the snake plasmas were not affected by treatment. Inhibitors of the contact system were detected in Bj but not in Wm plasma since the decrease observed in R plasma kininogen concentration was inhibited only by Bj plasma.

Fig. 7. Lack of release of active substance(s) by addition of kaolin (10 mg/ml of plasma) to chloroform-treated (1:1 v/v) and kininase-free *Bothrops jararaca* (Bj) plasma. Incubation of Bj plasma (a), kaolin-treated Bj plasma (b), chloroform plus kaolin-treated Bj plasma (c) or trypsinized (1 mg/ml) Bj plasma (d) at 37°C for 12 (a, b, c) or 30 (d) min. Reactions stopped with boiling ethanol; drying of the soluble material; residue dissolved in 2 ml of 0.9% NaCl; assay on Bj isolated uterus. Doses of acetylcholine (ACh) in μg and of the incubates in ml of Bj plasma. Addition of samples to the uterus every 6 minutes. No active substance, similar to that released by trypsin, was detected on Bj uterus after activation of Bj plasma with kaolin even after previous treatment with chloroform.

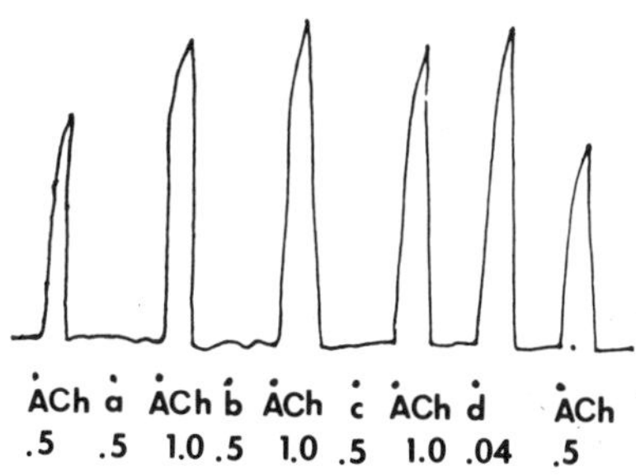

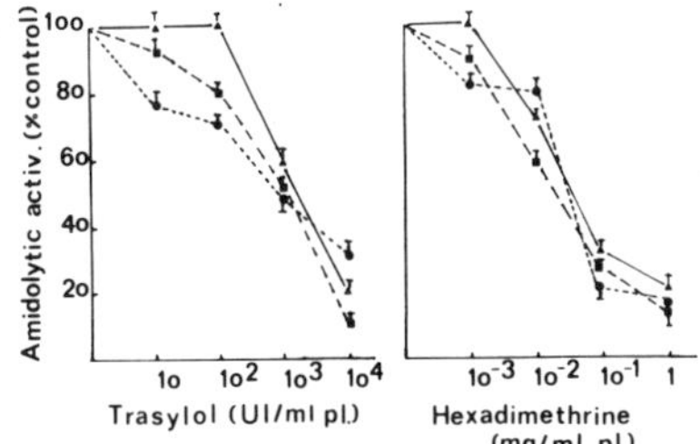

Fig. 8. Influence of the enzymatic inhibitors Trasylol and hexadimethrine bromide on human (•—•), *Waglerophys merremii* (▲—▲) and *Crotalus durissus* (—) kaolin-treated plasma hydrolytic activity on Ac-Phe-Arg-Nan, following incubation at 37°C and pH 7.65 during 120 min (snake plasma) and 15 min (human plasma). The inhibition of the hydrolytic activity by Trasylol and hexadimethrine indicates the presence of factor XII- and prekallikrein-like substances in such plasmas.

Table 1. Properties of the substance(s) released by incubating *Bothrops jararaca* plasma (BjP) with trypsin in comparison with those of bradykinin.

Procedure	pH	Time	Released Subst. (s)	Bradykinin
Dialysis against 0.9% NaCl, at 4°C	6.5	24 h	D	D
Heating at 98°C	1.5 – 2.0	30 – 60 min	S	S
	10.0 – 11.0	5 – 10 min	U	U
Incubation, at 37°C, with:				
Chymotrypsin (37 μg/ml)	6.5	5 min	I	I
Trypsin (110 μg/ml)	6.5	60 min	R	R
BjP (1:25)	7.4	15 min	I	I
ACE*	7.4	15 min	I	I
BjP (1:25) + Capt (170 μg/ml)	7.4	15 min	R	R
ACE + Capt (13.5 μg/ml)	7.4	15 min	R	R

D – dialysable; S – stable; U – unstable; I – inactivated; R – resistant.
*ACE – a purified kininase II, hydrolysing 83.3 μg of bradykinin/min/ml, obtained from BjP.
Capt – captopril (CAPOTEN, Sq 14225).

Table 2. Influence of kaolin treatment of human and snake plasmas on their amidolytic activity upon Ac-Phe-Arg-Nan. Incubation at pH 7.65 and 37°C during 120 minutes.

Plasma	Amidolytic activity (n moles/ml)	
	Control	Kaolin-treated
Human	22.48 ± 6.54 (3)	150.10 ± 8.17 (3)*
Waglerophis merremii	0.91 ± 0.21 (6)	12.27 ± 0.34 (4)*
Crotalus durissus	0.89 ± 0.45 (2)	12.65 ± 0.84 (3)*
Bothrops jararaca	0.94 ± 0.41 (4)	0.93 ± 0.32 (5)
Bothrops moojeni	1.05 ± 0.52 (2)	1.08 ± 0.41 (2)
Oxyrophus trigeminus	0.90 ± 0.32 (2)	0.83 ± 0.40 (2)

Values are mean ± sem. Number of experiments in parentheses.
*Values are significantly different ($p < 0.05$, "t" test) compared with the respective controls.

snake plasma with trypsin or Bj venom were shown to contain a substance (or substances) which had practically no effect on rat blood pressure, rat uterus, pigeon oviduct and guinea-pig ileum, but which did act on Bj blood pressure and uterus. Some chemical properties of this substance (these substances) are similar to those of the mammalian kinins[19].

In addition, these findings indicate that a kininogen-like component is present in Bj plasma as well as in the plasma of the other snakes used. Corroborating these results, Chudzinski *et al.*[20] have shown that a protein which exhibits both a molecular weight similar to that of mammalian kininogen as well as cysteine-proteinase inhibitory activity can be isolated from Bj or Wm plasma.

The impossibility of activating the kallikrein-kinin system in the plasma of Bj, Bm and Ot cannot be due to the high rate of destruction of the released substance by plasma kininases, since the experiments, wherever necessary, were done in the presence of kininase inhibitors. Inhibitors of factor XII and prekallikrein do not seem to be responsible for these results either, since pretreatment of Bj and Wm plasma with chloroform, a process which eliminates such inhibitors, did not change the negative results obtained with kaolin. Absence of factor XII and/or prekallikrein in such plasmas could explain these results. Nevertheless, it is necessary to consider that in Wm and Cd plasma, kaolin was able to produce amidolytic activity, which although 100 times weaker than that found in human plasma, was time, pH and temperature dependent and blocked by hexadimethrine, an inhibitor of factor XII, as well as by Trasylol, a kallikrein inhibitor. Therefore, this activity seems to be enzymatically-generated and dependent on factor XII and/or kallikrein; it is however, so low that it only can be revealed via assay of the amidolytic activity of the resulting kallikrein. The activation of the kallikrein-kinin system in the plasma of Bj, Bm and Ot may be even slower, so that even this assay method was unable to reveal it. Therefore, the results obtained in Bj, Bm and Ot may be due, either to the absence of factor XII and/or kallikrein, or to the use of a method incapable of detecting their activation.

Differences between animals species similar to those reported here, have been observed in turtles[4], fishes[21], lizards[22] and even mammals[23]; they render snakes interesting models for the study of blood clotting, fibrinolysis and the C_1 complement system.

Acknowledgements

Research supported by CNPq (Grants nos. 400324/81, 403415/82 and 1020/5/83) and FAPESP (Grant no. 84/0708-0). FMFA has scholarships from FUNDAP and FEDIB. The authors wish to thank Miss Wanda R.C. da Silva for technical assistance and typing of the manuscript.

References

1. Rocha e Silva, M., W.T. Beraldo and G. Rosenfeld, Bradykinin, a hypotensive and smooth muscle stimulating factor released from plasma globulin by snake venom and by trypsin, Am. J. Physiol. 156, 261-273 (1949).

2. Suzuki, T., and S. Iwanaga, Snake venoms. In: Bradykinin, Kallidin and Kallikrein. Handb. Exp. Pharmacol. XXV, 193-212 (Ed. E.G. Erdös). Springer, Heidelberg 1970.

3. Lavras, A.A.C., M. Fichman, E. Hiraichi, M.A. Boucault, T. Tobo, P. Schmuziger, L. Nahas and Z.P. Picarelli, Deficiency of kallikrein-kinin system and presence of potent kininase activity in the plasma of *Bothrops jararaca* (Serpentes. Crotalinae), Ciência e Cultura 31, 168-174 (1979).

4. Ratnoff, O.D., The biology and pathology of the initial stages of blood coagulation, Progr. Hematol. 15, 204-245 (1966).

5. Erdös, E.G., I. Miwa and W.J. Graham, Studies on the evolution of plasma kinins: reptilian and avian blood, Life Sci. 6, 2433-2439 (1967).

6. Seki, T., I. Miwa, T. Nakajima and E.G. Erdös, Plasma kallikrein-kinin system in nonmammalian blood: evolutionary aspects, Am. J. Physiol. 224, 1425-1430 (1973).

7. Werle, E., und J. Hürter. Über Ornitho-kallikrein. I-Mitteilung über kreislaufaktive Substanzen der Vögel, Biochem. Z. 285, 175-191 (1936).

8. Werle, E., und G. Leysath, Über das Molekulargewicht des Plasmakinins von Vögeln, Z. Physiol. Chem. 348, 352-353 (1967).

9. Kimura, M., T. Sueyoshi, K. Takada, K. Tanaka, T. Morita and S. Iwanaga, Isolation and characterization of ornithokininogen, Eur. J. Biochem. 168, 493-501 (1987).

10. Kaplan, A.P., and K.F. Austen, A pre-albumin activator of prekallikrein, J. Immunol. 105, 802-811 (1970).

11. Claesson, G., L. Aurell, P. Friberger, S. Gustavsson and G. Karlsson, Designing of peptide substrates. Different approaches exemplified by new chromogenic substrates for kallikreins and urokinase, Haemostasis 7, 62-68 (1978).

12. Prezoto, B.C., E. Hiraichi, F.M.F. Abdalla and Z.P. Picarelli, Activation of the kallikrein-kinin system in the plasma of some Brazilian snakes, Comp. Biochem. Physiol. 99C, 135-139 (1991).

13. Abdalla, F.M.F., E. Hiraichi, Z.P. Picarelli and B.C. Prezoto, Kallikrein-kinin system in the plasma of the snake *Bothrops jararaca*, Br. J. Pharmac. 98, 252-258 (1989).

14. Hamberg, U., and M. Rocha e Silva, On the release of bradykinin by tripsin and snake venoms, Arch. Int. Pharmacodyn. 110, 222-238 (1957).

15. Diniz, C.R., and I.F. Carvalho, A micromethod for determination of bradykininogen under several conditions, Ann. N.Y. Acad. Sci. 104, 77-89 (1963).

16. Gautvik, K.M., and H. Rugstard, Kinin formation and kininogen depletion in rats after intravenous injection of ellagic acid, Br. J. Pharmac. 31, 390-400 (1967).

17. Komissarova, N.V., and O.A. Gomazkov, Contact activation of kallikrein and plasmin systems of rabbit blood, Bull. exp. Biol. Med. 81, 390-392 (1976).

18. Kluft, C., Determination of prekallikrein in human plasma: optimal conditions for activating prekallikrein, J. Lab. Clin. Med. 91, 83-95 (1978).

19. Prado, J.L., R. Monier, E.S. Prado and C. Fromageot, Pharmacological active polypeptide formed from blood globulin by a cysteine – activated protease from *Clostridium hystolyticum*, Biochim. Biophys. Acta 22, 87-95 (1956).

20. Chudzinski, A.M., M.U. Sampaio, M.L.V. Oliva and C.A.M. Sampaio, A *Bothrops jararaca* plasma cysteine-proteinase inhibitor related to mammalian kininogen, Braz. J. Med. Biol. Res. 22, 945-948 (1989).

21. Doolittle, R.F., and D.M. Surgenor, Blood coagulation in fish, Am. J. Physiol. 203, 964-970 (1962).

22. Hackett, E., and C. Hann, Slow clotting of reptile blood, J. Comp. Path. 77, 175-180 (1967).

23. Robinson, A.J., M. Kropatkin and P.M. Aggeler. Hageman factor (Factor XII) deficiency in marine mammals, Science 166, 1420-1422 (1969).

AAS 36
Contributions to
Autacoid Pharmacology

THE ROLE OF HISTAMINE ON THE CONTROL OF THYROTROPIN SECRETION IN RATS

J.D.B. Silva

Department of Physiology and Biophysics, Institute of Biological Sciences, Federal University of Minas Gerais, 31270 Belo Horizonte, MG, BRazil

M.T. Nunes

Department of Physiology and Biophysics, Institute of Biological Sciences, University of São Paulo, SP, BRazil

Abstract

The presence of histamine (HA) in the hypothalamus, especially in its median eminence, as well as results of previous studies from this laboratory, suggest a participation of this amine in the regulation of TSH (thyroid stimulating hormone, thyrotropin) secretion. In the present investigation, rats were treated with a single injection of cimetidine (CIM – 100 mg/kg ip), an H_2–HA receptor antagonist. *In vitro* release of TSH in response to hypothalamic extracts from control animals, was approximately 20% smaller when evoked from pituitaries obtained from CIM-treated, rather than control animals. The addition of hypothalamic extracts from CIM-treated rats to incubates of pituitaries from either control or CIM treated rats did not significantly change basal TSH secretion, suggesting that TRH (thyrotropin releasing hormone) content was decreased by the anti-histamine treatment. These results point towards a facilitatory role of HA on TSH secretion both at the hypothalamic level where it may interfere with TRH synthesis, as well as at the pituitary level where it may modify TSH response to TRH.

Introduction

The mechanisms influencing central neurotransmitter control of thyrotropin secretion, although well studied, are still not completely understood. The system consists of a stimulatory input represented by the hypothalamic thyrotropin-releasing hormone and probably three inhibitory inputs represented in turn by the feed back effect of thyroid hormones and by the inhibitory effects of hypothalamic somatostatin and dopamine, whose release is also under neurotransmitter control[1,2].

Histamine is unevenly distributed in the hypothalamus. Large amounts are found in the median eminence and lesser quantities in the premamilary, suprachiasmatic and arcuate nuclei. The histidine decarboxylase (HD) content of hypothalamic nuclei correlates closely with their histamine content (high HD/HA ratio). However, in the median eminence most, if not all histamine can be found within mast cells whose histidine decarboxylase activity is very low[3]. These data point towards the existence of at least two hypothalamic pools of histamine which could be distinguished from each other by their rate of HA synthesis[3,4,5]. The presence of mast cells containing histamine in the median eminence suggests a possible physiological role of these cells in the control of TSH secretion.

Nunes and Britto[6] demonstrated that intracerebroventricular injection of BW 48/80, a drug that induces mast cell degranulation, increases TSH serum levels. This effect is blocked by disodium cromoglycate, a compound which specifically blocks mast cell degranulation, as well as by cimetidine, a H_2-histamine receptor antagonist. These data suggest that HA released by mast cell degranulation may play a stimulatory role on TSH secretion.

The present work studies the participation of HA on TSH secretion by evaluating the effect of the blockade of H_2 receptors on such secretion, thus attempting to complement related studies by others[7,8,9].

Materials and Methods

Animal treatment. Male Wistar rats weighing 250±30 g were used. The animals were conventionally kept, under controlled temperature (25±1°C) and a dark-light cycle (10/14 h), with free access to food and water.

Part of the animals (CIM), received a single injection of cimetidine (Smith Kline French Laboratory, Brazil), 100 mg/kg, i.p., 1 h prior to sacrifice. Control animals (C), received an equivalent volume of saline, i.p.

TSH determination. Serum and pituitary TSH as well as TSH secreted *in vitro* in response to hypothalamic extracts were determined by radioimmunoassay with reagents obtained from the National Institute of Health, Bethesda, MD.

Preparation of hypothalamic extracts. Immediately after the sacrifice of the animals by decapitation, brains were removed and quickly frozen on dry ice. Blocks of 4×4×3 mm of hypothalamic tissue were cut and homogenized in 225 μl of 0,1 N HCl. The homogenates were immersed for 10 min in a boiling water bath in order to destroy any TSH which might be present in the extracts, and centrifuged for 30 min at 2000 rpm. 200 μl of the supernatant were removed and stored at −20°C, usually for not longer than 24 h[10].

Preparation of pituitary homogenates. Pituitaries were removed from freshly-killed rats and divided in two halves. One of them was homogenized in 2 ml of saline and centrifuged at 3000 rpm for 15 min. TSH was determined in the supernate[11].

"In vitro" pituitary TSH response to hypothalamic extracts. The second halves of 5 pituitaries were pooled and placed in Erlenmeyer flasks containing 2 ml of tissue culture medium # 199 for the *in vitro* study of TSH secretion. After 30 min of preincubation in a Dubnoff Shaker at 37°C in an atmosphere of 95% O_2 and 5% CO_2, media were collected for determination of basal TSH levels; they were then replaced with the same volume of media containing 200 μl of hypothalamic extract. Incubations were continued for 180 min, media were collected, centrifuged at 2000 rpm for 30 min and TSH determined in the supernatants.

Statistical analyses were performed using Student t test; a value of $p < 0.05$ was considered to indicate a significant effect of treatment.

Results and Discussion

Cimetidine treatment led to a statistically significant decrease in both serum and pituitary TSH concentration (Fig. 1). Such blockade by an anti-histaminic drug suggests that histamine has a facilitatory role on the synthesis and/or secretion of TSH.

The *in vitro* study demonstrated that pituitaries from both C and CIM treated animals increase their TSH secretion under the influence of hypothalamic extracts (Fig. 2). The relative response from pituitaries of CIM-treated animals, was however approximately 20% smaller than that observed from the pituitaries of control animals. This result was consistently observed, suggesting that some action of HA at the pituitary level might exist. It deserves further investigation. When hypothalamic extracts from CIM-treated animals were incubated with pituitaries from either C or CIM-treated animals, TSH secretion was not significantly different from basal secretion observed prior to the addition of the extracts (Fig. 2). This suggests that TRH content may have decreased in the CIM-treated animals.

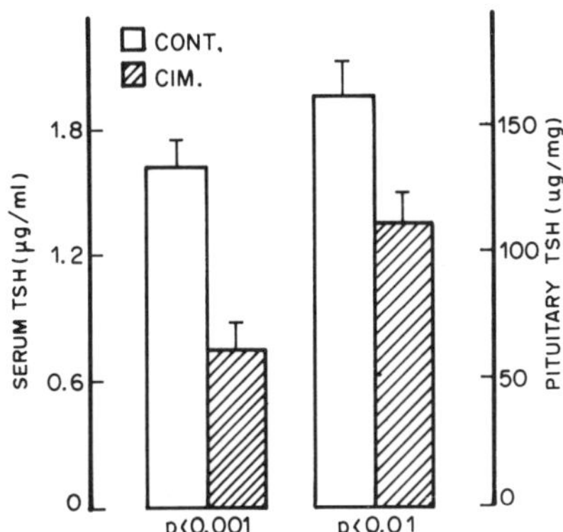

Fig. 1. Effect of treatment with cimetidine (CIM) (100 mg/kg), 1 h before sacrifice on serum and pituitary TSH of rats. The results are expressed as mean ±SEM for 20 animals of each group.

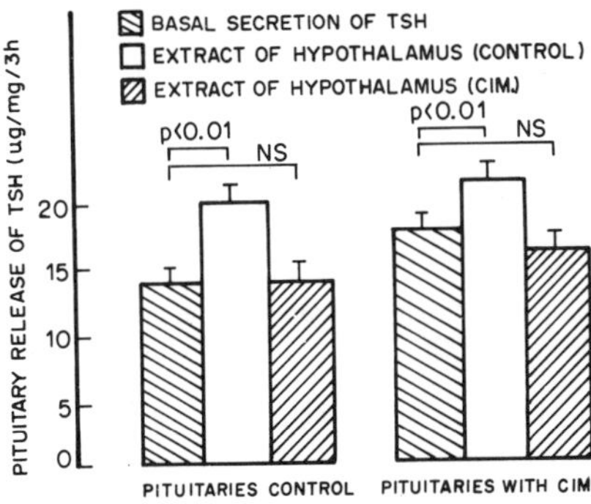

Fig. 2. *In vitro* TSH secretion from pituitaries of control and cimetidine (CIM)-treated rats in response to hypothalamic extracts obtained from control and cimetidine (CIM)-treated animals. Note that the relative increase in TSH secretion from pituitaries of control rats appeared somewhat larger than that evoked from pituitaries of CIM rats.

These results are in agreement with those of Bravo *et al.*[7], and support the hypothesis of a facilitatory role of HA on TSH secretion both at the hypothalamic level, where it may interfere with TRH synthesis, as well as at the pituitary level where it may modify the TSH secretion in response to TRH.

Acknowledgments

The authors thank Manuel José de Oliveira for technical assistance, and Maria Célia S. Costa for typing the manuscript.

References

1. Martin, J.B., Regulation of the pituitary thyroid axis, In: International Review of Science, Physiology, Series 1, vol. 5, pp. 67-107 (Ed. S.M. McCann). Butterworth, London 1974.

2. Scanlon, M.F., B. Ress Smith and R. Hall, Thyroid stimulating hormone: neuroregulation and clinical applications, Clin. Sci. Mol. Med. 55, 1-10, 129-138 (1978).

3. Pollard, H., S. Bischoff, C. Llorens-Cortes and Schwartz, J.C., Histidine descarboxylase and histamine in discrete nuclei of rat hypothalamus and the evidence of mast cells in the median eminence, Brain Res. 118, 509-513 (1976).

4. Brownstein, M.J., J.M. Saavendra, M. Palkovitz and J. Axelrod, Histamine content of hypothalamic nuclei in the rat, Brain Res. 77, 151-156 (1974).

5. Hough, L.B., Cellular localization and possible functions for brain histamine: recent progress, Prog. Neurobiol. 30, 469-505 (1988).

6. Nunes, M.T. and L.R.G. Britto, Mast cell degranulation acutely increases thyrotropin serum levels in the rat, Neuroendocrinol. Lett. 11, 131-137 (1989).

7. Joseph-Bravo, P., J.L. Charli, J.M. Palacios, and C. Kordon, Effect of neurotransmitters on the *in vitro* release of immunoreactive thyrotropin-releasing hormone from rat mediobasal hypothalamus, Endocrinology 104, 801-806 (1979).

8. Weiner, R.I. and W.F. Ganong, Role of brain monoamines and histamine in regulation of anterior pituitary secretion, Physiol. Rev. 58, 905-976 (1978).

9. Charli, J.L., P. Joseph-Bravo, J.M. Palacios and C. Kordon, Histamine-induced release of thyrotropin releasing hormone from hypothalamic slices, Eur. J. Pharm. 52, 401-403 (1978).

10. Krulich, L., M. Quijada, E. Hefco and D.K. Sundberg, Localization of thyrothropin-releasing factor (TRF) in the hypothalamus of the rat, Endocrinology 95, 9-17 (1974).

11. Hefco, E., L. Krulich, P. Illner and P.R. Larsen, Effect of acute exposure to cold on the hypothalamic-pituitary-thyroid system, Endocrinology 97, 1185-1195 (1975).